WO500
10/11

Anaesthesia, intensive care, and pain management for the cancer patient

Edited by

Dr Paul Farquhar-Smith

Dr Tim Wigmore

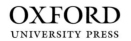

OXFORD

UNIVERSITY PRESS

OXFORD
UNIVERSITY PRESS

Great Clarendon Street, Oxford ox2 6DP

Oxford University Press is a department of the University of Oxford.
It furthers the University's objective of excellence in research, scholarship,
and education by publishing worldwide in

Oxford New York

Athens Auckland Bangkok Bogotá Buenos Aires Cape-Town
Chennai Dar-es-Salaam Delhi Florence Hong-Kong Istanbul Karachi
Kolkata Kuala-Lumpur Madrid Melbourne Mexico-City Mumbai Nairobi
Paris São-Paulo Shanghai Singapore Taipei Tokyo Toronto Warsaw

with associated companies in Berlin Ibadan

Oxford is a registered trade mark of Oxford University Press
in the UK and in certain other countries

Published in the United States
by Oxford University Press Inc., New York

British Library Cataloguing in Publication Data
Data available

Library of Congress Cataloguing in Publication Data
Data available

Typeset in Minion by Glyph International, Bangalore, India
Printed in Great Britain
on acid-free paper by
CPI Antony Rowe, Chippenham, Wiltshire

ISBN 978–0–19–958464–2

10 9 8 7 6 5 4 3 2 1

Oxford University Press makes no representation, express or implied, that the drug dosages in
this book are correct. Readers must therefore always check the product information and clinical
procedures with the most up-to-date published product information and data sheets provided by
the manufacturers and the most recent codes of conduct and safety regulations. The authors and the
publishers do not accept responsibility or legal liability for any errors in the text or for the misuse
or misapplication of material in this work. Except where otherwise stated, drug dosages and
recommendations are for the non-pregnant adult who is not breastfeeding.

Foreword

Both the medicine and the science of treating cancer have changed impressively over the last decade and continue to evolve at a rapid rate. As a direct consequence, a wide range of disparate diseases under the general title of malignancy now have very different treatments, and hence prognosis, as new developments in chemotherapy, radiotherapy immunotherapy, and surgery have been refined. Keeping up to date with each or any of these areas even for a single disease would be hard and would rightly be considered the domain of the specialists in that field, and outside of the perceived pertinent knowledge base for a practicing anaesthetist, pain clinician, or intensivist.

Yet under the umbrella of anaesthesia 'the specialty', almost all anaesthetists, pain clinicians, and intensivists regularly treat patients with malignant diseases. It is incumbent on us to have a working knowledge of the field with which we are interacting, and failing this then ready access to relevant information would be sensible. In practice, detailed current information on particular treatments or on prognosis in a user-friendly and relevant format is difficult or even impossible to locate. There is therefore a clear and obvious need for a resource that allows easy access to this kind of information.

In the UK there are specialist centres that focus entirely on cancer treatment such as the Royal Marsden Hospital, and where better to find a sensible, up-to-date, pragmatic approach to the problems that may occur in treating patients with malignancy. An holistic approach would cover not only the special anaesthetic requirements of particular types of surgery but also all of the other aspects of patient care that relate to anaesthesia in its broadest sense. This will range from preoperative assessment and risk benefit analysis, through the pharmacology of old and new chemotherapeutic regimens, and hence the implications of potential side effects and interactions. It needs to consider not just the role of intensive care in postoperative management but also in terms of what critical care can offer and what can benefit the critically ill patient with malignancy. It must embrace the whole panoply of pain management issues that are crucial in treatment in a wide range of settings which will include postoperative pain as just one component of the pain team's role.

There are many simple and practical aspects of care that would be immediately beneficial such as easy access to the nomenclature of chemotherapy regimens with ready reference to the problems they carry with them. For the intensivist, a pragmatic way of balancing the triad of expectation, clinical efficacy, and prognosis with relevant background information focused on these issues. An all-encompassing text would include the significant role of alternative medicine as a useful and positive aspect of the comprehensive management of these patients. Clearly an understanding of the ethics involved is also important. General guidance on the range of pain management available for the different circumstances that may be encountered and the issues around practical difficulties in pain management should also be considered.

Maybe a key element in arguing the case for such a book is recognition that this is in reality a specialist area of practice in which many work occasionally and in which few are real experts. Until now there has been no such book. In fact there has been an identifiable void in the recent literature yet there is no doubt that a book which successfully pulls all of these strings together will be a wonderfully useful resource in any hospital. This is that book, written by experts in the field who do this kind of work all the time, and it is pragmatic and hence easy to use. Of course it is inevitable that both the science and the medicine of the treatment of malignancy will continue to evolve but this book lays solid foundations for the core roles of anaesthesia, pain, and intensive care in malignant disease.

Neil Soni
MBChB FANZCA FRCA FCICM MD FFICM
Consultant in Intensive Care and Anaesthesia,
Chelsea and Westminster Hospital and Clinical Senior Lecturer
Department of Surgery & Cancer, Imperial College London

Contents

Contributors

Ravishankar Rao Baikady
Consultant Anaesthetist
Royal Marsden NHS Foundation Trust

Desmond P.J. Barton
Consultant Surgeon
Royal Marsden NHS Foundation Trust

Katie Blightman
Specialist Registrar in Anaesthetics
Royal Marsden NHS Foundation Trust

James Burrow
Specialist Registrar in Anaesthetics
Royal Marsden NHS Foundation Trust

Craig Carr
Consultant in Intensive Care Medicine
Royal Marsden NHS Foundation Trust

Deanne Cheyne
Specialist Registrar in Anaesthetics
Royal Marsden NHS Foundation Trust

David Chisholm
Consultant Anaesthetist
Royal Marsden NHS Foundation Trust

Laurie Cohen
Specialist Registrar in Anaesthetics
Royal Marsden NHS Foundation Trust

Andrew N. Davies
Consultant in Palliative Medicine
Royal Marsden NHS Foundation Trust

Joanne Droney
Specialist Registrar in Palliative Medicine
Royal Marsden NHS Foundation Trust

Mark Edwards
Specialist Registrar in Anaesthetics
Royal Marsden NHS Foundation Trust

Paul Farquhar-Smith
Consultant in Pain, Anaesthetics and
Intensive Care
Royal Marsden NHS Foundation Trust

Jacqueline Filshie
Consultant in Pain Management
Royal Marsden NHS Foundation Trust

Stefan J. Friedrichsdorf
Medical Director
Pain Medicine, Palliative Care and
Integrative Medicine
Children's Hospitals and Clinics of
Minnesota
Minneapolis, MN, USA

Elisabeth Grey-Davies
Specialist Registrar in Haematology
Royal Marsden NHS Foundation Trust

Matthew Hacking
Consultant Anaesthetist
Royal Marsden NHS Foundation Trust

Selena Haque
Specialist Registrar in Anaesthesia
Royal Marsden NHS Foundation Trust

Rachel Harrison
Core Trainee in Surgery
Royal Free Hospital

Colm Irving
Consultant Anaesthetist
Royal Marsden NHS Foundation Trust

Paul Kelly
Consultant Anaesthetist
Guy's and St Thomas' NHS Foundation
Trust

Andrew Lawson
Honorary Senior Lecturer in Medical
Ethics, Imperial College, and Consultant
in Pain Medicine.

Enrique Lopez
Theatre Manager
Royal Marsden NHS Foundation Trust

Andrew McLeod
Consultant Anaesthetist
Royal Marsden NHS Foundation Trust

Anna Minchom
Specialist Registrar in Medical Oncology
Royal Marsden NHS Foundation Trust

Olivia Mingo
Consultant Anaesthetist
Royal Marsden NHS Foundation Trust

Joanna Moore
Consultant Anaesthetist
Kings College Hospital

Charlotte Moss
Specialist Registrar in Anaesthesia
Royal Marsden NHS Foundation Trust

Alex Oliver
Consultant Anaesthetist
Royal Marsden NHS Foundation Trust

David O'Regan
Core Trainee Year in Liaison Psychiatry
Guy's Hospital

Mike Potter
Consultant Haematologist
Royal Marsden NHS Foundation Trust

Julia Riley
Consultant in Palliative Medicine
Royal Marsden NHS Foundation Trust

Naureen Starling
Specialist Registrar in Medical Oncology
Royal Marsden NHS Foundation Trust

Richard Stümpfle
Consultant in Anaesthesia and
Intensive Care
Hammersmith Hospital

Charles Swanton
Consultant Medical Oncologist
Royal Marsden Hospital
MRC Senior Clinical Research Fellow
CR-UK London Research Institute

Catherine Urch
Lead Palliative Medicine Consultant
Imperial College NHS Trust

Ajit Walunj
Specialist Registrar in Anaesthetics
Imperial School of Anaesthesia

Kate Wessels
Specialist Registrar in Anaesthetics
Royal Marsden NHS Foundation Trust

Tim Wigmore
Consultant in Anaesthesia and
Intensive Care
Royal Marsden NHS Foundation Trust

John E. Williams
Consultant Anaesthetist
Royal Marsden NHS Foundation Trust

Jonathan T.C. Yen
Advanced Pain Trainee
Royal Marsden NHS Foundation Trust

Abbreviations

AML	acute myeloid leukaemia	EPO	erythropoietin
ACTH	adrenocorticotropic hormone	ET	essential thrombocythaemia
ADH	antidiuretic hormone	FEV_1	forced expiratory volume in 1 second
ALL	acute lymphoblastic leukaemia	FOI	fibreoptic intubation
ARDS	acute respiratory distress syndrome	GCSF	granulocyte colony-stimulating factor
ARF	acute renal failure	GI	gastrointestinal
AT	anaerobic threshold	GIST	gastrointestinal stromal tumour
ATN	acute tubular necrosis	GIT	gastrointestinal tract
ATRA	all-trans retinoic acid	GM-CSF	granulocyte macrophage colony stimulating factor
BAL	bronchoalveolar lavage		
BMA	British Medical Association	GTN	glyceryl trinitrate
BMI	body mass index	GvHD	graft-versus-host disease
BTCP	breakthrough cancer pain	HCC	hepatocellular carcinoma
CAM	complementary and alternative medicine	HIFU	high-intensity focused ultrasound
		HLA	human leukocyte antigen
CDK	cyclin-dependent kinase	HPA	hypothalamic–pituitary–adrenal
CIBP	cancer-induced bone pain	HPV	hypoxic pulmonary vasoconstriction
CIPN	chemotherapy-induced peripheral neuropathy	HSCT	haematopoietic stem cell transplantation
CLL	chronic lymphocytic leukaemia	IASP	International Association for the Study of Pain
CML	chronic myeloid leukaemia		
CMV	cytomegalovirus	ICS	intraoperative cell salvage
CNS	central nervous system	ICU	intensive care unit
CO	cardiac output	IGF	insulin-like growth factor
CO_2	carbon dioxide	IJV	internal jugular vein
COX	cyclo-oxygenase	IL	interleukin
CPAP	continuous positive airway pressure	IPI	International Prognostic Index
CPEX	cardiopulmonary exercise testing	IPSS	International Prognostic Scoring System
CPR	cardiopulmonary resuscitation		
CRC	colorectal cancer	IV	intravenous
CRT	capillary refill time	IVC	inferior vena cava
CT	computed tomography	IVCF	inferior vena cava filter
CTL	cuff-tip length	LA	local anaesthesia
CVP	central venous pressure	LMA	laryngeal mask airway
CXR	chest X-ray	LMWH	low-molecular-weight heparin
DLBCL	diffuse large B-cell lymphoma	mAb	monoclonal antibody
DLT	double-lumen tube	MAHA	microangiopathic haemolytic anaemia
EBV	Epstein–Barr virus	MAP	mean arterial pressure
EGF	epidermal growth factor	MBC	metastatic breast cancer
EGFR	epidermal growth factor receptor	MDS	myelodysplastic syndromes

MDT	multidisciplinary team	RCT	randomized controlled trial
MGUS	monoclonal gammopathy of unknown significance	RFA	radiofrequency ablation
		RSV	respiratory syncytial virus
MM	multiple myeloma	SCCHN	squamous cell carcinoma of the head and neck
MODS	multiple organ dysfunction syndrome		
MRI	magnetic resonance imaging	SIRS	systemic inflammatory response syndrome
NHL	non-Hodgkin's lymphoma		
NHS	National Health Service	SV	stroke volume
NICE	National Institute for Health and Clinical Excellence	SVC	superior vena cava
		SWT	shuttle walk test
NIV	non-invasive ventilation	TBI	total body irradiation
NPC	nasopharyngeal cancer	TEA	thoracic epidural analgesia
NSCLC	non-small-cell lung cancer	TIVA	total intravenous anaesthesia
OLV	one-lung ventilation	TKI	tyrosine kinase inhibitor
PAC	pulmonary artery catheter	TNF	tumour necrosis factor
PARP	poly(ADP ribose) polymerase	TOD	transoesophageal Doppler
PBCSP	post-breast cancer surgery pain	TPN	total parenteral nutrition
PEEP	positive end-expiratory pressure	TRAM	transverse rectus abdominis muscle
PET	positron emission tomography	TTP	thrombotic thrombocytopenic purpura
PICC	peripherally inserted central venous catheter		
		TUR	transurethral resection
PP	pulse pressure	TV	tidal volume
PPV	pulse pressure variation	VEGF	vascular endothelial growth factor
PRES	posterior reversible encephalopathy	VOD	veno-occlusive disease
PRV	polycythaemia rubra vera	VTE	venous thromboembolism
PVB	paravertebral blockade	WCC	white cell count
PVR	pulmonary vascular resistance	WHO	World Health Organization
QALY	quality-adjusted life year		

Part 1

Cancer

Chapter 1

Haematological malignancy: a rough guide

Elisabeth Grey-Davies and Mike Potter

Introduction

Haematological malignancies arise from uncontrolled expansion of cells of the blood and lymphatic system and their precursors. These are either:

◆ Myeloid—arising from the myeloid progenitor cell which gives rise to neutrophils, monocytes, platelets, and erythrocytes or

◆ Lymphoid—arising from the lymphoid stem cell which gives rise to B and T lymphocytes, natural killer cells, and plasma cells.

The World Health Organization (WHO) classification of malignant haematological diseases lists over 140 separate disorders. This chapter focuses on the most common ones and those with particular clinical significance.

The leukaemias

The term leukaemia, derived from the Greek meaning 'white blood', refers to those conditions where there is uncontrolled proliferation of the white blood cells. In addition to a high circulating white cell count, symptoms related to either bone marrow failure or tissue infiltration by leukaemic cells are often present. Typical presenting features include:

◆ Anaemia

◆ Neutropenia

◆ Thrombocytopenia

◆ Hepatosplenomegaly

◆ Lymphadenopathy

◆ Skin infiltration

◆ Swollen gums

◆ Hyperviscosity

◆ Deranged coagulation.

Diagnosis is made by examination of the peripheral blood and bone marrow (confirming >20% blasts), immunophenotyping (to identify specific cell surface markers), and cytogenetic and molecular genetic analysis. The acute leukaemias are derived from immature precursors or blast cells and the chronic leukaemias from mature white blood cells.

Acute myeloid leukaemia

Acute myeloid leukaemia (AML) arises from immature myeloid precursors. In the original FAB (French–American–British) classification AML was divided into eight groups (M0–M7) according to blast morphology, but this was neither prognostic nor useful in defining treatment strategies. The revised WHO classification subdivides AML into:

◆ AML with recurrent translocations

◆ AML with multilineage dysplasia

◆ AML therapy-related and

◆ AML not otherwise specified

AML arising from previous myelodysplasia or secondary to previous chemotherapy has a poor prognosis. Specific clinical presentations are associated with distinct molecular subtypes and understanding the molecular basis of AML is important in risk stratification, defining new therapeutic strategies, and understanding the genetic abnormalities underlying leukaemogenesis.

AML is stratified into three risk groups according to the presence or absence of certain cytogenetic abnormalities. The good prognostic group (5-year survival 75–80%) includes acute promyelocytic leukaemia (APML, M3 in the FAB classification). This subtype has characteristic morphology with hypergranular promyelocytes packed with Auer rods and the PML-RARA fusion protein. It has an excellent long-term outlook but a high early mortality from bleeding. Leukaemic promyelocytes release thromboplastins resulting in disseminated intravascular coagulation. Patients require correction of coagulopathies even in the absence of clinical bleeding. Introduction of all-trans retinoic acid (ATRA), which induces differentiation of promyelocytes into mature granulocytes, has revolutionized the treatment and prognosis of this condition. It is crucial that ATRA is commenced as soon as APML is suspected.

The incidence of AML rises exponentially with age and the elderly have a poor prognosis. This partly relates to the biology of the disease, with adverse cytogenetics more frequent, but also treatment options are often limited by comorbidities. Quality of life is a key consideration for patients in the poor prognostic group and palliative care may be appropriate.

Treatment

The standard of care for fit patients with non-APML AML is induction treatment with daunorubicin and cytosine arabinoside, with which 60–90% will achieve a complete remission dependent on age and cytogenetics. The major cause of treatment failure in AML is disease relapse and those patients who achieve remission are consolidated with either further high-dose chemotherapy or allogeneic transplant. Understanding of the pathogenesis of AML has led to targeted therapies, for example, the monoclonal anti-CD33 agent gemtuzumab.

Allogeneic transplant remains the most potent antileukaemic strategy in AML through the administration of myeloablative chemotherapy and the graft-versus-leukaemia effect. Reduced intensity conditioning regimens have allowed transplants for older patients. There is a convincing evidence base for allogeneic transplant in first remission in those patients with standard risk AML under the age of 40 with a suitable sibling or matched unrelated donor, but outside this group careful patient selection is vital. Transplant-related mortality is significant and the morbidity of post-transplant infections and graft-versus-host disease must not be underestimated.

Acute lymphoblastic leukaemia

Acute lymphoblastic leukaemia (ALL) is an aggressive malignant disorder of lymphoid progenitor cells. It is most common in childhood, with a peak incidence between the ages of 2–5 years, and a further peak in old age. Paediatric ALL is a success story of modern haematology with 5-year survival of 85–90%, in contrast to the often poor outlook for adults. This partly reflects the biology of the disease, yet adolescents and young adults treated with paediatric protocols may have a better outcome than with adult protocols. Thus in the UK the under 25s are generally treated on paediatric regimens and in dedicated adolescent units. High white cell counts at presentation (>30 for B-ALL, >100 for T-ALL) and the presence of the Philadelphia chromosome are poor prognostic features. The incidence of this and other adverse cytogenetic abnormalities increases with age.

Treatment

ALL is treated with intensive 'induction' chemotherapy including steroids, vincristine, L-asparaginase and anthracycline, often with cyclophosphamide or cytarabine. Central nervous system (CNS) directed therapy with either intrathecal chemotherapy or irradiation is an important component as the induction chemotherapy has poor CNS penetration. Remission is consolidated with either an allogeneic transplant or maintenance chemotherapy for a further 2–3 years. Long-term remission rates in adult ALL are of the order of 30–35% and therefore most are offered an allogeneic transplant in first remission if fit. The treatment of ALL in the elderly remains a challenge and elderly patients are excluded from most clinical trials.

Chronic lymphocytic leukaemia

Chronic lymphocytic leukaemia (CLL) is the most common form of leukaemia in the Western world. It is generally a disease of the middle-aged and elderly, with a median age at diagnosis of 65–70 years and a male predominance. Symptomatic patients present with: bone marrow suppression, lymphadenopathy, hepatosplenomegaly, weight loss, night sweats, recurrent infection, and immune complications (immune thrombocytopenia or autoimmune haemolytic anaemia). Herpes zoster and pneumococcal pneumonia are particularly prevalent, together with long-term complications such as bronchiectasis. A long asymptomatic phase means diagnosis of CLL is often from a full blood count done for another reason.

CLL cells have characteristic morphology in the peripheral blood and the diagnosis can be confirmed by using flow cytometry to define a specific set of cell surface markers and derive the 'CLL score'. The Binet staging system is the most widely employed:

◆ Stage C: Hb <10g/dl or a platelet count of <100 × 10 ^{9}/l

◆ Stage B: involvement of >3 lymphoid areas

◆ Stage A: neither of the above.

The natural history of the illness is very variable. Recently identified prognostic markers (e.g. unmutated IgVH genes) can be used to define a high-risk group although these remain predominantly research based. The transformation (Richter's transformation) to diffuse large B-cell lymphoma is associated with a poor prognosis (median survival of <1 year).

Treatment

CLL is a low-grade, generally incurable malignancy. Treatment decisions depend on a balance between symptoms and side effects of treatment. Median survival is 7–10 years. Patients with Stage C or progressive Stage B disease are usually recommended treatment. First line includes a purine analogue in combination with the monoclonal anti-CD20 agent rituximab (CD20 is a B-cell surface marker). The current UK approach is fludarabine, cyclophosphamide, and rituximab in combination. Alemtuzumab, a monoclonal antibody targeting CD52, is useful in refractory and resistant cases. Allogeneic transplantation may be appropriate for a carefully selected group of younger patients with high-risk disease.

The myeloproliferative disorders

Chronic myeloid leukaemia

Chronic myeloid leukaemia (CML) was the first human disease to be linked to a single acquired genetic abnormality: the balanced translocation between chromosome 9 and chromosome 22, the Philadelphia chromosome. This fusion gene leads to the formation of BCR-ABL, a tyrosine protein kinase which causes uncontrolled proliferation of both mature and immature white blood cells in the blood and bone marrow.

Patients typically present with weight loss, splenomegaly, fatigue and fevers, and leuco-cytosis. Diagnosis can be made by peripheral blood film and confirmed by demonstrating the presence of either the Philadelphia chromosome or BCR-ABL transcripts in blood or bone marrow cells. CML has three recognized phases distinguished predominantly by the number of bone marrow blasts:

◆ Chronic phase

◆ Accelerated phase

◆ Blast crisis (similar to acute leukaemia).

Treatment

CML treatment has been revolutionized with the advent of specific molecular-targeted therapy and 5-year survival now exceeds 90%. Imatinib, the prototype tyrosine kinase inhibitor, and its successors inhibit the BCR-ABL tyrosine kinase by competitive binding at the ATP-binding site. Oral treatment results in complete cytogenetic remissions in up to 87%. Hence allogeneic transplantation is reserved for those patients who are resistant to tyrosine kinase inhibitors.

Essential thrombocythaemia, polycythaemia rubra vera, and idiopathic myelofibrosis

These myeloproliferative disorders are clonal, neoplastic conditions characterized by over-production of red cells (polycythaemia rubra vera, PRV), platelets (essential thrombocythaemia, ET), or by reactive bone marrow fibrosis in myelofibrosis. Patients with PRV are plethoric, often have splenomegaly, and may present with vascular complications such as cerebrovascular accident, myocardial infarction, peripheral ischaemia, and venous thromboembolism. Patients with ET present with similar vascular complications, headache, and bleeding (due to acquired von Willebrand disease). Clinical signs and symptoms of myelofibrosis are hepatosplenomegaly, which may be massive (due to extramedullary haemopoiesis) and in the latter stages weight loss and night sweats. In the 'cellular phase' there is neutrophilia and thrombocytosis but as the disease progresses patients develop pancytopenia with the associated symptoms and risk of infection.

The molecular basis of these myeloproliferative disorders is also being unravelled. One mutation of the *JAK2* gene is detected in 95% of cases of PRV and 50% of cases of ET and idiopathic myelofibrosis. Both ET and PRV can transform to myelofibrosis and all three have a tendency to transform to AML. Treatment is with cytoreductive agents such as hydroxycarbamide and anagrelide. Agents such as thalidomide can be used in myelofibrosis. Allogeneic transplantation may occasionally be appropriate, but targeted therapies may play an increasing role as the molecular basis is better understood.

Myelodysplasia

The myelodysplastic syndromes (MDS) are a heterogeneous group of haematological neoplasms characterized by ineffective and dysplastic haemopoiesis. Patients present with symptoms related to isolated cytopenias or pancytopenia. MDS can occur either *de novo* or as a consequence of previous chemotherapy or radiotherapy. The natural history is progression to AML, although the rate of progression is extremely variable. Disease factors which contribute to prognosis have been combined to produce an International Prognostic Scoring System (IPSS) which includes: number of blasts in the bone marrow, karyotype, and number of cytopenias. Median survival ranges from 0.4 months to 5.7 years. Cytogenetic abnormalities are present in 40–60% of patients and are more frequent in aggressive disease. The incidence of MDS rises with age. Allogeneic transplantation is recommended for fit patients with high-risk disease and the demethylating agent 5-azacytidine is the only agent to have demonstrated a survival benefit in MDS. The majority of patients are managed with supportive care.

The lymphomas

Lymphomas are neoplasms of B, T, or NK lymphoid cells and their precursors, broadly divided into Hodgkin's disease and Non-Hodgkin's lymphoma (NHL). NHL is further classified into high grade and low grade according to the proliferation rate. In general, the high-grade lymphomas are aggressive but chemosensitive malignancies, whereas the low-grade lymphomas follow a more indolent course but are generally not curable.

Presenting symptoms common to all subtypes of lymphoma are lymphadenopathy, 'B' symptoms (drenching night sweats, fever, and weight loss of >10% body weight in 6 months), hypercalcaemia, pruritis, and symptoms of organ infiltration. HIV infection is a significant risk factor for lymphoma of all subtypes and all patients should be offered testing.

The Ann Arbour staging system is widely employed.

- Stage 1: involvement of a single lymph node group
- Stage 2: >1 lymph node group on the same side of the diaphragm
- Stage 3: lymph node involvement on both sides of the diaphragm
- Stage 4: disseminated extra-lymphatic spread.

These are designated A or B according to the absence or presence of 'B' symptoms.

All lymphoma subtypes generally respond well to steroids, which may be used as a holding measure (ideally after taking histological samples) in the acutely unwell patient until full histological subtype is available and definitive treatment can start.

Hodgkin's lymphoma

Hodgkin's lymphoma is a neoplasm of the germinal centre B cell and is defined histologically by the presence of characteristic Reed–Sternberg cells. Most patients are young adults (more males) presenting with lymphadenopathy (often cervical). Early-stage disease (I–IIa) is typically treated with a short course of chemotherapy followed by local radiotherapy and more advanced disease (Stage IIb–IV) with longer courses of chemotherapy. First-line chemotherapy is usually with ABVD (doxorubicin, bleomycin, vinblastine, and dacarbazine) and response rates are excellent (80–95%). Since the majority of patients are curable with current therapy, limiting treatment-related toxicity has become a major focus for research. Positron emission tomography (PET) is an excellent imaging modality in Hodgkin's lymphoma, both in improving accuracy of disease staging and assessing response to treatment.

Non-Hodgkin's lymphoma

High-grade lymphoma

Burkitt's lymphoma is a highly aggressive tumour with overexpression of the *C-MYC* oncogene and a proliferation rate approaching 100%. It is highly chemoresponsive, with current 5-year survival rates greater than 90%, but patients are often extremely unwell with advanced stage disease at presentation, and may require intensive care support. There is a significant early mortality and hence making the diagnosis and initiating treatment is a medical emergency.

There are three subtypes of Burkitt's lymphoma:

- Sporadic (most common in the West): typically affects children and young adults, is associated with Epstein–Barr virus (EBV) in 10% of cases and often involves the gastrointestinal tract.
- Endemic: common in Africa and where malaria is hyperendemic, is strongly correlated with EBV infection, and usually affects children, often presenting as a mass in the jaw.
- HIV associated.

Treatment is with intensive combination chemotherapy regimens including cyclophosphamide, anthracycline, cytarabine, methotrexate, and rituximab, and CNS-directed therapy is an important component. The risk of tumour lysis syndrome is extremely high and rasburicase prophylaxis is usually recommended.

Diffuse large B-cell lymphoma (DLBCL) encompasses a heterogeneous group of disorders, all characterized by diffuse tissue infiltration by mature B cells. It is potentially curable, with a 5-year survival of around 60%, and typically affects adults of middle age or the elderly. DLBCL may occur *de novo* or after transformation of a low-grade NHL, where the prognosis is less favourable. The International Prognostic Index (IPI) combines adverse prognostic factors at diagnosis (advanced age, elevated lactate dehydrogenase, poor performance status, advanced stage disease) to stratify patients into prognostic groups. An activated B-cell type, as opposed to a germinal centre type (distinguished by immunophenotyping), is also an adverse prognostic factor. The incidence is markedly increased in patients with concurrent HIV infection.

Treatment is with chemotherapy in combination with rituximab, the addition of which has significantly improved both progression-free survival and overall survival. The standard first-line chemotherapy regimen is CHOP (cyclophosphamide, doxorubicin, vincristine, prednisolone) which may be followed by targeted or 'involved field' radiotherapy. Second-line therapy is usually high-dose chemotherapy supported by autologous stem cell transplant in fit patients although a palliative approach may be appropriate in some cases.

Low-grade lymphoma

This encompasses a heterogeneous group of disorders which have a relatively indolent clinical course but are generally considered incurable with conventional chemotherapy. Allogeneic transplantation following non-myeloablative conditioning may be considered for younger patients. They all have a variable tendency to transform to high-grade lymphomas, in which case they may be refractory to treatment. Key features of a number of the more common low-grade lymphomas are summarized in Table 1.1.

Myeloma and plasma cell dyscrasias

Plasma cell malignancies involve uncontrolled proliferation of a clone of immunoglobulin-secreting B lymphocytes which typically produce a single homogeneous (monoclonal)

Table 1.1 Key characteristics of the more common low-grade lymphomas

Name	Pathological features	Clinical features
Follicular lymphoma	Germinal centre B cells Usually presents with stage IV disease FLIPI scoring system prognostic Grades 1–3a indolent lymphomas, but grade 3b behaves like a high-grade lymphoma	More common in women 'Watch and wait' is the recommended strategy for asymptomatic patients FCR (fludarabine, cyclophosphamide, rituximab) recommended first-line therapy Benefit from maintenance rituximab Median survival 9–10 years
Mantle cell lymphoma	Characteristic translocation t(11;14) leading to dysregulation of cyclin D1 Grade of malignancy indeterminate between DLBCL and follicular NHL	Middle-aged to older individuals Marked male predominance Clinically heterogenous—from the aggressive blastic subtype to a more indolent form Median survival 3 years
Extranodal marginal zone lymphoma of mucosa-associated lymphoid tissue (MALT lymphoma)	Antigenic stimulation may play an important role, e.g. *Helicobacter pylori* in gastric MALT T(11;18) associated with a poorer prognosis	Gastric MALT may regress following *Helicobacter* eradication Usually very indolent
Nodal marginal zone lymphoma	Similar to above, but nodal disease only	
Splenic marginal zone lymphoma	Usually significant splenomegaly with minimal lymphadenopathy Peripheral blood lymphocytosis—lymphocytes may have distinctive villous projections	Splenectomy may result in long remissions Median survival >8 years
Lymphoplasmacytic lymphoma (Waldenström macroglobulinaemia)	IgM paraprotein Lymphoplasmacytoid morphology	Can present with symptoms of hyperviscosity Usually has a very indolent course

immunoglobulin, although 15% of myelomas do not produce immunoglobulin. These 'paraproteins' are identified by protein electrophoresis or immunofixation and are key to both the diagnosis and monitoring of myeloma and other plasma cell disorders. A monoclonal paraprotein identified without other features of myeloma is termed a monoclonal gammopathy of unknown significance (MGUS), and may precede the development of myeloma. Sometimes just the immunoglobulin light chain is produced and this can be detected in the urine as Bence Jones protein or in the serum by a free light chain assay.

Myeloma

Patients with myeloma present with anaemia and more rarely other cytopenias due to replacement of bone marrow by malignant plasma cells. Excess monoclonal light chains in the serum and urine leads to saturation of the glomerular reabsorption capacity, leading to light chain precipitation in the renal tubules, cast nephropathy, and resulting in acute or chronic renal failure. Hypercalcaemia and amyloidosis can also be important contributing factors. Renal impairment in a myeloma patient is a medical emergency, with the chance of renal recovery diminishing in proportion to the duration of the insult. Dexamethasone can temporarily switch off light chain production and therefore protect the kidneys prior to the introduction of definitive therapy. Myeloma plasma cells secrete cytokines which upregulate osteoclast activity, leading to lytic bone disease with pain, deformity, and the risk of pathological fracture. Bisphosphonates play an important role in preventing lytic bone disease. Recurrent infection is also an important feature of myeloma as well as symptoms of hyperviscosity (sluggishness, bleeding, visual disturbance due to retinal haemorrhage). Rarely, patients present with extramedullary deposits of myeloma known as plasmocytomas. Adverse prognostic features include anaemia, renal failure, elevated β_2 microglobulin, elevated C-reactive protein, low serum albumin, and the presence of certain cytogenetic abnormalities.

Treatment

The treatment and outlook of myeloma has improved significantly in recent years with the advent of new therapies. Use of the novel agents thalidomide, bortezomib, and lenalidomide during the last 10 years have meant median overall survival from diagnosis is now approximately 9 years. First-line therapy is generally with thalidomide-based regimens, but neuropathy and increased risk of venous thromboembolism are key toxicities. Once in remission, progression-free survival is prolonged by a median of 9–18 months by consolidation with high-dose melphan and stem cell rescue—an 'autograft'. In the UK the proteosome inhibitor bortezomib is generally used at first relapse, again with neuropathy (both sensorimotor and autonomic) a potentially dose-limiting toxicity. Lenalidomide, a thalidomide analogue with an immunomodulatory mechanism of action, is used at second relapse or beyond and has a role in the maintenance setting. Myelosuppression and risk of infection are key risks. The optimum schedule for use of the new antimyeloma agents is the subject of ongoing research and UK treatment protocols are driven by cost-effectiveness as well as clinical efficacy.

Conclusion

There has been huge progress in the outlook of haematological malignancies in the past 40 years with the improvement in both therapeutic agents and supportive care. As the understanding of the molecular pathogenesis of the haematological malignancies is unravelled, treatment will increasingly move towards specific and targeted therapy. The use of imatinib in CML was the prototype. However most haematological malignancies have a more complex pathogenesis dependent on multiple genetic hits and a microenvironment that encourages oncogenesis, hence research is key to improving prognosis further for the next generation of patients.

Bibliography

1. Burnett AK, Wheatley K, Goldstone AH, *et al.* (2002). The value of allogeneic bone marrow transplant in patients with acute myeloid leukaemia at differing risk of relapse: results of the UK MRC AML 10 trial. *Br J Haematol* **118**(2):385–400.

2. Child JA, Morgan GJ, Davies FE, *et al.* (2003). High-dose chemotherapy with hematopoietic stem-cell rescue for multiple myeloma. *N Engl J Med* **348**(19):1875–83.

3. Coiffier B, Lepage E, Briere J, *et al.* (2002). CHOP chemotherapy plus rituximab compared with CHOP alone in elderly patients with diffuse large-B-cell lymphoma. *N Engl J Med* **346**(4):235–42.

4. Dimopoulos M, Spencer A, Attal M, *et al.* (2007). Lenalidomide plus dexamethasone for relapsed or refractory multiple myeloma. *N Engl J Med* **357**(21):2123–32.

5. Gallamini A, Hutchings M, Rigacci L, *et al.* (2007). Early interim 2-[18F]fluoro-2-deoxy-D-glucose positron emission tomography is prognostically superior to international prognostic score in advanced-stage Hodgkin's lymphoma: a report from a joint Italian-Danish study. *J Clin Oncol* **25**(24):3746–52.

6. Hallek M, Fischer K, Fingerle-Rowson G, *et al.* (2010). Addition of rituximab to fludarabine and cyclophosphamide in patients with chronic lymphocytic leukaemia: a randomised, open-label, phase 3 trial. *Lancet* **376**(9747):1164–74.

7. O'Brien SG, Guilhot F, Larson RA, *et al.* (2003). Imatinib compared with interferon and low-dose cytarabine for newly diagnosed chronic-phase chronic myeloid leukemia. *N Engl J Med* **348**(11): 994–1004.

8. Palumbo A, Bringhen S, Caravita T, *et al.* (2006). Oral melphalan and prednisone chemotherapy plus thalidomide compared with melphalan and prednisone alone in elderly patients with multiple myeloma: randomised controlled trial. *Lancet* **367**:825–31.

9. Richardson PG, Sonneveld P, Schuster MW, *et al.* (2005). Bortezomib or high-dose dexamethasone for relapsed multiple myeloma. *N Engl J Med* **352**(24):2487–98.

10. Scott LM, Campbell PJ, Baxter EJ, *et al.* (2005). The V617F JAK2 mutation is uncommon in cancers and in myeloid malignancies other than the classic myeloproliferative disorders. *Blood* **106**(8):2920–1.

11. Swerdlow SH, Campi E, Harris N, *et al.* (2008). *WHO Classification of Tumours of Haemopoietic and Lymphoid Tissues*, 4th Edition. Geneva: WHO Press.

Chapter 2

Cancer biology and treatment: a molecular and therapeutic overview

Anna Minchom, Naureen Starling, and
Charles Swanton

Introduction

More than a quarter of a million people are diagnosed with cancer in the UK each year and one in four people in the UK will die of cancer. There are over 200 types of solid cancer, classified according to the tissue of origin (Table 2.1). The vast majority of human cancers originate from epithelial tissues, known as carcinomas. These can be further subdivided into squamous cell carcinomas that arise from epithelial cells and adenocarcinomas that arise from the cells of the glandular ducts within the epithelial surfaces. Cancer development may result from the breakdown of normal cellular growth control mechanisms and is a multistep process that can involve DNA damage to a normal cell resulting from ultraviolet (UV) radiation, pollutants, or dietary carcinogens. Errors in the normal DNA replication processes also cause DNA alterations. Repair processes attempt to minimize and reverse this damage. Later stages of malignant progression involve the acquisition of accelerated growth characteristics dependent on access to nutrients and oxygen through the development of new blood vessels (angiogenesis) and invasion through local tissues and metastasis. Cancer cells differ in their physiology and behaviour from normal cells in fundamental ways, defined by Weinberg and Hanahan:

- Self-sufficiency in growth signals
- Insensitivity to growth-inhibitory signals
- Loss of capacity for apoptosis—apoptosis, or programmed cell death, destroys cells that have potentially harmful genetic errors
- Loss of capacity for senescence (ageing), rendering them immortal
- Ability to initiate angiogenesis
- Ability to invade neighbouring tissues and metastasize to distant sites.

This chapter will focus on these key aspects of cancer biology and review their application to the development of successful therapeutic strategies in this disease.

Table 2.1 Classification of solid tumours

Tissue of origin	Name	Examples
Epithelial	Carcinoma (squamous cell)	Skin, nasal cavity, oropharynx, larynx, lung, oesophagus, cervix
	Carcinoma (adeno)	Lung, colon, breast, pancreas, stomach, oesophagus, prostate, endometrium, ovary
Connective tissues/ mesenchymal	Sarcomas	Bone (osteosarcomas), blood vessels (angiosarcomas), fat (liposarcomas), skeletal muscle (rhabdomyosarcoma), smooth muscle (leimyosarcoma)
Nervous system (neuroectodermal malignancies)		Gliomas, glioblastomas, neuroblastomas, schwannomas, medulloblastomas
Germ cell		Teratomas, seminoma, choriocarcinoma

Cellular signalling and oncogenes

Cellular response to signals transduced from the extracellular environment is an essential part of embryogenesis and tissue maintenance and can result in changes in cell metabolism, cell structure, or cell growth. Extracellular signals may be initiated through secreted polypeptide molecules known as cytokines or growth factors, such as epidermal growth factor (EGF) and vascular endothelial growth factor (VEGF). These growth factors and their cognate receptors are often deregulated in tumour development and malignant progression.

Growth factor receptors are classified according to their primary signal transduction mechanisms and are comprised of ligand-gated ion channels, GTPase (G-protein)-linked receptors, and protein-kinase-linked receptors. The majority of growth factors mediate their effects through binding to tyrosine kinase receptors (Figure 2.1). Growth factors such the EGF and VEGF growth factor family bind to the extracellular component of their cognate tyrosine kinase receptors resulting in receptor dimerization (bonding with a fellow receptor) and receptor activation via phosphorylation of cytoplasmic tyrosine residues. Ligand engagement by the receptor results in the initiation of diverse intracellular signalling pathway activity. Figure 2.1 gives the example of the intracellular signalling pathways. An end point of cellular signalling is the initiation of gene transcription from nuclear DNA. Growth factor signalling can lead to the initiation of processes such as growth, differentiation, migration, angiogenesis, and apoptosis.

An oncogene is a gene whose protein product when altered (e.g. mutation, truncation, or overexpression) contributes to cellular transformation and cancer progression. Oncogenes were discovered 25 years ago, encoded by viruses that caused tumours in chickens and rodents. Proto-oncogenes are involved in normal cellular processes such as cell signalling. Mutation of proto-oncogenes may result in acquisition of growth promoting activity through such mechanisms as expression of a constitutively activated form of a receptor (e.g. epidermal growth factor receptor, EGFR) or overexpression of the growth

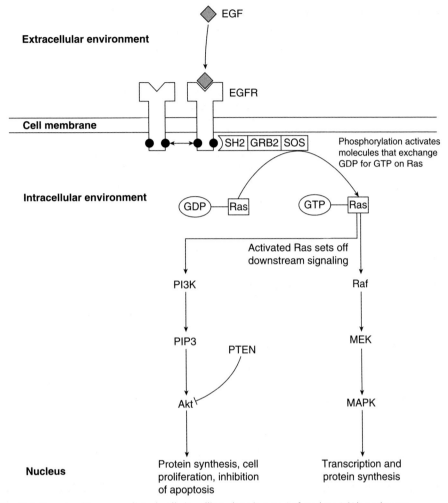

Fig. 2.1 Tyrosine kinase-mediated cell signalling showing ras/raf and ras/pi3k pathways.

factor receptor ligand. Activation of growth factors and their receptors is seen in many cancers. The EGFR family of receptors are commonly overexpressed, truncated, or mutated in glioblastoma, colorectal cancer (CRC), non-small-cell lung cancer (NSCLC), breast cancer, and ovarian cancer. VEGFR overexpression is seen in a variety of cancers including CRC and lung.

One of the best studied oncogenes is *Ras* that mediates signalling through the Raf-MAPK pathway (Figure 2.1). In normal cells Ras largely exists in an inactive state bound to GDP. It has been shown that activating mutations in *K-ras* occur in up to 30% of cancers including CRC and pancreatic cancer. An activating mutation will lead to constitutive activation of growth promoting pathways. Signal transduction pathways can also become deregulated through the loss of an inhibitory influence that negatively regulates pathway activity, for example, through inactivation of the phosphatase and tensin homologue, PTEN. Mutations in the *PTEN* gene have been found in melanoma, breast, prostate, endometrial, ovarian, and colorectal cancer.

The cell cycle

The cell cycle is divided into several phases (Figure 2.2). The majority of the cells in the body are in the quiescent G_0 phase. Transition between the phases is governed by activation of protein kinases (cyclin-dependent kinase (CDK) family) mediated by their cyclin partners. A cell cycle inhibitory protein, retinoblastoma (pRB), is progressively phosphorylated and inactivated by cyclins in the G_1 phase of the cell cycle leading to the transcriptional activation of genes required for S phase and DNA synthesis by the E2F family of transcription factors. CDK activity is kept in check by two families of CDK inhibitory proteins (CKIs): the p21 family and the p16 family.

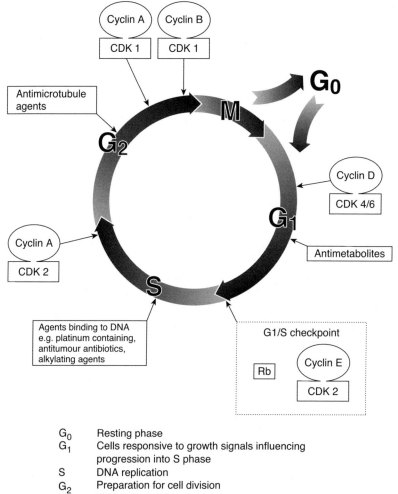

G_0	Resting phase
G_1	Cells responsive to growth signals influencing progression into S phase
S	DNA replication
G_2	Preparation for cell division
M	Mitosis (cell division)

Fig. 2.2 The cell cycle showing actions of chemotherapeutic agents.

Tumour suppressor genes

Tumour suppressor genes are able to inhibit cancer-specific characteristics such as enhanced proliferative capacity or resistance to cell death. They were originally identified in familial cancer syndromes through the inheritance of inactivating mutations (e.g. familial retino-blastoma and pRB). An important concept when considering tumour suppressor genes is that of 'loss of heterozygosity'. This occurs when one allele is subject to loss of function when the other allele is already inactivated. In some familial cancer syndromes, the first step involves the inactivation of one tumour suppressor allele in the germline with the second inactivating mutation occurring in somatic cells as a sporadic event. One tumour suppressor gene, *p53* is often referred to as the 'guardian of the genome', and controls DNA repair and cell proliferation. *Rb* (the retinoblastoma gene), is mutated in a variety of malignancies as a sporadic event in cancer cells or as a familial condition where one defective allele is inherited in the germline and the second mutation occurs as a sporadic event promoting the familial condition, retinoblastoma. Mutations in *Rb* allow unscheduled proliferation and cell division to occur through premature release of E2F from its inhibitory influence.

DNA repair mechanisms

There are complex cellular processes that function in normal cells to limit DNA mutation rate during replication and cell division. DNA polymerase is the enzyme that 'reads' the DNA strand using it as a template to synthesize new strands. It has a low error rate. If errors do occur other proteins correct this 'mismatch'. Errors in mismatch repair lead to hereditary cancer conditions.

There are a host of proteins that can repair established DNA damage. Repair pathways can occur through 'base excision' and 'nucleotide excision' repair. Base excision repair entails the removal of one base (the individual molecules making up DNA) and replacement with the correct one. Nucleotide excision repair removes a group of bases. Xeroderma pigmentosum is an autosomal recessive condition caused by faulty nucleotide excision repair. It results in increased sensitivity to UV light with skin cancers at a young age. The poly(ADP ribose) polymerase (PARP) family play an important role in base-excision repair. PARP-1 is activated following the detection of DNA breaks. Modification of nuclear proteins by PARP-mediated poly(ADP-ribosylation) occurs leading to attraction of DNA repair complexes.

Other DNA damage occurs in the form of 'double strand breaks'. Repair occurs in G_1 phase by a process known as 'non-homologous end-joining' or in S and G_2 by 'homologous recombination repair'. *BRCA1* and *-2* mutations are associated with compromised homologous recombination repair and familial breast and ovarian cancer.

Angiogenesis

Adequate blood supply is critical for tumour growth. Without an independent blood supply tumours cannot grow larger than 0.2mm as hypoxia develops, nutrients decrease, and waste products accumulate. Angiogenesis is thought to be regulated by a number of pro-angiogenic factors (e.g. VEGF, EGF) and anti-angiogenic factors (e.g. thrombospondin-1).

Therapeutics of oncology

Chemotherapy

The first chemotherapy agent, nitrogen mustard, was introduced in the 1940s. Since then a wide range of chemotherapy drugs have been developed from natural and manufactured sources (Table 2.2). Chemotherapy agents affect processes involved in DNA synthesis, DNA structure, and metabolism and mechanisms associated with cell division. They are therefore relatively unselective in their action, attacking normal cells that are physiologically fast dividing. This includes cells in the bone marrow (resulting in immunosuppression), gastrointestinal system (resulting in mucositis), and hair follicles (resulting in alopecia). Other side effects are more specific to each class of chemotherapy (Table 2.2).

Targeted therapeutics and personalized cancer medicine

The exploitation of processes in cancer biology has led to useful therapeutic strategies. The rationale for such pathway-directed drug therapy is to target critical cellular processes that a cancer is dependent on for growth and progression. In theory this allows the delivery of therapy tailored to the characteristics of the tumour (so-called personalized cancer medicine) that may result in less toxicity compared to standard chemotherapy with therapeutic benefit in molecularly pre-defined patient cohorts. Despite the potential tumour-specific nature of targeted therapeutics there are well recognized, potentially life-threatening side effects associated with defined agents that relate to their mechanism of action. Furthermore, despite the target-driven nature of their development (e.g. the anti-angiogenesis agents), defined and accurate predictive biomarkers to identify responding patient cohorts in some cases are lacking.

Table 2.3 gives some examples of important drug targets to which biological therapies have been developed and which are further discussed below. The drugs fall into two categories: tyrosine kinase inhibitors (TKIs) and monoclonal antibodies (mAbs).

Endothelial growth factor receptor

EGFR is thought to play an important role in the pathogenesis of many tumour types including NSCLC, CRC, and head and neck cancer. EGFR can be targeted by TKIs directed against the intracellular domain or by mAbs directed against the extracellular component. The goal of both is the abrogation of EGFR-directed growth signalling. Examples of anti-EGFR TKIs furthest in their clinical development are gefitinib and erlotinib. EGFR-directed mAbs include cetuximab and panitumumab.

EGFR overexpression is found in approximately 62% of NSCLC. Erlotinib monotherapy improves survival in relapsed NSCLC. Patients with mutation in the tyrosine kinase domain of EGFR appear to be preferentially sensitive to erlotinib. Erlotinib is orally administered and adverse effects include skin rashes, diarrhoea, nausea, and transient

Table 2.2 Chemotherapeutic agents

Chemotherapy group	Examples	Mode of action	Tumour types	Toxicities
Platinum-containing drugs	Cisplatin, carboplatin, oxaliplatin	Causes DNA cross links inhibiting replication and causing apoptosis	Lung, colon, oesophagus, stomach, head and neck, breast, ovarian, cervix, endometrial, bladder, testis	Renal toxicity, peripheral neuropathy, ototoxicity
Antimicrotubule agent	Vinca alkaloids, e.g. vinblastine, vinorelbine	Bind to microtubules. Microtubules are part of cellular framework required for cell division. Cells arrest at G_2M phase of cell cycle.	Melanoma, breast, lung leukaemia, lymphoma	Alopecia, immunosuppression, abdominal cramps, neuropathy
	Taxanes, e.g. paclitaxel, docetaxel		Breast, ovarian, non-small-cell lung cancer, prostate	Immunosuppression, nausea, alopecia, neuropathy, muscle pain
Antimetabolites	Pyrimidine antimetabolites, e.g. 5-FU, gemcitabine. Purine antimetabolites, e.g. mercaptopurine.	Chemical structures similar to DNA precursor. Prevent precursors becoming incorporated into DNA during synthesis (S phase). Also affect RNA synthesis	MTX: breast, lung, head and neck, oesophagus, bladder leukaemias, lymphomas	MTX: immunosuppression, hepatotoxicity, mucositis, nausea
	Antifolates, e.g. methotrexate (MTX). Thymidylate synthase inhibitors. Adenosine deaminase inhibitors. Ribonucleotide reductase inhibitors		5-FU: gastric, oesophagus colon, anal, breast, head and neck	5-FU: immunosuppression, mucositis, diarrhoea, rashes

(continued)

Table 2.2 (*Continued*)

Chemotherapy group	Examples	Mode of action	Tumour types	Toxicities
Antitumour antibiotics	Anthracyclines, e.g. doxorubicin, daunorubicin. Bleomycin. Mitomycin C. Actinomycin C. Podofyllotoxins, e.g. etoposide. Camptothecins, e.g. irinotecan	Interact with DNA. Interactions differ between group Doxorubicin has antitopoisomerase action. Topoisomerase is involved in the coiling structure of DNA Bleomycin generates DNA double-strand breaks	Doxorubicin: breast, ovarian, lung, gastric, sarcomas, thyroid, lymphomas Bleomycin: colon, melanoma, squamous cell carcinoma skin	Doxorubicin: cardiotoxicity, alopecia, nausea Bleomycin: pulmonary toxicities, nausea, alopecia, skin toxicities
Alkylating agents	Cyclophosphamide. Melphalan. Nitrosoureas, e.g. carmustine. Alkane sulfonates, e.g. busulphan.	Forms covalent link with DNA causing cross links and apoptosis	Cyclophosphamide: breast, lung, endometrial, ovarian, cervix, bladder, testes, brain	Cyclophosphamide: haemorrhagic cystitis, nausea, mucositis

Table 2.3 Targeted agents

Target	Agents	
	Monoclonal antibodies	**Tyrosine kinase inhibitors**
EGFR	Cetuximab, panitumumab	Gefitinib, erlotinib
HER2	Trastuzumab (Herceptin)	Lapatinib
VEGF	Bevacizumab	
Multitargeted TKIs (activity against platelet-derived growth factor receptors, VEGFR, and others)		Imatinib, sunitinib, sorafenib, axitinib

liver function test abnormalities. Rarely corneal ulceration and interstitial pneumonitis have been reported.

Cetuximab and panitumumab have been licensed for the treatment of pre-treated metastatic CRC and in the first-line treatment of head and neck cancer. In head and neck cancers, cetuximab in combination with high-dose radiotherapy improves loco-regional control and confers a significant survival gain. In patients with relapsed, irinotecan-refractory, metastatic CRC, cetuximab in combination with chemotherapy or as mono-therapy improves response rates and results in a modest survival advantage. Up to 40% of patients with metastatic CRC have activating *K-ras* tumour mutations and 60% of patients have *K-ras* 'wild-type' tumours. Recent studies have demonstrated that *K-ras* mutations are predictive of lack of response to anti-EGFR antibodies and tumour *K-ras* mutation status is now routinely tested before starting anti-EGFR mAb therapy. Common side effects of all the anti-EGFR mAbs include rash and diarrhoea. There are data to suggest rash correlates with response. Infusion reactions including angio-oedema occurred in up to 20% of trial patients. Hypomagnesaemia has also been reported and is thought to be an effect of the mAbs on the distal renal tubules.

Human epidermal growth factor receptor 2

Human epidermal growth factor receptor 2 (HER2) is overexpressed in 25–30% of breast cancers. Trastuzumab (Herceptin) is a mAb that blocks the extracellular domain of the HER2 receptor. When trastuzumab is used in the post-surgery (adjuvant) treatment of breast cancer it confers a significant survival benefit and a reduction in the risk of relapse of over 50%. This magnitude of benefit demonstrates a targeted therapy that has added in a very meaningful way to patient outcomes. In the adjuvant treatment of breast cancer, trastuzumab is given sequentially or concurrently with taxane-based chemotherapy and continued for 1 year. In the treatment of metastatic breast cancer (MBC), it is often continued as monotherapy until disease progression and there are data to suggest additional benefit for continuing treatment beyond progression of disease.

Up to 20% of gastric cancers overexpress HER2. The addition of trastuzumab to chemotherapy in untreated HER2-positive gastric cancer improved median survival by approximately 2 months, an important survival increment in a disease with poor prognosis.

Trastuzumab can be cardiotoxic, especially when administered with anthracycline chemotherapy, due to suppression of cardiac remodelling. Cardiac function monitoring is recommended whilst on treatment. Infusion reactions occur and have been fatal. Following the first loading dose, patients are monitored for several hours. Pneumonitis or pulmonary infiltrates have been reported in less than 1% of patients.

Vascular endothelial growth factor signalling

Angiogenesis is critical for tumour development and VEGF is a vital modulator of angiogenesis. Drugs that target VEGF have been shown to increase response when used in combination with standard chemotherapy in certain tumour types. Bevacizumab is a mAb against VEGF that provides a modest improvement in survival when used in combination with chemotherapy in metastatic colorectal cancer and enhances progression-free survival in the treatment of MBC. Both bevacizumab and sunitinib (a multitargeted TKI with VEGFR as one of its targets) are approved for treatment of renal cell carcinoma.

Common side effects of bevacizumab include hypertension (10%), bleeding, thrombosis, and delayed wound healing. Gastrointestinal perforation has been reported in approximately 2% of patients. In view of wound healing and bleeding consequences of bevacizumab, elective surgery should be delayed by 4–6 weeks following the last dose.

Imatinib and gastrointestinal stromal tumour

Imatinib is a TKI that inhibits multiple tyrosine kinases such as the Kit receptor. Kit receptor is mutated in gastrointestinal stromal tumour (GIST), a rare sarcoma of the stomach. In clinical studies, 75–90% of patients with advanced GISTs treated with imatinib experienced a clinical response. Patients with *KIT* exon 11-mutant GIST have a higher response rate and a significantly better survival compared with patients who do not have mutant GIST. The most commonly side effects of imatinib are mild nausea, diarrhoea, fatigue, myalgia, muscle cramps, and rash. In patients with unresectable or metastatic GIST, gastrointestinal and intra-tumoural haemorrhages have been reported. Mild perioribital and leg oedemas were a common finding in studies.

PARP inhibitors

PARP are a group of proteins involved in base-excision repair. PARP inhibitors have proven efficacy in BRCA1 and -2 defective cancers since cells lacking BRCA1 and -2 appear to survive by depending on PARP as a backup system to maintain DNA repair. BRCA1 and -2 deficient cells have been found to be sensitive to PARP-1 inhibitors.

Conclusion

In conclusion the development of cancer is a multistep process. Oncogenes affect cell signalling pathways that may enhance cell proliferation or inhibit differentiation and apoptosis. Tumour suppressor genes have an array of protective functions including the recognition and repair of DNA damage (BRCA1/2), cell cycle inhibitory functions (e.g. pRB/p16), cell signalling inhibitory properties (e.g. PTEN), and apoptotic pathway initiation.

An improved knowledge of cancer molecular biology acquired through modern high-throughput 'functional genomics' approaches combined with rigorous laboratory and clinical validation will enable the development of the next generation of effective pathway-driven anticancer therapies to improve clinical outcome across many tumour types.

Bibliography

1. Amado RG, Wolf M, Peeters M, *et al.* (2008). Wild-type KRAS is required for panitumumab efficacy in patients with metastatic colorectal cancer. *J Clin Oncol* **26**(10):1626–34.

2. Bonner JA, Harari PM, Giralt J, *et al.* (2006) Radiotherapy plus cetuximab for squamous-cell carcinoma of the head and neck. *N Engl J Med* **354**(6):567–78.

3. Bos JL (1989). Ras oncogenes in human cancer: a review. *Cancer Res* **49**(17):4682–9.

4. Cancer Research UK. *Cancer Stats Key Facts on Cancer.* Available at: http://info.cancerresearchuk.org/cancerstats/keyfacts/index.htm (accessed 16 December 2009).

5. Cunningham D, Humblet Y, Siena S, *et al.* (2004). Cetuximab monotherapy and cetuximab plus irinotecan in irinotecan refractory metastatic colo-rectal cancer. *N Engl J Med* **351**(4):337–45.

6. Demetri GD, von Mehren M, Blanke CD, *et al.* (2002). Efficacy and safety of imatinib mesylate in advanced gastrointestinal stromal tumors. *N Engl J Med* **347**(7):472–80.

7. Downward J, Parker P, Waterfield MD (1984a). Autophosphorylation sites on the epidermal growth factor receptor. *Nature* **311**(5985):483–5.

8. Downward J, Yarden Y, Mayes E, *et al.* (1984b). Close similarity of epidermal growth factor receptor and v-erb-B oncogene protein sequences. *Nature* **307**(5951):521–7.

9. Escudier B, Pluzanska A, Koralewski P, *et al.* (2007). Bevacizumab plus interferon alfa-2a for treatment of metastatic renal cell carcinoma: a randomised, double-blind phase III trial. *Lancet* **370**(9605):2103–11.

10. Farmer H, McCabe N, Lord CJ, *et al.* (2005). Targeting the DNA repair defect in BRCA mutant cells as a therapeutic strategy. *Nature* **434**(7035):917–21.

11. Ferrara N, Gerber HP, LeCouter J (2003). The biology of VEGF and its receptors. *Nat Med* **6**:669–76.

12. Fong PC, Boss DS, Yap TA, *et al.* (2009). Inhibition of poly(ADP-ribose) polymerase in tumors from BRCA mutation carriers. *N Engl J Med* **361**(2):123–34.

13. Gudmundsdottir K, Ashworth A (2006). The roles of BRCA1 and BRCA2 and associated proteins in the maintenance of genomic instability. *Oncogene* **25**(43):5864–74.

14. Hanahan D, Weinberg RA (2000). The hallmarks of cancer. *Cell* **100**(1):57–70.

15. Harfe BD, Jinks-Robertson S (2000). DNA mismatch repair and genetic instability. *Annu Rev Gen* **34**:359–99.

16. Heinrich MC, Corless CL, Demetri GD, *et al.* (2003). Kinase mutations and imatinib response in patients with metastatic gastrointestinal stromal tumor. *J Clin Oncol* **21**(23):4342–9.

17. Hoeijmakers JH (2001). Genomic maintenance mechanisms for preventing cancer. *Nature* **411**(6835):366–74.

18. Hurwitz H, Fehrenbacher L, Novotny W, *et al.* (2004). Bevacizumab plus irinotecan, fluorouracil, and leucovorin for metastatic colorectal cancer *N Engl J Med* **350**(23):2335–42.

19. Jonker DJ, O'Callaghan CJ, Karapetis CS, *et al.* (2007). Cetuximab for the treatment of colorectal cancer. *N Engl J Med* **357**(20):2040–48.

20. Karapetis CS, Khambata-Ford S, Jonker DJ, *et al.* (2008). K-ras mutations and benefit from cetuximab in advanced colorectal cancer. *N Engl J Med* **359**(17):1757–65.

21. Li J, Yen C, Liaw D, *et al.* (1997). PTEN, a putative protein tyrosine phosphatase gene mutated in human brain, breast, and prostate cancer. *Science* **275**(5308):1943–7.

22. Mok TS, Wu Y-L, Thongprasert S, *et al.* (2009). Gefitinib or carboplatin–paclitaxel in pulmonary adenocarcinoma. *N Engl J Med* **361**(10):947–57.

23. Motzer RJ, Michaelson MD, Rosenberg J, *et al.* (2007). Sunitinib efficacy against advanced renal cell carcinoma. *J Urol* **178**(5):1883–7.

24. Robert HJ, Dieras V, Glaspy J, *et al.* (2009). RIBBON-1: Randomized, double-blind, placebo-controlled, phase III trial of chemotherapy with or without bevacizumab (B) for first-line treatment of HER2-negative locally recurrent or metastatic breast cancer (MBC). *J Clin Oncol, ASCO Annual Meeting Proceedings (Post-Meeting Edition)* **27**(15S):1005.

25. Rosell R, Moran T, Queralt C, *et al.* (2009). Screening for epidermal growth factor receptor mutations in lung cancer. *N Engl J Med* **361**(10):958–67.

26. Sharma, SV, Bell, DW, Settleman J, Haber DA (2007). Epidermal growth factor receptor mutations in lung cancer. *Nat Rev Cancer* **7**(3):169–81.

27. Shepherd FA, Rodrigues Pereira J, Ciuleanu T, *et al.* (2005). Erlotinib in previously treated non-small cell lung cancer. *N Engl J Med* **353**(2):123–32.

28. Smith I, Procter M, Gelber RD *et al* (2007). HERA study team. 2-year follow-up of trastuzumab after adjuvant chemotherapy in HER-2 positive breast cancer: a randomised controlled trial. *Lancet*, **369**(9555):29–36.

29. Sobrero AF, Maurel J, Fehrenbacher L, *et al.* (2008). EPIC: phase III trial of cetuximab plus irinotecan after fluoropyrimidine and oxaliplatin failure in patients with metastatic colorectal cancer. *J Clin Oncol* **26**(14):2311–19.

30. Steck PA, Pershouse MA, Jasser SA, *et al.* (1997). Identification of a candidate tumour suppressor gene, MMAC1, at chromosome 10q23.3 that is mutated in multiple advanced cancers. *Nat Genet* **15**(4):356–62.

31. Swanton C (2004). Cell-cycle targeted therapies. *Lancet Oncol* **5**(1):27–36.

32. The electronic Medicines Compendium. *Bevacizumab*. Available at: http://emc.medicines.org.uk/medicine/15748/SPC/Avastin (accessed 17 December 2009).

33. The electronic Medicines Compendium. *Cetuximab*. Available at: (http://emc.medicines.org.uk/medicine/19595/SPC/Erbitux (accessed 17 December 2009).

34. The electronic Medicines Compendium. *Erlotinib*. Available at: http://emc.medicines.org.uk/medicine/16781/SPC/Tarceva (accessed 17 December 2009).

35. The electronic Medicines Compendium. *Imatinib*. Available at: (http://emc.medicines.org.uk/medicine/14954/XPIL/GLIVEC (accessed 17 December 2009).

36. The electronic Medicines Compendium. *Trastuzumab*. Available at: http://emc.medicines.org.uk/medicine/3567/SPC/Herceptin (accessed 17 December 2009).

37. Van Cutsem E, Kang YK, Chung HC, *et al.* (2009a). Efficacy results from the ToGA trial: a phase III study of trastuzumab added to standard chemotherapy in first-line human epidermal growth factor receptor 2 (HER2)-positive advanced gastric cancer. *J Clin Oncol* **27**(15S):204.

38. Van Cutsem CE, Kohne CH, Hitre E, *et al.* (2009b). Cetuximab and chemotherapy as initial treatment for metastatic colorectal cancer. *N Engl J Med* **360**(14):1408–17.

39. Verweij J, Casali PG, Zalcberg J, *et al.* (2004). Progression-free survival in gastrointestinal stromal tumours with high-dose imatinib: randomised trial. *Lancet* **364**(9440):1127–34.

40. von Minckwitz G, du Bois A, Schmidt M, *et al.* (2009). Trastuzumab beyond progression in human epidermal growth factor receptor 2-positive advanced breast cancer: a german breast group 26/breast international group 03–05 study. *J Clin Oncol* **27**(12):1999–2006.

41. World Health Organization. WHO Anatomical Therapeutic Chemical (ATC) Classification System. Available at: http://www.who.int/classifications/atcddd/en (accessed 17 December 2009).

Part 2

Anaesthesia for specific surgeries and other interventions

Chapter 3

Preassessment for major cancer surgery

Kate Wessels and Tim Wigmore

Introduction

Within the UK, there are on average 288,000 newly diagnosed cases of cancer each year of which approximately 68% present for elective surgery with curative intent per year. Cancer presents a number of unique challenges that should be recognized preoperatively to enable suitable preoptimization, intraoperative preparation, and identification of appropriate postoperative location.

There are a range of issues to consider in assessment of a patient's fitness for major cancer surgery and these are discussed in the following sections.

Premorbid conditions

Patients affected by cancer are often elderly and may be long-term smokers or alcohol abusers. Varying degrees of chronic obstructive airways disease and emphysema are common, together with associated ischaemic heart disease, cardiac failure, and myocardial dysfunction.

Obesity is associated with an increased risk of endometrial cancer, and obesity itself may be associated with diabetes or varying degrees of insulin resistance, malnutrition, and the cardiorespiratory effects of long-term obstructive sleep apnoea.

Effects of anticancer treatments

Chemotherapeutic agents are increasingly administered preoperatively to render tumours resectable (neoadjuvant chemotherapy). They may be the cause of significant side effects and adverse reactions. The reader is referred to Chapter 15 for greater detail, but a brief overview of systemic effects is given in Table 3.1.

Radiotherapy and brachytherapy—severe fibrosis secondary to localized therapy may occur. For patients with head and neck cancers this may result in very difficult airway manipulation. Localized radiotherapy may also result in coronary artery fibrosis and cardiac ischaemia. Appropriate investigations may include coronary angiography prior to definitive cancer surgery.

Table 3.1 Overview of systemic side effects of chemotherapeutic agents

System	Chemotherapeutic agents	Effect
Cardiovascular	Anthracyclines (e.g. doxorubicin, adriamycin) Trastuzumab (Herceptin)	Dose-related cardiomyopathy and heart failure Direct cardiotoxic effect
Respiratory	Methotrexate Cyclophosphamide Bleomycin	Pneumonitis Fibrosing alveolitis exacerbated by the use of high FiO_2
Gastrointestinal	Many	Nausea, vomiting, mucositis, colitis, bowel perforation (particularly with bevacizumab)
Renal	Cisplatin Carboplatin	Nephrotoxic—chronic renal dysfunction Reversible renal dysfunction
Electrolyte	Cisplatin Cyclophosphamide Vincristine	Chronic hypomagnesaemia Life-threatening hyponatraemia
Bone marrow	Many	Anaemia, thrombocytopenia, and neutropenia

Cancer attributable effects

Systemic effects

Weight loss

Many patients, particularly those with bowel, pancreatic, and ovarian cancers, have poor nutritional status and weight loss. Although weight per se is a poor measure of nutritional assessment (due to the influence of ascites, oedema, or extensive tumour mass), it may highlight the need for dietetic input and preoperative supplementation if necessary.

A range of scoring systems have been used in an attempt to quantify nutritional status and the need for supplementation:

◆ The Prognostic Nutrition Index comprises a number of markers including serum albumin, serum transferrin, triceps skinfold measurement, and skin testing for delayed hypersensitivity reactions and has been used to prospectively predict the risk of postoperative complications in gastrointestinal surgical patients. It has been utilized in a wider surgical population and proved reliable, but is not widely used clinically.

◆ The Subjective Global Assessment. This system categorizes patients as well nourished, malnourished, or severely malnourished based on measurements of muscle wasting, loss of subcutaneous tissue, and weight loss. The severely malnourished group have been shown to have significantly higher rates of infection and longer hospital stays.

◆ Laboratory tests of nutritional status measure visceral protein levels although the effect of non-nutritional factors (fluid status and liver function) on these levels needs to be borne in mind. Hypoalbuminaemia is associated with an increased incidence of poor wound healing, anastomotic breakdown, and mortality amongst surgical patients. Serum transferrin levels are thought to be a more sensitive marker of a patient's response to nutritional support due to its shorter half-life. Prealbumin has also been used as a measure of short-term changes in nutrition.

A number of studies have been carried out regarding the value of preoperative total parenteral nutrition (TPN). Of note was the Veterans Affairs TPN Cooperative study which included 395 malnourished patients undergoing non-emergency laparotomies or thoracotomies. Patients were randomized to receive TPN for 7–15 days before surgery and 3 days after, or no perioperative TPN. At 90 days, there was found to be a slightly higher incidence of infectious complications (pneumonia and bacteraemia) amongst the TPN group (thought to be attributable to hyperglycaemia in these patients), but there was a far lower incidence of cardiovascular events and respiratory failure. Similarly, a meta-analysis of 22 studies found that malnourished patients receiving TPN for 7–10 days before surgery had a 10% absolute reduction in postoperative complications.

Anaemia

Anaemia may occur secondary to marrow infiltration, blood loss, or erythropoietin (EPO) deficiency. If presenting in adequate time preoperatively, iron ± EPO should be used. Following reports of an association between erythropoietic-stimulating agent therapy and the potential for either thrombotic cardiovascular events or more rapid tumour progression in some cancers, EPO use has diminished.

Intravenous iron preparations are increasingly being used either with or without EPO supplementation. Intravenous iron is proven to be safe, is more efficacious than oral, and modern preparations come with a low risk of anaphylaxis.

Paraneoplastic syndromes

There are numerous syndromes that occur as a result of substances secreted by tumours. Those of significance to anaesthesia are summarized in Tables 3.2 and 3.3.

Table 3.2 Endocrine abnormalities

Hormone secreted	Typical tumour type	Anaesthetic implication
Adrenocorticotropic hormone (ACTH)	Many but lung particularly	Cushing's syndrome, Hypokalaemia
Antidiuretic hormone (ADH)	Lung, head, and neck	Hyponatraemia, oliguria
Parathyroid hormone-related peptides	Lung, head and neck, kidney, pancreas	Hypercalcaemia
Parathyroid hormone	Tumours with bony metastases (e.g. breast and prostate)	Hypercalcaemia
Insulin-like growth factors 1 and 2	Pituitary	Hypoglycaemia
Erythropoietin (EPO)	Lung, kidney, liver, central nervous system	Erythrocytosis

Table 3.3 Neurological syndromes

Syndrome	Typical tumour type	Anaesthetic implication
Myasthenia gravis	Thymoma	Risk of prolonged respiratory depression Hypersensitivity to non-depolarizing muscle relaxants Risk of cholinergic crisis
Lambert–Eaton syndrome	Small-cell lung, lymphoma, thymoma, breast, kidney, prostate, uterus, bowel	Hypersensitivity to all muscle relaxants No response to neostigmine

Localized effects

◆ *Head and neck masses*: head and neck tumours may cause supra- or infraglottic airway obstruction, recurrent laryngeal nerve damage, and superior vena caval obstruction. In the last case, positive pressure ventilation can result in complete vascular obstruction. The preassessment clinic is an opportunity to plan airway management and devise alternative strategies that may be required.

◆ *Mediastinal masses*: patients, particularly children, with mediastinal masses secondary to cancers such as Hodgkin's lymphoma, T-cell acute lymphoblastic leukemia, and T-cell non-Hodgkin's lymphoma can present major problems. These can cause tracheobronchial, cardiac, and great vessel compression to such an extent that induction of anaesthesia may result in an unventilatable patient or a catastrophic reduction in cardiac output and consequent death (see Chapter 5).

◆ *Abdominal masses*: sarcomas and ovarian cancers in particular may present with massive abdominal masses. These may cause diaphragmatic splinting and reduced gastric emptying and venous return. In addition their proximity to major intra-abdominal vessels may raise the possibility of significant intraoperative blood loss.

◆ *Ascites, pleural fluid collections, pericardial collections*: depending on the location of tumours and their extent of metastatic spread, extravascular fluid accumulation can be significant. Large-volume ascites is common amongst patients with ovarian cancers and may cause significant diaphragmatic splinting, respiratory embarrassment, and a reduction in venous return with cardiovascular collapse. Similarly, pericardial and pleural effusions may severely compromise cardiorespiratory function. The extent of fluid collections should be assessed prior to surgery commencing as large volume drainage may be necessary to avoid significant cardiovascular or respiratory complications intraoperatively.

Investigations

In addition to the routine preoperative measurement of full blood count, biochemistry, coagulation, electrocardiogram, and chest X-ray there are a number of studies particularly relevant to the patient with cancer:

◆ *Echocardiography:* of utility if there is clinical suspicion of impaired function either premorbidly or secondary to cardiotoxic chemotherapy or for identification/quantification of a pericardial effusion.

- *Cardiopulmonary exercise testing (CPEX):* CPEX is a non-invasive method of testing the ability of the combined respiratory and cardiovascular systems to increase oxygen delivery to the point demanded by major surgery. Its performance results in the generation of a number of variables, the most widely quoted of which is the anaerobic threshold (AT). Work by Older and colleagues demonstrated an AT of less than 11ml/kg/min was associated with an increased mortality (18%) versus those with greater than 11ml/kg/min (0.8%) in patients undergoing major surgery. Increased intervention in the low AT group (particularly with respect to preoptimization and postoperative intensive care) has been associated with improved survival. Peak oxygen consumption (VO_2) has also been shown to correlate with outcomes following surgery, with a peak VO_2 less than of 800ml/min/m^2 suggesting postoperative cardiovascular morbidity following oesophagogastrectomy.

- *Lung function testing:* spirometry is used to help define intra- versus extrathoracic airway obstruction (through flow volume loops), and to quantify degree of respiratory and ventilatory impairment. The most common routine preoperative test of lung function is forced expiratory volume. Results are expressed as that in one second (FEV_1), and as a percentage of total vital capacity. An FEV_1 below 70% of expected value for patient age and weight has been accepted as increased risk of developing postoperative pulmonary complications. Blood gas analysis should also be taken into account however, as a $PaCO_2$ above 6.7kPa often indicates the need for postoperative ventilation, prolonged intubation, or the need for tracheostomy which is not detected by FEV_1 alone. Postoperative ventilation requirements should be discussed during the patient's preoperative assessment visit.

- *Radiology:* Computed tomography (CT) scans in particular are often a vital aid in planning the anaesthetic technique and anticipating potential problems. The CT required obviously depends on the tumour site:
  - *Head and neck*: demonstrates airway compromise and allows planning of airway management
  - *Chest*: demonstration of mediastinal masses, and cardiac, great vessel, and airway compression. Additionally allows assessment of pleural effusions and lung disease
  - *Abdominal*: demonstration of ascites, abdominal masses, and proximity of those masses to major vessels.

Risk estimation

A variety of risk scoring systems exist but scoring systems specific to surgical oncology patients are limited. Identifying which risk prediction tools are most appropriate to an individual hospital practice and recalibrating each tool (particularly CPEX testing) to give valid figures for institutional outcomes, is the key to informing both clinicians and patients.

Lee's score for enumerating cardiac risk in non-cardiac surgery and the American College of Physicians risk of postoperative respiratory complications score are non-oncology specific. The POSSUM score (Physiological and Operative Severity for enUmeration of

Morality and morbidity) has been used for risk stratification to identify patients likely to benefit from postoperative level two or level three care but is more accurate for a general group of surgical patients. More specific versions have been produced (O-POSSUM for oesphagogastric and CR-POSSUM for colorectal surgery). The Association of Coloproctology of Great Britain and Ireland Colorectal cancer (ACPGBI CRC) Model and Malignant Large Bowel obstruction models offer other options for colorectal cancer.

The Karnofsky and Zubrod score are the most widely measures of performance status in oncology patients. They are used to quantify general well-being and can be used to compare effectiveness of different therapies and to assess the quality of life and prognosis in individual patients. The Karnofsky score runs from 100 to 0, where 100 is 'perfect' health and 0 is death. The lower the Karnofsky score, the worse the survival for most serious illnesses.

Whilst it is appropriate to inform patients of the risk of proceeding with surgery, and to ameliorate those risks than can be, it should never be forgotten that in the majority of cases there is an opportunity cost to delay. Tumours will continue to grow and in some cases spread while investigative delays occur and allowing a resectable neoplasm to become unresectable is a highly undesirable outcome.

Optimization

Adequate optimization and planning prior to major surgery ensures both that the patient is properly investigated and prepared, and that all necessary equipment, surgical skill (often a combination of surgical teams and specialities), and resources (postoperative intensive care beds) are available.

Patients can best be preoptimized using a systems-based approach. Multiple disciplines, both medical and allied health professionals, are involved in patient management.

Patients requiring cardiorespiratory work-up prior to surgery should have their medications (antihypertensives, beta blockers or bronchodilators, preoperative short-course steroids or antibiotics) optimized and additionally often benefit from physiotherapy input. Physiotherapy is a vital part of maximizing respiratory function and conducting patient education regarding the prevention of postoperative respiratory tract infections and complications associated with long-term immobility. Providing the urgency of the case allows, establishing a graded preoperative exercise programme before surgery can improve a patient's functional capacity (as evidenced by an improved CPEX result)

Other allied health professionals in the form of occupational therapists and speech and language therapists are invaluable in long-term rehabilitation especially following limb sarcoma surgery and head and neck oncology patients. Presurgery patient education by these groups of professionals ensures greater success and compliance with treatment and rehabilitation in the postsurgical period.

Dietetics plays a major role in nutritional support and supplementation preoperatively. Malnourished patients are known to be at greater risk for morbidity and mortality pre- and postoperatively in comparison with well-nourished patients. Guidelines suggest that preoperative nutritional support for 7–10 days is beneficial in severely malnourished patients in whom surgery can be delayed. In addition, nutritional supplementation should also be considered in postoperative patients who cannot eat within 7–10 days after surgery. A debate remains as to whether enteral or parenteral nutrition is preferred, as comparative studies have shown that outcomes are similar with either route. Parenteral nutritional support carries the risks of catheter sepsis, hyperglycaemia, electrolyte abnormalities, and liver dysfunction. As a result, in patients with adequate digestive and absorptive capacity of the gastrointestinal tract, enteral nutrition is preferred. Immunonutrition involves the use of immune-enhancing formulas containing arginine, RNA, and omega-3 fatty acids to boost immune system function in surgically stressed or immunocompromised patients. The addition of glutamine to parenteral nutrition has been shown in a number of studies to improve nitrogen balance, preserve intestinal mucosal integrity and absorption, and thus have an effect more comparable with enteral feeding than standard parenteral feeds. Shortened hospital stays have been demonstrated in patients after major surgery.

Oncology patients under the care of hepatic or renal physicians should be optimized in consultation with these specialist medical teams. Patients requiring chronic dialysis, be it haemo- or peritoneal, should have a management plan arranged before surgery regarding dialysis in the postoperative period, especially if surgery is performed in a setting in which dialysis facilities are not available. Haemodialysis patients may require the insertion of a tunnelled venous exchange catheter prior to surgery, as dialysis access may become problematic postoperatively.

Conclusion

The multisystem involvement of many cancers and their treatments poses significant challenges to the anaesthetist. Many of these challenges may however be surmounted with careful preassessment and preoptimization.

Bibliography

1. Atabek U, Alvarez R, Pello MJ, *et al.* (1995). Erythropoetin accelerates hematocrit recovery in post-surgical anaemia. *Am Surg* **61**(1):74–7.
2. Binder RK, Wonisch M, Corra U, *et al.* (2008). Methodological approach to the first and second lactate threshold in incremental cardiopulmonary exercise testing. *Eur J Cardiovasc Prev Rehabil* **15**:726–34.
3. Boyd O, Jackson N (2005). Clinical review: How is risk defined in high-risk surgical patient management? *Crit Care* **4**:390–6.
4. Buccheri G, Ferrigno D, Tamburini M (1996). Karnofsky and ECOG performance status scoring in lung cancer. *Eur J Cancer* **32A**(7):1135–41.
5. Carr C, Ng J, Wigmore T (2008). The side effects of chemotherapeutic agents. *Curr Anaesth Crit Care* **19**:70–9.
6. Davies S, Wilson R (2007). CPX testing for the surgical patient. *Care Crit Ill* **23**:4.
7. den Boer S, de Keizer NF, de Jonge E (2005). Performance of prognostic models in critically ill cancer patients–a review. *Crit Care* **9**(4):458–63.
8. Lansky SB, List MA, Lansky LL, Ritter-Sterr C, Miller DR (1987). The measurement of performance in childhood cancer patients. *Cancer* **60**(7):1651–6.
9. Moore J, McLeod A (2009). Anaesthesia for Gynacological oncology surgery. *Curr Anaesth Crit Care* **20**:8–12.

10. Morlion BJ, Stehle P, Wachtler P, *et al.* (1998). Total parenteral nutrition with glutamine dipeptide after major abdominal surgery. A randomised, double-blind, controlled study. *Ann Surgery* **227**:302–8.

11. Office for National Statistics (2007). Annual Update: Cancer incidence and mortality in the United Kingdom and constituent countries. *Health Stat Q* **35**:78–83.

12. Older P, Hall A (2004). Clinical review: How to identify high-risk surgical patients. *Crit Care* **8**:369–72.

13. Older P, Hall A, Hader R (1999). Cardiopulmonary exercise testing as a screening test for perioperative management of major surgery in the elderly. *Chest* **116**:355–62.

14. Ramesh HSJ, Pope D, Gennari R, Audisio RA (2005). Optimising surgical management of elderly cancer patients. *World J Surg Oncol* **3**:17.

15. Salvino RM, Dechicco RS, Seidner DL (2004). Perioperative nutrition support: Who and how. *Cleve Clin J Med* **71**(4):345–51.

16. Shander A, Spence RK, Auerbach M (2010). Can intravenous iron therapy meet the unmet needs created by the new restrictions on erythropoietic stimulation agents? *Transfusion* **50**(3):719–32.

17. Wu GH, Liu ZH, Wu ZG (2006). Perioperative artificial nutrition in malnourished gastrointestinal cancer patients. *World J Gastroenterol* **12**(15):2441–4.

Chapter 4

Perioperative fluid management for major cancer surgery

Mark Edwards and Tim Wigmore

Introduction

The management of perioperative fluid has been the subject of heated debate for many years. The choices of fluid and required volume have been contested, and much of the evidence is derived from oncological surgery. The aims of the chapter are to briefly refresh basic physiology and outline the goals of a fluid administration strategy and how, with reference to the literature, these goals can be met. Finally we will outline approaches to various procedure specific situations.

Basic physiology

Fluid compartments and their barriers

In the adult, total body water represents approximately 60% of body weight. Of this water, two-thirds are intracellular and one-third extracellular. Of the extracellular fluid, one-fifth is intravascular, just under four-fifths are interstitial, with the remainder trans-cellular (e.g. cerebrospinal fluid, aqueous humour). The barrier between the intravascular and interstitial compartments is the intact vascular endothelium. Electrolytes and water can pass freely, but there is limited permeability to larger molecules. The resultant oncotic pressure gradient helps to limit the net flow of capillary fluid into the interstitium caused by the higher intravascular hydrostatic pressure. The cell membrane forms a barrier between the interstitial and intracellular compartments. Whilst water may still pass freely, electrolyte concentration gradients are maintained across the cell wall by energy-consuming ATPase ion pumps.

Hypotonic fluids will redistribute throughout all fluid compartments, isotonic fluids through the extracellular compartment, while colloids will remain predominantly in the intravascular compartment for some time (the actual time depending upon the endothelial permeability coefficient).

Pathophysiology

Disruptions to normal fluid compartments

Fluid compartments can be disturbed by various insults during surgery, commencing with the depletion of all compartments that may be seen with preoperative starvation or following bowel preparation, and continuing with direct blood loss from penetration of the intravascular space.

The barrier function of the vascular endothelium itself may be also be compromised by an inflammatory response to surgical trauma, tissue ischaemia, and sepsis. The glycocalyx, a crucial determinant of endothelial permeability, can also be degraded by atrial natriuretic peptide which may be elevated by iatrogenic acute hypervolaemia. Increased endothelial permeability may lead to oedema formation and reduces the plasma volume expansion effect of administered colloids.

The significance of the so-called 'third space' has been widely debated. Its definition is any compartment outside the intravascular, interstitial, and intracellular spaces (e.g. the bowel lumen, pleural space or peritoneum, or traumatized tissue) where fluid can collect. Fluid sequestered here is lost from the other compartments.

Stress response and effect on fluid balance

Major surgery causes considerable physiological stress. Increased endogenous catecholamines, cortisol, and antidiuretic hormone (ADH) secretion in the immediate postoperative period can all cause renal water retention and a reduced urine output despite normovolaemia.

Influence of underlying cancer

The underlying disease can also affect perioperative fluid balance. Malignant fluid collections such as pleural effusions and ascites represent examples of third-space loss, and rapid drainage can lead to major compartment shifts. Treatments can be similarly problematic; cardiotoxic chemotherapy such as Herceptin or anthracyclines may reduce ventricular performance and result in cardiac failure. The impaired nutritional status of many patients, who may have low levels of circulating plasma proteins with a subsequent reduction in plasma oncotic pressure, can also result in a tendency to oedema.

Effects of perioperative hypo- and hypervolaemia

Hypovolaemia

Adequate volume is key in maintaining organ perfusion. The typical response to a reduced effective circulating volume is to divert flow from the gut, skin, and kidneys to the heart and brain. If intravascular fluid replacement is insufficient, tissue oxygen delivery is reduced and anaerobic metabolism supervenes.

Gastrointestinal tract hypoperfusion in particular appears crucial in the subsequent development of multiorgan failure (MOF). The countercurrent blood supply to the intestinal villi tends to shunt blood away from superficial mucosa during periods of inadequate flow resulting in mucosal necrosis. This is compounded by damage from gut bile salts, acids, digestive enzymes, and luminal bacteria. At this stage the barrier function of the gut is compromised and the passage of bacterial endotoxin into the systemic circulation activates a cytokine cascade that leads to the systemic and metabolic features of the systemic inflammatory response syndrome. Translocation of viable gut bacteria across impaired bowel mucosa causes systemic infection and further inflammatory response. Reperfusion of compromised bowel leads to the release of oxygen free radicals. Activation of the cytokine cascade, cellular and humoral immune systems, complement and fibrino-lytic systems can lead to diffuse tissue injury and MOF. Several studies have demonstrated that inadequate gut perfusion as measured by gastric tonometry is associated with worse outcome and giving fluid challenges to increase stroke volume has been shown to nor-malize gastric mucosal pH (as measured by tonometry) and reduce adverse outcomes.

Gut anastomoses are also vulnerable. Hypoperfusion here, contributed to by hypovol-aemia and vasoconstriction, reduces the local tissue oxygen tension leading to poor anastomotic healing and breakdown.

Excess fluid administration

Excessive fluid administration also has potential associated morbidity.

Oedema can be caused by any type of intravascular fluid administration. Whilst the redistribution of crystalloids from the intravascular to interstitial space is well recognized, it also occurs with colloids, particularly if capillary permeability is increased. Oedema in general reduces tissue oxygenation and impairs organ function. Gut oedema reduces gas-trointestinal motility and nutrient absorption, and oedema at a surgical anastomosis can reduce its integrity, with potentially catastrophic complications. Pulmonary oedema may lead to respiratory failure and chest infections.

Other side effects of excessive fluid include dilutional coagulopathy, with increased blood loss, and hypothermia.

Appropriate physiological targets for fluid therapy

It has long been suggested that the ability of a patient to attain certain physiological tar-gets either spontaneously or with fluid and pharmacological augmentation is associated with improved outcomes following major surgery. Strategies to achieve these parameters form the basis of preoperative optimization and 'goal-directed' fluid therapy. However, not all physiological variables are easy to measure and therefore may not be suitable tar-gets for goal-directed therapy. In addition, it should be noted that fluids form only one part of goal-directed therapy, and that many approaches require manipulation of the cardiovascular system by inotropic agents.

Increasing cardiac output, oxygen delivery, and oxygen uptake

Shoemaker showed in the 1970s that survivors of high-risk surgery had a higher cardiac index (CI), higher oxygen delivery (DO_2), and higher oxygen uptake (VO_2). This initial study was followed by trials demonstrating improved survival when patients were randomized to protocols where these parameters were manipulated both pre- and intraoperatively, particularly if DO_2 was raised to greater than 600ml/min/m^2.

This approach is not without problems. First, there are resource implications— monitoring and achieving these parameters requires a critical care setting which may not be readily available. Second, measuring them has until recently required the placement of a pulmonary artery catheter (PAC). The PAC has fallen out of use in the vast majority of UK centres, with a consequent drop in familiarity with catheter insertion and data interpretation (see later). However, this data can now in part be derived from measurements made using newer, less invasive devices explored later in this chapter.

Adequate tissue perfusion and oxygenation

This is the most obvious goal of fluid administration, and relies on sufficient tissue blood flow and oxygen content. Direct measurement of tissue oxygenation is not currently a reality in clinical care. Various techniques, including near-infrared spectroscopy, microdialysis catheters, transcutaneous oxygen measurement, and gastrointestinal mucosal pH measurement have been used experimentally to relate local surgical and global tissue oxygenation to outcome. Of these, the only device to be used in randomized interventional studies is the gastric tonometer, and no significant improvement in perioperative mortality has been shown.

Measuring the success of fluid administration

The question remains as to what tools should be used to measure the success of a fluid administration strategy in a practical setting. No single measurement or clinical sign can reliably predict the volume status of a patient and not all devices will be appropriate or usable in all situations.

The options include:

◆ *Clinical signs:* physical examination is the starting point in assessing volume status. It may help to make a diagnosis of hypovolaemia or fluid overload, but can be misleading if taken in isolation. There are many causes of tachycardia other than fluid balance, normal blood pressure does not exclude hypovolaemia, and urine output is not a reliable indicator of intravascular volume due to the increase in ADH secretion seen with the stress response.

◆ *Invasive monitoring:* invasive arterial and central venous pressure (CVP) monitoring have limitations in guiding perioperative fluid administration. Nevertheless, they can give information which can form part of a goal-directed approach and have numerous other uses which may make them indispensable during high risk surgery:

1. Invasive blood pressure

   Placing an arterial catheter should be an easy and low morbidity intervention. Continuous blood pressure measurement aids the rapid detection of overt hypovolaemia, and a clinical assessment of systolic pressure or pulse pressure variation (the 'swing' in the arterial trace) can be an approximate indicator of intravascular depletion. In addition, the ability to perform serial arterial blood gas analyses allows the trend in lactate and base excess to be monitored closely.

   However, when used in isolation, blood pressure is a poor indicator of fluid requirements. Intravascular pressure depends on cardiac output (CO)—in turn dependent on stroke volume (SV) and heart rate—and vascular tone, not just blood volume. The result is that 'normal' blood pressure does not exclude hypovolaemia. In addition the relationship between blood pressure and tissue blood flow is not consistent and in some circumstances tissue perfusion can be adequate despite apparently low systemic blood pressure.

2. Central venous pressure

Measuring CVP has traditionally been a fundamental part of fluid management. Low CVP often reflects intravascular depletion. Central venous blood oxygen saturation (whilst not strictly mixed venous saturation) can also indicate tissue hypoperfusion, where saturations below 70% may represent increased tissue oxygen extraction due to low oxygen supply.

Whilst CVP response to fluid challenges may be a useful guide to therapy, the assumption that right atrial pressure represents left atrial pressure, and therefore left ventricular end-diastolic volume, is flawed. Aside from the influence of cardiac valvular disease, pulmonary disease, and ventricular impairment, pressure is proportional to volume divided by compliance. A rise in CVP can be seen due to venoconstriction by vasopressors; isolated CVP is not an indicator of fluid responsiveness and strategies targeting static CVP figures have worse outcomes than those targeting blood flow.

3. The pulmonary artery catheter (PAC)

The PAC was historically seen as the 'gold standard' for measuring left heart filling pressures and CO together with derived parameters such as DO_2 and VO_2 and was used in early studies on preoperative optimization.

The use of the PAC increased enormously in the USA in the 1970s, until the publication of a group of papers questioning the necessity and safety of such widespread placement. The turning point was the Connors et al. study, a large retrospective analysis suggesting higher 30-day mortality and resource utilization with PAC use.

The PAC-Man study, a large randomized controlled trial (RCT) in intensive care patients, showed no difference in outcome with PAC use. Critics of PACs argue that they should be abandoned; there are inherent risks but no outcome benefits. Others reason that it is treatments, not devices, which lead to benefits and therefore as a tool that can steer fluid management without any excess mortality, the PAC should still be used to monitor CO.

When looking at outcomes after major surgery where the PAC has been used, one large RCT showed no benefit from the use of a PAC and goal-directed therapy, albeit with methodological flaws. But when high-risk patients are specifically targeted and DO_2 greater than 600ml/min/m² is achieved, most studies show improved survival.

Meanwhile a more practical problem has emerged. Following years of controversy, PAC usage has fallen significantly in most centres. The result is that expertise in PAC insertion and ongoing management is declining, and practitioners are unable to accurately interpret the numbers generated. It seems that these factors are most likely to sound the death knell for the PAC.

4. Doppler

The transoesophageal Doppler (TOD) is a relatively recent device that derives SV and CO figures from blood flow in the descending aorta. Red blood cell velocity is measured via an ultrasound transmitter/receiver in the probe tip. The estimated cross-sectional area of the aorta is used to calculate blood flow (in ml/sec). The waveform generated is analysed to give figures for SV, CO, CI and the corrected flow time (FTc, which is considered to be a 'static' preload index). In addition, systemic vascular resistance (SVR) and systemic vascular resistance index (SVRI) can be calculated.

TOD has many advantages. Probe insertion is simple and interpretation of the figures generated is straightforward. Whilst not entirely non-invasive, morbidity from the use of this device is low. It is also the most widely studied device used in goal-directed therapy since the PAC. The available trial protocols focus on giving fluid boluses at intervals until there is no further rise in SV, rather than aiming for a prescribed SV value. Most have shown a reduction in hospital or ICU length of stay and an earlier return to enteral feeding. Two meta-analyses of the use of Doppler for goal-directed therapy in major abdominal surgery also showed a reduction in postoperative complications, but no mortality difference has been shown.

There are limitations of TOD. The quality of the Doppler waveform obtained is operator-dependent and even the probes designed for use in awake patients can cause discomfort and TOD is therefore seldom used postoperatively. TOD probes are contraindicated in oesophageal surgery and in patients with oesophageal or pharyngeal tumours.

5. Haemodynamic monitors based on the arterial waveform

i. Pulse pressure-based, e.g. FloTrac

This device samples arterial pressure at 100Hz and calculates the standard deviation of each of these points to give a 'whole waveform' measure of the pulse pressure (PP). In a constant vasculature, PP is proportional to SV, and estimates for SV are generated by this device every 20sec.

Other similar devices do not generate SV figures, but focus on measuring pulse pressure variation (PPV), i.e. the variations in PP due to the cyclical variations in SV with respiration. PPV is maximal when the left ventricle is on the steep part of the Frank–Starling curve, so intravascular filling reduces PPV by maximizing SV. Systolic pressure variation (SPV) has been shown to be a poor predictor of response to fluid in cardiac surgery, however there has been some success in predicting fluid responsiveness in sepsis by targeting PPV.

In addition, a small pilot RCT using this technique to guide intraoperative fluid administration during high risk surgery (aiming for PPV <10%) has shown a reduction in the number of postoperative complications, shorter duration of mechanical ventilation, and reduced length of ITU stay.

ii. Pulse contour/pulse power analysis, e.g. LiDCO, PiCCO

These devices also analyse the arterial waveform, having first been calibrated to generate a figure for CO using either lithium dilution (LiDCO) or thermodilution (PiCCO). Various parameters are then derived continuously, including CO, SVR, and PPV. The advantage here is that the calibration step aims to correct for interpatient variations in vascular compliance, and the manufacturers claim a good correlation between their devices and the numbers derived from PAC measurements. A recent RCT used the LiDCO device to obtain figures for CO and DO_2, and used these in a postoperative goal-directed therapy protocol following major general surgery. They found a reduction in postoperative complications and shorter hospital stay in one of their protocol groups.

Devices based on arterial waveform analysis have many advantages. They utilize devices (CVC and arterial cannula) that are often used during major surgery anyway. There is therefore little additional risk to the patient, and these devices can be used in awake preoperative or postoperative patients. Despite small numbers, there is some emerging evidence of improved outcomes when these devices are used to target PPV, CO, or DO_2 as part of a goal-directed fluid strategy.

The drawbacks are that regular recalibration is required for the LiDCO and PiCCO systems, and that these devices all rely on a good quality arterial waveform. Lastly, the numbers of published trials using these devices to date is small, and so the evidence base for using these tools is not as strong as for TOD.

Real-world approach to fluid administration

An increasing body of evidence backs up the theories that appropriate fluid administration can improve postoperative outcome.

When fluid is given very liberally as per a traditional 'recipe' there is an excess of respiratory and wound complications and more anastomotic breakdown. Other studies have also demonstrated differences in surgical and cardiopulmonary complications and return of enteral function with either 'liberal', 'restricted', or 'standard' fluid administration. A clear message here is that the evidence for recipe-based fluid strategies is not consistent and that fluid administration should be individualized to a patient in a particular clinical situation, with specific physiological goals.

Fluid studies targeting morbidity such as postoperative nausea and vomiting have typically been conducted in relatively minor surgery. Their findings do not translate easily to patients undergoing major cancer surgery.

A typical approach is therefore to monitor CO with an TOD intraoperatively, giving 200ml colloid boluses with the aim of increasing SV by 10%. Fluid challenges are continued until no further increments in SV are obtained, and restarted if there is blood loss or a progressive fall in SV. Regular clinical assessment and measurement of base excess and lactate provide further evidence of adequate tissue perfusion. Postoperatively, the TOD may be continued, or an alternative device used in awake patients. A period of ongoing goal-directed therapy in the early postoperative phase aims to maximize tissue perfusion at a time of ongoing major fluid shifts.

This fluid strategy may be modified depending on the operation being performed, and this is covered elsewhere in this book. For example, in oesophagogastrectomies, retrospective studies have shown reduced pulmonary complications and even mortality with a less positive overall fluid balance. Other surgeries with specific fluid requirements include:

- Liver resection surgery: restricting fluid administration during the resection phase may reduce blood loss, without adverse effects on renal or liver function.

- Free flap surgery: tissue flaps are particularly vulnerable to oedema, so large volumes of crystalloid are avoided.

Conclusion

- Fluid administration has a bearing on both minor and major morbidity following surgery. Ensuring adequate gut perfusion is particularly important during and after major surgery.

- Both excessive and inadequate fluids can cause harm, however knowing a patient's intravascular volume status is not always easy. Giving fluids simply by recipe is unlikely to have the best outcome for all patients.

- Tailoring fluid administration to an individual by measuring and titrating to parameters such as SV or oxygen delivery probably improves outcome.

- There is no consensus on the best device for measuring these physiological variables, although currently the best evidence base is for oesophageal Doppler used in goal-directed therapy. Nevertheless, many patients undergoing major cancer surgery are likely to require CVC and arterial cannula placement, and consideration should be given to cardiac output monitoring devices which use these lines.

- Whilst starting optimization preoperatively may not be possible in reality, continuing goal-directed therapy in the early postoperative period may be beneficial.

- Simply using a device which measures cardiac output or PPV does not automatically lead to improved outcomes. They must be used as tools to facilitate a defined goal-directed fluid strategy.

- Many major cancer operations require the fluid strategy to be modified according to the surgical and physiological insult.

Bibliography

1. Abbas SM, Hill AG (2008). Systematic review of the literature for the use of oesophageal Doppler monitor for fluid replacement in major abdominal surgery. *Anaesthesia* **63**(1):44–51.

2. Bennett-Guerrero E, Welsby I, Dunn TJ, *et al.* (1999). The use of a postoperative morbidity survey to evaluate patients with prolonged hospitalization after routine, moderate-risk, elective surgery. *Anesth Analg* **89**(2):514.

3. Boyd O, Grounds RM, Bennett ED (1993). A randomized clinical trial of the effect of deliberate perioperative increase of oxygen delivery on mortality in high-risk surgical patients. *JAMA* **270**(22):2699–707.

4. Brandstrup B, Tønnesen H, Beier-Holgersen R, *et al.* (2003). Effects of intravenous fluid restriction on postoperative complications: comparison of two perioperative fluid regimens: a randomized assessor-blinded multicenter trial. *Ann Surg* **238**(5):641–8.

5. Connors AF, Speroff T, Dawson NV, et al. (1996). The effectiveness of right heart catheterization in the initial care of critically ill patients. SUPPORT Investigators. *JAMA* **276**(11):889–97.

6. Grocott MPW, Mythen MG, Gan TJ (2005). Perioperative fluid management and clinical outcomes in adults. *Anesth Analg* **100**(4):1093–106.

7. Harvey S, Harrison DA, Singer M, *et al.* (2005). Assessment of the clinical effectiveness of pulmonary artery catheters in management of patients in intensive care (PAC-Man): a randomised controlled trial. *Lancet* **366**(9484):472–7.

8. Lopes M, Oliveira M, Pereira V, *et al.* (2007). Goal-directed fluid management based on pulse pressure variation monitoring during high-risk surgery: a pilot randomized controlled trial. *Critical Care* **11**(5):R100.

9. Mythen MG, Webb AR (1994). Intra-operative gut mucosal hypoperfusion is associated with increased post-operative complications and cost. *Intensive Care Med* **20**(2):99–104.

10. Pearse R, Dawson D, Fawcett J, *et al.* (2005). Early goal-directed therapy after major surgery reduces complications and duration of hospital stay. A randomised, controlled trial [ISRCTN38797445]. *Critical Care* **9**(6):R687–93.

11. Polonen P, Ruokonen E, Hippelainen M, Poyhonen M, Takala J (2000). A prospective, randomized study of goal-oriented hemodynamic therapy in cardiac surgical patients. *Anesth Analg* **90**(5):1052–9.

12. Shoemaker WC, Montgomery ES, Kaplan E, Elwyn DH (1973). Physiologic patterns in surviving and nonsurviving shock patients. Use of sequential cardiorespiratory variables in defining criteria for therapeutic goals and early warning of death. *Arch Surg* **106**(5):630–6.

13. Walsh SR, Tang T, Bass S, Gaunt ME (2008). Doppler-guided intra-operative fluid management during major abdominal surgery: systematic review and meta-analysis. *Int J Clin Pract* **62**(3):466–70.

14. Wilson J, Woods I, Fawcett J, *et al.* (1999). Reducing the risk of major elective surgery: randomised controlled trial of preoperative optimisation of oxygen delivery. *BMJ* **318**(7191):1099–103.

Chapter 5

Anaesthesia for paediatric oncology

David Chisholm and Alex Oliver

Introduction

Cancer is uncommon in children with an incidence of around 1500 new cases per annum in the UK. It accounts for 1 in 5 deaths in children aged 0–14 years. The commonest cancers in children are acute myeloid leukaemia (AML) and acute lymphoblastic leukaemia (ALL), lymphomas, and central nervous system (CNS) tumours which make up two-thirds of all paediatric cancers. The incidence of leukaemia is highest in the 0–9 years age group accounting for one-third of all cancers. Lymphoma is commoner than leukaemia in teenagers and CNS tumours make up around 20% of cancers in the 0–14 years group. Less common are the embryonal tumours that form from proliferation of embryonic tissue. These tumours include neuroblastoma, Wilm's tumour (nephroblastoma), hepatoblastoma, medulloblastoma, retinoblastoma, and embryonal rhabdomyosarcoma. Germ cell tumours and malignant bone tumours occur in all age groups but their incidence increases with age. Carcinomas and other malignant epithelial tumours are very rare in children under 10 years but incidence increases with age to make up 20% of cancers in the 15–19 years age group.

Survival rates for paediatric cancers have improved dramatically over the last 30 years: 80% of children survive more than 5 years after diagnosis. The majority of these children will be cured of their original disease but often at some cost to their long-term health. In over 10,000 childhood cancer survivors from USA treated between 1970 and 1986 (mean age 26 years at follow-up), over two-thirds had a chronic health condition. Among survivors the cumulative incidence of chronic poor health reached 73% at 30 years post cancer diagnosis with 42% experiencing severe, disabling, life-threatening conditions or death due to a chronic condition. This was more than eight times the incidence in their siblings who had not been treated for cancer. The three groups at the highest risk were survivors of bone tumours, Hodgkin's lymphoma, and CNS tumours.

Clinical presentation of cancer in children

Anaesthesia and sedation are regularly required to make the diagnosis of cancer in children such as for diagnostic imaging (computed tomography (CT) and magnetic resonance imaging (MRI)) where infants and small children will require anaesthesia to ensure high-quality images. Painful diagnostic procedures such as bone marrow aspiration, lumbar puncture, and needle biopsy will nearly always require a short anaesthetic. These children will often have been unwell for a number of days or weeks and will require careful preoperative assessment prior to what many non-anaesthetists would consider a brief low-risk anaesthetic.

Symptoms and signs of cancer in infants and children are often non-specific and delay in diagnosis is unfortunately quite common. Clinical presentation of acute leukaemia is determined by the degree of leukaemic infiltration of the bone marrow causing a decrease in number/function of blood cells from the three haemopoietic cell lines. Anaemia, fever, infections, bone pain, and bruising are typical.

- All children with leukaemia should have a full blood count on the day of the procedure as changes in acute leukaemia can be very rapid. A haemoglobin concentration of greater than 7g/dl is usually acceptable with a platelet count of greater than 25×10^9/L for bone marrow aspiration and 50×10^9/L for lumbar puncture although levels as low as 10×10^9/L have been reported as safe.

- A coagulation screen is required as consumptive coagulopathy can be a feature of acute leukaemia especially AML.

- A biochemical profile should also be performed as there may be evidence of increased cell turnover or renal impairment.

Signs of sepsis must be identified as clinical deterioration with anaesthesia can be sudden. Children with suspected acute leukaemia should be started on first-line antibiotics as they are presumed to have a functional abnormality of neutrophils. Persistent pyrexia is common, often a consequence of disease rather than infection. Although leukaemia is primarily a disease of the bone marrow, extramedullary infiltration of lymph nodes may cause mass effects especially in the mediastinum. Leukaemic infiltration of the tonsils may cause massive enlargement with associated snoring and sleep apnoea.

Anaesthetic considerations of specific tumour effects

Non-Hodgkin's lymphomas (NHL) are characterized by rapid growth of extranodal disease, typically in the abdomen and mediastinum. Mediastinal disease may also be present in ALL (Figure 5.1). NHL may also present as masses in the retropharynx and nasopharyngeal space causing airway compromise. Rapid dissemination to the bone marrow causes similar signs and symptoms to acute leukaemia.

Hodgkin's lymphoma presents as painless lymphadenopathy often with constitutional symptoms. Up to 60% will have mediastinal disease at presentation. Children are at particular risk of airway compression as the cartilage rings in the major bronchi are less rigid compared to adults. Up to 20% of children with anterior mediastinal masses have complications under general anaesthesia with 5% having serious life-threatening problems. The presence of unrecognized anterior mediastinal masses have led to numerous reports of fatal cardiorespiratory collapse at induction of anaesthesia. Stridor is the only sign predictive of complications under general anaesthesia. Cough and wheeze are also common and have often been misdiagnosed as asthma. All children with a suspected

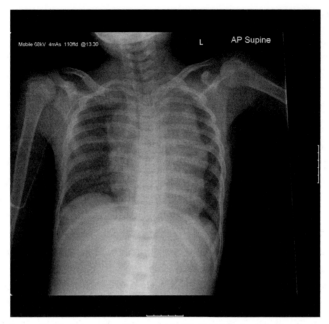

Fig. 5.1 X-ray of a mediastinal mass in a 10-year-old with T-ALL demonstrating tracheal compression and deviation.

diagnosis of acute leukaemia or lymphoma must have a recent chest radiograph (CXR) prior to anaesthesia. Echocardiogram and CT scan should be performed if the CXR is abnormal as there are often associated large pleural and pericardial effusions. A cross-sectional tracheal area of less than 30% of normal or bronchial compression is predictive of perioperative respiratory problems. All centres should have local guidelines on the management of children with anterior mediastinal masses. It may be safer to pretreat with steroids based on the most likely diagnosis to reduce the size of the mass. The response to chemotherapy is often dramatic and anaesthesia can safely be administered within a few days.

CNS tumours are associated with greatest delay in diagnosis as the symptoms and signs are quite subtle often until an advanced stage. Mood and behavioural changes are common with headaches and visual disturbances and infants may have regression of milestones. Raised intracranial pressure may be seen as bulging of the fontanelles in infants. Neuroblastomas typically present as an abdominal mass but the tumour can appear anywhere in the sympathetic chain or as metastases. These tumours often secrete catecholamines which can cause marked hypertension, and surgical manipulation can cause adrenergic crisis in the untreated child. Catecholamines should be measured preoperatively. Wilm's tumours also present usually in infants as large abdominal masses and may be associated with hypertension secondary to increased renin production. Abdominal neuroblastomas and Wilm's tumours may cause marked splinting of the diaphragm with associated ventilatory impairment. Raised intra-abdominal pressure may increase the risk of regurgitation and pulmonary aspiration.

ANAESTHESIA FOR DIAGNOSTIC PROCEDURES AND IMAGING | 47

Anaesthesia for diagnostic procedures and imaging

Although pain is common among children with cancer, highest pain scores are related to diagnostic procedures without general anaesthesia. These children are often frightened and traumatized by admission to hospital, repeated blood tests, and cannulation. The presence of a reassuring and friendly child-centred anaesthetic team can make a substantial difference both to the child and parents.

Anaesthetics may be given outside the theatre environment (e.g. in a procedure room on the paediatric ward). The area must be fully equipped and appropriately staffed. The commonest procedures are lumbar puncture, bone marrow aspirate, and trephine. A non-intubated spontaneously breathing technique is usually appropriate if gastric stasis and vomiting are not present. Nearly all children will have vascular access established in advance of their anaesthetic and an intravenous induction is therefore preferred although an inhalation technique is acceptable. These children will often have repeated anaesthetics over many months or even years and most will not tolerate repeated inhalational inductions. Short-acting agents such as propofol and remifentanil are ideal for these procedures that are not associated with much postoperative pain. An effective technique is induction with propofol 3mg/kg and remifentanil 1mcg/kg often resulting in apnoea which will require a short period of assisted ventilation with oxygen. Supplemental doses of remifentanil 0.5–1.0mcg/kg and propofol 0.5–1.0mg/kg are given if there is any movement or response to painful stimuli. This technique ensures a smooth induction with minimal movement during the procedure. Although bradycardia might be anticipated with this technique, it is rarely seen in practice. Other agents that have been successfully used are fentanyl, alfentanil, midazolam, and ketamine. Volatile agents such as sevoflurane and isoflurane are associated with a higher incidence of postoperative nausea and vomiting.

If anaesthesia is required to establish the diagnosis in a child with significant mediastinal disease, this must be performed in the operating theatre with full cardiothoracic support immediately available. All centres looking after such children should have an agreed protocol for perioperative management. A spontaneously breathing technique that avoids paralysis is deemed to be safest. Inhalational induction and maintenance with a volatile agent has been used as have combinations of ketamine and midazolam. The use of supplementary local anaesthesia may be helpful. Anterior mediastinal masses often extend beyond the carina hence endotracheal intubation may not relieve the obstruction. Rigid bronchoscopy and selective bronchial intubation has been life saving in this situation. A change in position to lateral or prone may help relieve obstruction. With severe cardiorespiratory collapse immediate sternotomy and direct elevation of the tumour may be the only effective measure. Institution of femoral–femoral bypass has been advocated but the practicality of this in an emergency situation is doubtful. These patients should be monitored in an intensive care environment postoperatively.

Anaesthesia is often required for MRI scans especially in brain tumour patients. The suspected presence of raised intracranial pressure must be established preoperatively as the effects of hypercapnia associated with general anaesthesia may be deleterious. Providing safe anaesthesia in an MRI scanner is challenging due to the remote access and disastrous conse-quences of bringing ferromagnetic objects into the scanner. Local protocols must be estab-lished to ensure safe conduct in the vicinity of the scanner even in emergency situations. This usually involves inducing anaesthesia or conducting any resuscitation in an anteroom outside the scanner. Numerous safe anaesthetic techniques have been described for MRI scans including nurse-based intravenous sedation, deep sedation with target controlled propofol, spontaneously breathing inhalational anaesthesia with laryngeal mask airway (LMA) or neuromuscular blockade and endotracheal intubation with positive pressure ventilation. More important than the method is ensuring that everyone is accustomed to the technique and that local protocols are strictly implemented.

CT scans are preferred to MRI in the diagnosis and response to therapy in neuroblastoma and Wilm's tumours. Before treatment these tumours are often massive and can cause sig-nificant respiratory comprise under spontaneously breathing anaesthesia. Spiral CT scans also require a prolonged breath-hold for optimum picture quality. Endotracheal intubation with a short-acting neuromuscular blocker such as rocuronium is often the safest way to provide anaesthesia in these infants who are also at increased risk of regurgitation and aspi-ration. Associated hypertension should be identified and treated prior to anaesthesia.

Initiation and maintenance of cancer therapy

Many of the major advances in paediatric cancer have been made by the extensive use of randomized trials to investigate the benefits of established and new therapy combina-tions. All children should be discussed in a multidisciplinary meeting early in their treat-ment to ensure latest evidence-based therapies are used.

Chemotherapy is the mainstay of treatment in paediatric cancer. This usually involves an initial intensive induction period to induce remission followed by a prolonged period of maintenance therapy with periods of intensive consolidation. Pulsed treatment maxi-mizes antitumour effects while potentially reducing the detrimental effects on healthy tissue and organs. Reliable vascular access is often required early in the induction phase of chemotherapy. Repeated blood tests and peripheral vascular cannulas can cause signifi-cant distress and phobic behaviour. A long-term central venous catheter such as a tun-nelled Hickman catheter or a subcutaneous Portacath system are usually inserted early after diagnosis (see Chapter 6). Peripherally inserted central venous catheters (PICCs) are sometimes inserted at diagnosis but they are rarely sufficient for long-term treatment. In ALL, central access is avoided if possible during the induction phase as L-asparaginase (one of the induction chemotherapy agents) causes a pro-thrombotic tendency associated with a high incidence of central vein thrombosis. A Portacath is usually inserted after induction during the first maintenance phase of chemotherapy.

The provision of a vascular access service provides a significant proportion of the anaesthetic requirements in a paediatric cancer centre. It is often safest to incorporate an anaesthetic technique that includes endotracheal intubation and positive pressure venti-lation for surgery for long-term central venous catheters. Patients are usually positioned head down and if breathing spontaneously may generate significant negative intrathoracic pressure causing a substantial risk of air embolism into open central veins. LMAs may also distort the anatomy of the central veins in the neck causing difficulty with surgical access.

Paediatric tumour lysis syndrome

Rapidly dividing tumours such the acute leukaemias and high-grade lymphomas may have a large volume of cancer cells that are acutely sensitive to the initiation of anticancer therapy. The sudden death and disruption of the cancer cells releases larges amounts of intracellular contents into the extracellular space and circulation. If not anticipated and prophylactic measures started in advance of therapy, this can result in a potentially fatal condition known as tumour lysis syndrome. This syndrome has also been caused by surgery in untreated patients and the use of dexamethasone as an antiemetic with fatal outcomes. Steroids are very potent anticancer drugs in this context. Metabolic derangements include hyperkalaemia, hyperphosphateamia, hyperuricaemia, and hypocalaemia. The rise in the extracellular potassium is much more rapid than that seen in renal failure alone as it is secondary to massive intracellular release as opposed to delayed excretion, hence supportive measures must be instituted rapidly to avoid hyperkalaemic cardiac arrest. This includes the acute control of potassium with dextrose and insulin, correction of hypocalcaemia and hyperhydration to prevent urate nephropathy. Continuous haemodiafiltration may be necessary. The patients should be managed on a paediatric intensive care unit. Patients at risk of tumour lysis syndrome should be identified in advance of starting anticancer therapy and pretreated with hyperhydration and allopurinol. If patients are regarded as high risk the recombinant urate oxidase enzyme rasburicase should be used. Any general anaesthetic should be delayed until these preventative measures have been instituted.

Anticancer drug toxicities

Children on anticancer therapy may become acutely unwell secondary to toxicity of treatment, opportunistic infection, or progression of their disease. Treatment toxicity usually affects tissues that normally divided rapidly such as the bone marrow and gastrointestinal tract (GIT). Anaemia, neutropenia, and thrombocytopenia are all common and usually require supportive measures only. Mucositis is the commonest manifestation of damage to the GIT mucosa. This is an extremely unpleasant and painful condition that may cause difficulty with airway management secondary to crusting and sloughing mucosa in the oropharynx. The epithelial damage exists throughout the GIT and like an acute burn has been reported to cause acute hyperkalaemia with the use of suxamethonium. Acute cardiac, pulmonary, hepatic, and renal dysfunction are also seen during treatment with chemotherapy and a high index of suspicion must be maintained at all times.

Sepsis in paediatric cancer

Severe sepsis is probably the commonest treatment-related complication that anaesthetists are likely to be involved in when managing in paediatric cancer patients. Children with neoplasia account for about 13% of cases of severe sepsis in the 1–9 years age group and 17% in those aged 10–19 years. The mortality is 16% for those with cancer compared to 10% without. Treatment for leukaemia and lymphoma causes a prolonged period of immune dysfunction and an increased predisposition to opportunistic infection. The highest risk is in those children who have had bone marrow transplantation (particularly allogenic since in this case prolonged immunosuppression is required). Management is as for any paediatric patient with sepsis with oxygen, fluids, inotropes, and early endotracheal intubation and ventilatory support. The most appropriate antibiotic therapy should be managed in conjunction with the paediatric oncologists. Removal of any suspected infected central venous catheters should be delayed until the child has been stabilized.

Anaesthesia for radiotherapy

Radiotherapy is used in children mainly for the treatment of CNS tumours but is also part of the treatment protocol for some patients with lymphoma, rhabdomyosarcoma, and neuroblastoma. Total body irradiation (TBI) is also used in the conditioning of patients prior to bone marrow transplantation. To reduce the exposure of healthy tissue, conformal treatment is now the standard. This involves three-dimensional imaging to produce a radiation dose profile that mirrors the shape of the area to be treated. Fractionating the total dose over a number of days or weeks gives normal tissue a better chance to repair without reducing the anticancer effect of the radiotherapy.

During radiotherapy the patient must be completely immobile and in a position that is exactly reproducible over a number of treatment fractions. For CNS tumours this will nearly always involve the use of a shell or mould that holds the head and spine in reliable position. Although the treatments only last a few minutes and are not painful, young children often find the environment intimidating and the shell can be quite claustrophobic. Only the patient can be in the room during the radiotherapy exposure, with the staff in a distant control room with audiovisual monitoring. Children under 5 years will nearly always require a general anaesthetic. Older children will often manage without general anaesthesia with a combination of familiarization and play therapy.

Providing safe anaesthesia in a challenging area such as a radiotherapy suite requires careful planning and adequate staffing and equipment. Radiotherapy treatment areas are often in the basement of hospitals in isolated areas. Older facilities may not have piped oxygen or suction. Resuscitation facilities for all size of paediatric patients must be immediately available. There no proven best anaesthetic technique, however an ideal anaesthetic would involve rapid onset and offset with prompt recovery enabling early mobilization and discharge. Previously ketamine was considered the anaesthetic of choice. However, it is not ideal due to excess salivation, spontaneous movement, and detrimental effects on patients with increased intracranial pressure. Control of the airway with either a LMA or endotracheal tube is preferred by some with an inhalational anaesthetic used for maintenance. This technique is, however, associated with an increased incidence of nausea and vomiting, daily exposure to volatile agents, and problems with scavenging.

Total intravenous anaesthesia with propofol without routine use of any artificial airway is the preferred technique in our institution. This avoids the daily instrumentation of the airway, is associated with rapid awakening, and a low incidence of nausea and vomiting. Opiate analgesia is avoided as the treatment is not painful.

For CNS tumours the initial planning for radiotherapy requires a mould to be produced. This is made of a sheet of thermoplastic which has preformed holes for the mouth and nose. This is draped across the patient's face while warm and conformed to the shape of the face and head. As the sheet starts to harden at room temperature it is crucial that the child can maintain their airway without obstruction. A spacer is used between the teeth to enable room for the insertion of a LMA if this was to subsequently become necessary, though in reality this is rare. The mould is fixed to the radiotherapy treatment table by rapid release studs. For children having radiotherapy to the abdomen or other parts of the body the area to be treated is immobilized in a vacuumized bag and the head is supported to one side with a foam wedge. With conformal radiotherapy the requirement for children to be treated in the prone position has disappeared.

A bolus dose of propofol of 3–5mg/kg is given for induction. Although the aim is to maintain spontaneous respiration throughout the ability to manually ventilate must be immediately available as a brief period of apnoea can occur after induction. A continuous infusion is commenced at 10mg/kg/h and adjusted to response. Once the child is settled in the mould or in position there is very little stimulation and the infusion rate can often be reduced. The child is observed to ensure an unobstructed respiratory pattern. Oxygen is delivered by facemask and a section of narrow bore tubing with a Luer-lock connector is taped close to one nostril to sample carbon dioxide (Figure 5.2). Closed circuit television is used to observe both the patient and monitor from the control room (Figure 5.3). This technique is associated with rapid psychomotor recovery and discharge home can be as early as 30 minutes post procedure. Treatment can last up to 7 weeks and the patients

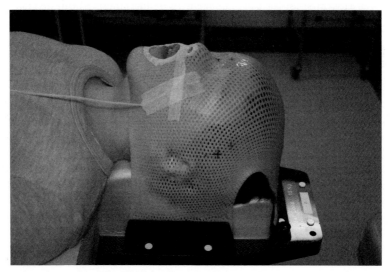

Fig. 5.2 Perinasal sampling of end-tidal carbon dioxide.

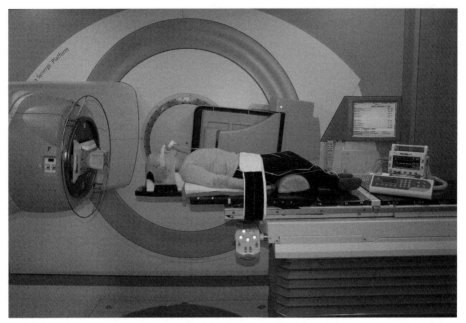

Fig. 5.3 Set-up of positioning and monitoring for radiotherapy.

require careful daily review as respiratory infections and treatment related complications are common.

Conclusion

Anaesthetists may be exposed to children with cancer in both the specialist and non-specialist settings. A working knowledge of both the effects of cancer and complications of therapy are essential for the safe management of anaesthesia in this diverse group of patients.

Bibliography

1. Al-Khafaji AH, Dewhirst WE, Cornell CJ Jr, Quill TJ (2001). Succinylcholine-induced hyperkalemia in a patient with mucositis secondary to chemotherapy. *Crit Care Med* **29**(6):1274–6.
2. Anghelescu DL, Burgoyne LL, Liu W, *et al.* (2008). Safe anesthesia for radiotherapy in pediatric oncology: St. Jude Children's Research Hospital Experience, 2004–2006. *Int J Radiat Oncol Biol Phys* **71**(2):491–7.
3. Culshaw V, Yule M, Lawson R (2003). Considerations for anaesthesia in children with haematological malignancy undergoing short procedures. *Paediatr Anaesth* **13**(5):375–83.
4. Farley-Hills E, Byrne AJ, Brennan L, Sartori P (2001). Tumour lysis syndrome during anaesthesia. *Paediatr Anaesth* **11**(2):233–6.
5. Ferrari LR, Bedford RF (1990). General anesthesia prior to treatment of anterior mediastinal masses in pediatric cancer patients. *Anesthesiology* **72**(6):991–5.
6. Glaisyer HR, Sury MR (2005). Recovery after anesthesia for short pediatric oncology procedures: propofol and remifentanil compared with propofol, nitrous oxide, and sevoflurane. *Anesth Analg* **100**(4):959–63.

7. Hack HA, Wright NB, Wynn RF (2008). The anaesthetic management of children with anterior mediastinal masses. *Anaesthesia* **63**(8):837–46.

8. Keidan I, Berkenstadt H, Sidi A, Perel A (2001). Propofol/remifentanil versus propofol alone for bone marrow aspiration in paediatric haemato-oncological patients. *Paediatr Anaesth* **11**(3):297–301.

9. Keidan I, Perel A, Shabtai EL, Pfeffer RM (2004). Children undergoing repeated exposures for radiation therapy do not develop tolerance to propofol: clinical and bispectral index data. *Anesthesiology* **100**(2):251–4.

10. Kutko MC, Calarco MP, Flaherty MB, *et al.* (2003). Mortality rates in pediatric septic shock with and without multiple organ system failure. *Pediatr Crit Care Med* **4**(3):333–7.

11. Latham GJ, Greenberg RS (2010a). Anesthetic considerations for the pediatric oncology patient—part 1: a review of antitumor therapy. *Paediatr Anaesth* **20**(4):295–304.

12. Latham GJ, Greenberg RS (2010b). Anesthetic considerations for the pediatric oncology patient—part 2: systems-based approach to anesthesia. *Paediatr Anaesth* **20**(5):396–420.

13. Latham GJ, Greenberg RS (2010c). Anesthetic considerations for the pediatric oncology patient—part 3: pain, cognitive dysfunction, and preoperative evaluation. *Paediatr Anaesth* **20**(6):479–89.

14. Lee MH, Cheng KI, Jang RC, Hsu JH, Dai ZK, Wu JR (2007). Tumour lysis syndrome developing during an operation. *Anaesthesia* **62**(1):85–7.

15. Oeffinger KC, Mertens AC, Sklar CA, *et al.*; Childhood Cancer Survivor Study (2006). Chronic health conditions in adult survivors of childhood cancer. *NEJM* **355**(15):1572–82.

16. Scheiber G, Ribeiro FC, Karpienski H, Strehl K (1996). Deep sedation with propofol in preschool children undergoing radiation therapy. *Paediatr Anaesth* **6**(3):209–13.

17. Serafini G, Zadra N (2008). Anaesthesia for MRI in the paediatric patient. *Curr Opin Anaesthesiol* **21**(4):499–503.

18. Viswanathan S, Campbell CE, Cork RC (1995). Asymptomatic undetected mediastinal mass: a death during ambulatory anesthesia. *J Clin Anesth* **7**(2):151–5.

Chapter 6

Vascular access in cancer

Ajit Walunj, Enrique Lopez, and Ravishankar
Rao Baikady

Introduction

The techniques of intravenous (IV) access and infusion were first described in 1665 by
Escholtz. IV infusion of saline and water were introduced successfully to treat cholera in
humans in 1832 using silver cannulas. Myers and Zimmermann reported separately in
1945 the use of plastic catheters for continuous vascular access. Roy and colleagues in
1967 used a long nylon catheter into central veins inserted initially by venous cut-down
and later percutaneously for chemotherapy. Dr Robert O. Hickman was a paediatric
nephrologist in Seattle and introduced further modifications such as subcutaneous tunnelling and the Dacron cuff to prevent spread of infection. Hickman promoted the use of
a modified right atrial catheter in 1979.

Peripherally inserted central venous catheters (PICCs) were introduced in 1975.
Hoshal used silicone elastomer catheters, placed in the superior vena cava via the basilic
or cephalic vein for IV nutrition and demonstrated the safety and efficacy of these
PICC lines.

Totally implantable ports were initially used in 1980s in cancer patients. The device had
a conical chamber with a self-sealing silicone rubber septum connected to a silastic catheter. A variety of anticancer drugs, blood and blood products, and antibiotics were
administered without difficulty and accepted by patients.

Short-term venous access

Short-term access involves central venous catheters placed percutaneously into the jugular, femoral, or subclavian veins. The site of insertion depends on operator and patient
preference, indication for insertion, and presence of coagulopathy or local infection and
disease characteristics (Table 6.1).

Although the right internal jugular is the first preference because of technical and anatomical reasons, compliance in ambulatory patients is poor. Also neck movements may
lead to catheter movement and the potential for bacterial migration and catheter-related
bloodstream infection (CRBSI). Jugular or femoral approach may be safer in patients
with coagulopathy as local compression can be used to stop bleeding.

Multiple lumens may be necessary for simultaneous administration of chemotherapy
and total parenteral nutrition (TPN), which requires dedicated access. Drugs administered

Table 6.1 Sites for vascular access

Site	Advantages	Disadvantages
Internal jugular vein (IJV)	◆ Straighter anatomical course (right IJV) ◆ Familiarity with the technique	◆ Poor compliance in ambulatory patients
Femoral vein	◆ Less complications such as pneumothorax and arrhythmias	◆ Higher infection risk ◆ Increased venous thrombosis ◆ Reduced mobility ◆ Inappropriate in post-transplant patients
Subclavian vein	◆ Comfortable for mobile patients, better compliance ◆ Reduced infection rate ◆ Reduced neurovascular problems	◆ Higher incidence of pneumothorax and haemorrhage ◆ Unable to compress if arterial puncture ◆ Higher incidence of late stenosis

into central veins are rapidly diluted by the circulating blood volume, ensuring systemic distribution and reducing local adverse effects.

Central venous catheters are usually made of polyurethane. They are relatively hydrophobic and stiff *in vitro* but soften when placed, thus facilitating easy insertion and endothelial protection. Catheters may also be made of polytetrafluoroethylene or silicone (Silastic), which is the most flexible. Silastic is hydrophobic, relatively non-thrombogenic, and minimally immunoreactive. Silastic catheters are usually inserted over guidewires or introducer sheaths because of their elasticity and impact resistance. Impregnation with antibiotic substance such as silver-sulphadiazine and chlorhexidine may lead to significant reduction in bacterial colonization and catheter-related infection.

Indications for vascular access for cancer

- IV administration of short-term chemotherapy and other drugs
- Long-term administration of antibiotics
- TPN
- Haemodialysis
- Marrow transfusion
- Peripheral blood stem-cell harvesting
- Fluid and electrolyte administration
- Treatment of graft-versus-host disease
- Access for frequent blood samples.

Long-term vascular access

Skin tunnelled venous access

Skin tunnelled catheters are commonly used for cancer treatment and are inserted by anaesthetists, surgeons, radiologists, and nurse practitioners. Insertion takes place in the

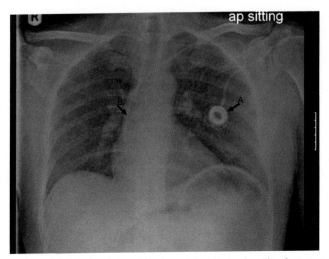

Fig. 6.1 Chest radiography showing left subclavian portacath *in situ*. Titanium port chamber in the chest wall (A) and catheter tip in the right atrium (B).

operating theatre or radiological suite with full aseptic precautions under local anaesthesia with conscious sedation or full general anaesthesia.

Portacath

Portacaths provide a permanent closed system for easy access for drug delivery and drawing blood. This provides a cosmetically acceptable option allowing the patient to bathe or swim. In the UK, their use is becoming increasingly common.

These are totally implantable devices consisting of two components (Figure 6.1). A titanium or plastic case is surgically implanted into the subcutaneous tissue (chest wall or upper arm) (Figure 6.1). Brachial ports have also been used reducing pneumothorax, but with a shorter lifetime and higher incidence of thrombosis. The case has a thick membrane, accessed by non-coring Huber-type needle.

The second component is the intravascular segment which is in continuum with the case and delivers the drugs (Figure 6.1). While the initial cost of insertion is high, they have low ongoing costs and are economically viable for prolonged use. They also have low rates of catheter-related infections and mechanical complications compared to external catheters.

The most common approach is through the internal jugular or subclavian vein under ultrasound guidance. The placement of the wire in the right atrium is confirmed by image intensifier. The portacath chamber is placed in the chest wall via a skin incision. The catheter is tunnelled from the port to the vein access site. Correct placement is confirmed by X-ray imaging throughout the procedure. The tip of the catheter should be in the mid to apex of the right atrium so that the catheter is always in the moving bloodstream to avoid erosion of the vessel wall.

Removal involves making an incision into the dense fibrous sac that forms around the port in long term. There are typically three to four anchoring sutures that go through the holes in the port to deeper tissues.

Access needles have a fine bore restricting the flow rate and must be inserted vertically to avoid bending the tip. More than 2000 punctures can be made using a non-coring Huber needle which can be kept in for 3 days but should be replaced after 24 hours when administering blood products or lipid emulsions. Most devices are single lumen only for limited, short-term access on an outpatient basis. They are not suitable for bone marrow transplant, when a multilumen skin tunnelled (Hickman) catheter is the preferred option. They are also useful for induction of anaesthesia in children undergoing repeated procedures such as lumbar puncture.

The portacath should be flushed with heparinized saline once a month to check the patency when not accessed regularly for treatment. Removal of portacath can be done under local anaesthesia.

Skin tunnelled multilumen catheters

These are commonly used devices, available in various sizes, for adults and children, with one, two, or three lumens. They are manufactured from soft silicone rubber or PVC and are characterized by the presence of a Dacron cuff. The cuff provides anchorage by stimulating growth of fibrous tissue around the cuff. The cuff may act as an antimicrobial barrier, however definite evidence is lacking. It should ideally be placed at least 2 weeks prior to the commencement of chemotherapy, to allow adequate fibroblastic response to the cuff.

Specialized procedures like aphaeresis, which involves removal of a particular component and peripheral blood stem cell collection (PBSCC) demand higher flows and an 'aphaeresis catheter' with a wider lumen and increased rigidity, is the preferred option. Long-term silicone (LTS) catheters are preferred for stem cell harvest. They have a 12.5F diameter and 28-cm fixed length dual lumen catheter with staggered tip. In the UK most of the skin tunnelled catheters are supplied by BARD® and KIMAL®.

Hickman lines are also inserted in children for frequent blood sampling or administration of repeated blood transfusion, chemotherapy, and fluid therapy.

Insertion

Insertion should be carried out in the operating theatre under strict aseptic control and fluoroscopic guidance. Full routine monitoring is recommended, particularly electrocardiography for detection of arrhythmias. Sedation with propofol, midazolam, or remifentanil or general anaesthesia may be used.

Insertion is percutaneous using a Seldinger technique directly into the subclavian vein or internal jugular vein (IJV). A surgical cut-down is used in children under 7 years to avoid potential damage to the vessels from the stiff dilators. The aim is to place the catheter tip in the upper quadrant of the right atrium or at the junction of the superior vena cava and right atrium.

Preoperative chest X-ray is essential to identify any mediastinal mass or distortion of anatomy relevant to the access placement. A coagulation screen and platelet count must be carried out and abnormalities corrected. Platelet count should be 50,000 or more. Local site infection and uncontrolled bacteraemia are contraindications to the procedure. Fever, infection at another site, and neutropenia are not absolute contraindications.

The role of prophylactic antibiotics is unclear and they are not routinely administered in most centres.

Percutaneous technique

- The patient is placed in the Trendelenburg position, skin is prepared with 2% chlorhexidine at the site, and a sterile drape placed. For subclavian access, insertion too close to the clavicle may lead to difficulty in introduction of the catheter and the introducer whereas a very medial approach may cause kinking of the introducer and sharp angulation. The catheter can get pinched between the clavicle and first rib leading to catheter malfunction or breakage. The IJV is accessed in the lower part of the anterior neck above the clavicle (Figure 6.2).

- The exit site is on the anterior chest wall above the nipple line. In females breast tissue should be avoided for cosmetic reasons. Relatively large volumes of local anaesthetic (30–40ml) with adrenaline are injected at the insertion, exit sites, and along the subcutaneous tunnel with a long spinal needle.

- The vein is identified under ultrasound guidance with a 16G or 18G needle or cannulae through which a J-wire is introduced. The position is confirmed radiographically (Figure 6.2).

- A 5-mm incision is made at the entry and the exit sites. Tunnelling is done from exit site to entry site with the catheter attached (Figure 6.3). Perforating branches of the internal mammary artery may be damaged if the tunnelling extends deeper than subcutaneous tissue. For subclavian access the tunnel is best kept medial in the immobile tissues near the sternum to avoid catheter retraction following movement. Lateral tunnelling is preferred for IJV access to avoid acute angulations (Figure 6.3). The Dacron cuff should be placed in mid-tunnel position at least 3–5cm from the exit site. For internal jugular catheters the cuff site should be below the clavicle for ease of catheter removal. The tunnel length may vary from 5–12cm.

- The catheter is cut to the required length after checking the X-ray image to confirm the wire position and measuring the length of the wire outside the vein (Figure 6.4).

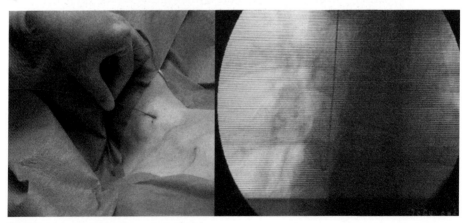

Fig. 6.2 J-wire in right atrium via right IJV.

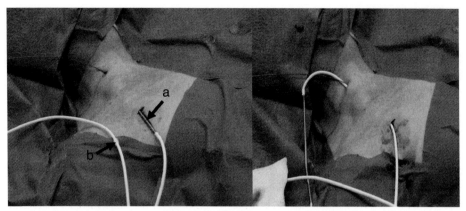

Fig. 6.3 Tunelling the catheter from exit site to entry with a metallic tuneller (a) and Dacron cuff (b).

It can also be done by surface marking of the right atrium, at the third or fourth intercostal space as the final tip position and measuring the length along the track using X-ray image. Once cut the catheter is primed with heparinized saline.

♦ The splitting sheath with dilator is advanced over the wire (Figure 6.5). Once the sheath is introduced the dilator and the wire are removed together by pinching the sheath firmly to avoid air embolism and blood loss. The catheter is passed through the sheath with non-toothed forceps (Figure 6.5). Once confirmation of the location of the catheter tip is confirmed, the sheath is removed (Figure 6.6). The split sheath is then slowly split apart with the catheter remaining in place (Figure 6.6). Catheter placement is also confirmed by blood aspiration through all lumens.

♦ The venous puncture site is closed with a single skin suture and the catheter is secured at the tunnel exit site to the skin. The suture is removed after 3 weeks when the Dacron cuff fibrous sheath will hold the catheter firmly to the skin. A post-insertion chest X-ray is performed.

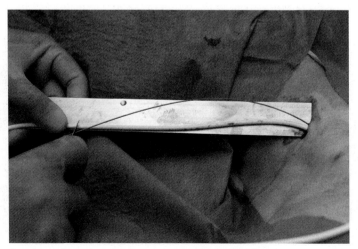

Fig. 6.4 Cutting the catheter length after measuring with the ruler.

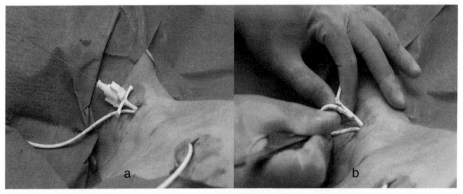

Fig. 6.5 a) Dilator with sheath introduced through the wire. b) Catheter is inserted with non-tooth forceps after removal of dilator and J-wire.

Catheter removal

Recently inserted catheters may be removed by traction alone, but long-term ones may need a surgical cut-down procedure under local anaesthesia. The fibrous sheath formed around the Dacron cuff may need dissection. Potential problems of incorrect removal are catheter damage, embolization, infection, or poor cosmetic results. Rarely, part of the sheath during insertion or split catheter during removal may be left in the right atrium or right ventricle.

Peripherally inserted venous access

PICC line

These are soft thin-walled catheters inserted at the antecubital fossa and passed into a central vein via the axillary and the subclavian veins, so that the tip of the catheter is in the superior vena cava (SVC). They are relatively straightforward to insert, and can be inserted in procedure suites or fluoroscopy room under local anaesthesia (or general anaesthesia in paediatrics). The catheter is tolerated well by most patients. The basilic vein is generally preferred as it is usually larger and straighter than the medial cubital vein and cephalic vein. Ultrasound is increasingly used to identify the vein.

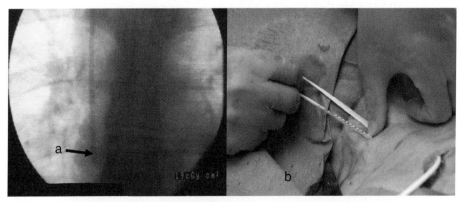

Fig. 6.6 a) Final position of the catheter in right atrium. b) Technique to remove the sheath while firmly holding the catheter with thumb.

Insertion technique

- The site is cleaned with 2% chlorhexidine. Local anaesthesia is injected at the venepuncture site.
- If fluoroscopy is not used then the catheter is measured from the insertion site to second rib on the sternum and cut accordingly. A fine guidewire from the kit is introduced into the catheter.
- A cannula is inserted into a vein near the elbow and the needle is removed. The PICC catheter is advanced through the cannula. The cannula is then pulled back and peeled away from the catheter.
- The catheter is advanced further into the vein (under fluoroscopy if available) until it reaches its terminating point. The wire is removed.

The position of the tip is confirmed with chest X-ray (Figure 6.7):

- In the modified Seldinger technique, a guidewire is passed several centimetres into the cannula. The cannula is removed leaving the guidewire in place. The guidewire is not advanced past the shoulder. An introducer sheath with a dilator is introduced over the guidewire after a small incision is made on the skin near the wire. The guidewire and dilator are removed. The catheter is advanced through the introducer sheath. The introducer is then pulled back and removed.
- The position of the tip of the catheter is confirmed with chest X-ray. Fluoroscopic dye injection can also identify the catheter tip.

The arm may need to be abducted during difficult catheter insertion. The catheter is aspirated for blood and heparinized saline is flushed to maintain the patency. The incidence of correct positioning of tip of the catheter is up to 65% in blind insertion technique and under fluoroscopy this may be improved up to 90%.

PICC lines are well tolerated. However, it has a single small-diameter lumen and increased incidence of line blockade and axillary vein thrombosis compared to other long-term venous access.

Complications of long-term venous access

Insertion-related complications

- During venepuncture:
  - Haematoma/bleeding (up to 20%)
  - Venous laceration (rare)
  - Arterial puncture (rare if ultrasound is used)
  - Pneumothorax (<1%)
  - Haemo/chylothorax (rare)
  - Arrhythmias (usually self-limiting)
  - Nerve injury (rare)
  - Difficult wire positioning (up to 10%)

- Tunnel catheter insertion:
  - Bleeding and haematoma (<5%)
  - Arrhythmias (self-limiting)
  - Displacement of wire by dilator (<1%)
  - Air embolus (insignificant, <0.5%)
  - Perforation of vessel (rare)
  - Damage/kinking/loss of guidewire (rare).

Incidence of pleural injury is commoner after subclavian vein puncture, but use of ultrasound has reduced the incidence to less than 1%. Most pnemothoraces are self-limiting and rarely require drainage.

Line-related complications

- Infection:
  - Exit site (up to 5%)
  - Tunnel (1–3%)
  - Bacteraemia (up to 20%)
  - Infected thrombophlebitis (up to 2%)
  - Endocarditis (rare)
- Thrombosis:
  - Fibrin sheath
  - Catheter occlusion
  - Large vessel thrombosis (up to 2%)
  - Right atrial thrombosis (up to 1%)
  - Pulmonary thromboembolism (rare)
- Unusual complications:
  - Arrhythmias (up to 1%)
  - Migration of tip or cuff extrusion (up to 2%)
  - Positional functioning
  - Material failure or breakage
  - Lymphorrhoea—chyle leak
  - Port getting lost in the chest wall.

Infection

Catheter related infection rate ranges from 0.6–2.7% depending on the site of insertion, type of catheter, and patient immunological status. The incidence of infection-related complications are less after portacath compared to other skin tunnelled catheters.

Possible mechanisms of infection include:

- Migration of skin organisms along the catheter surface

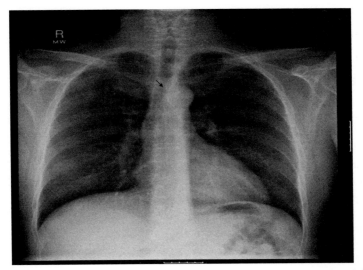

Fig. 6.7 Chest radiograph after insertion of the PICC line. Arrows show the course of the line and the tip in SVC.

- Contamination at insertion
- Contamination of catheter hub by administered substances
- Haematogenous spread from a distant source.

The common organisms implicated are coagulase-negative *Staphylococcus*, *Staphylococcus aureus*, and *Candida* species.

Thromboembolism

Placement of a central venous access further increases the pre-existing risk of venous thrombosis in cancer patients. Possible mechanisms implicated are prothrombotic effects of the malignancy, increased venous stasis, endothelial injury, and the effects of chemotherapy.

Venous thrombosis may present as limb swelling or pain or may be asymptomatic and occlusion of the catheter may be partial or complete. The incidence may range from 12–66%, depending on diagnostic methodology.

There is no clear evidence to support prophylactic anticoagulation in cancer patients with venous catheters to prevent thrombosis induced by long-term catheters. Equally, presence of only catheter tip thrombosis where flushing is possible but aspiration is not, presents a similar dilemma. Administration of a small dose of heparin over 24 hours using a perfusor system has been tried successfully to regain patency of the port.

Conclusion

Establishing and maintenance of long-term venous access devices is a crucial component of managing cancer patients. The choice of catheter and insertion technique depends on clinical expertise, patient preference, and the therapy planned. Subcutaneous ports are becoming increasingly common with lower infection and higher patient acceptance rates.

Specialized teams are increasingly being developed and utilized for insertion, management, and removal. Knowledge of various aspects of these devices is imperative for anaesthetists and intensive care physicians involved in the care of cancer patients.

Bibliography

1. Bach A, Böhrer H, Motsch J, Martin E, Geiss HK, Sonntag HG (1994). Prevention of bacterial colonization of intravenous catheters by antiseptic impregnation of polyurethane polymers. *J Antimicrob Chemother* **33**:969–78.

2. Brooks AJ, Alfredson M, Pettigrew B, Morris DL (2005). Ultrasound-guided insertion of subclavian venous access ports. *Ann R Coll Surg Engl* **87**:25–7.

3. Broviac JW, Cole JJ, Scribner BH (1973). A silicone rubber atrial catheter for prolonged parenteral alimentation. *Surg Gynecol Obstet* **136**(4):602–6.

4. Cosnett JE (1989). The origins of intravenous fluid therapy. *Lancet* **1**:768–71.

5. De Cicco M, Panarello G, Chiaradia V, *et al.* (1989). Source and route of microbial colonisation of parenteral nutrition catheters. *Lancet* **2**:1258–61.

6. Galloway S, Bodenham A (2004). Long-term central venous access. *Br J Anaesth* **92**:722–34.

7. Gilsdorf JR, Wilson K, Beals TF (1989). Bacterial colonization of intravenous catheter materials in vitro and in vivo. *Surgery* **106**(1):37–44.

8. Hacking MB, Brown J, Chisholm DG (2003). Position dependent ventricular tachycardia in two children with peripherally inserted central catheters (PICCs). *Paediatr Anaesth* **13**(6):527–9.

9. Hickman RO, Buckner CD, Clift RA, *et al.* (1979). A modified right atrial catheter for access to the venous system in marrow transplant recipient. *Surg Gynecol Obstet* **148**:871–5.

10. Hind D, Calvert N, McWilliams R, *et al.* (2003). Ultrasonic locating devices for central venous cannulation: meta-analysis. *BMJ* **327**:361–8.

11. Hoshal VL Jr (1975). Total intravenous nutrition with peripherally inserted silicone elastomer central venous catheters. *Arch Surg* **110**:644–6.

12. Kuriakose J, Colon-Otero G, Paz-Fumagalli R (2002). Risk of deep vein thrombosis associated with chest versus arm central venous subcutaneous port catheters; a 5-year single institution retrospective study. *J Vasc Interv Radiol* **13**:179–84.

13. Merrell SW, Peatross BG, Grossman MD, Sullivan JJ, Harker WG (1994). Peripherally inserted central venous catheters. Low risk alternatives for ongoing venous access. *West J Med* **160**:25–30.

14. Meyers L (1945). Intravenous catheterization. *Am J Nurs* **45**:930–1.

15. Niederhuber JE, Ensminger W, Gyves JW, *et al* (1982). Totally implanted venous and arterial access system to replace external catheter in cancer treatment. *Surgery* **92**:706–12.

16. Nightingale CE, Norman A, Cunningham D, Young J, Webb A, Fishie J (1997). A prospective analysis of 949 long-term central venous access catheters for ambulatory chemotherapy in patients with gastrointestinal malignancy. *Eur J Cancer* **33**:398–403.

17. O'Grady NP, Alexander M, Dellinger EP, *et al.* (2008). Guidelines for prevention of intravascular catheter related infections. *Am J Infect Control* 2002; **30**:476–89.

18. Pratt RJ, Pellowe CM, Wilson JA, *et al.* (2007). epic2: Guidelines for Preventing Healthcare-Associated Infections in NHS Hospitals. *J Hosp Infect* **65S**:S1–S64.

19. Press OW, Ramsey PG, Larson EB, Fefer A, Hickman RO (1984). Hickman catheter infections in patients with malignancies. *Medicine (Baltimore)* **63**:189–200.

20. Randolph AG, Gonzales CA, Pribble CG (1996). Ultrasound guidance for placement of central venous access catheters *Crit Care Med* **24**:2053–8.

21. Ray S, Stacey R, Imrie M, Filshie J (1996). A review of 560 Hickman catheter insertions. *Anaesthesia* **51**:981–5.

22. Roy RB, Wilkinson RH, Bayliss CE (1967). The utilization of long nylon catheters for prolonged intravenous infusions. *Can Med Assoc J* **96**:94–7.

23. Selby Jr JB, Cohn DJ, Koenig G (2001). Peripherally inserted tunnelled catheters: a new option for venous access. *Min Invas Ther & Allied Technol* **10**(4/5):231–4.

24. Venkatesan T, Sen N, Korula PJ, *et al.* (2007). Blind placements of peripherally inserted antecubital central catheters: initial catheter tip position in relation to carina. *Br J Anaesth* **98**(1):83–8.

25. Vescia S, Baumgärtner AK, Jacobs VR, *et al.* (2008). Management of venous port systems in oncology: a review of current evidence. *Ann Oncol* **19**:9–15.

26. Wendt JR (1992). Avoiding serious complications with central venous access. *Surg Rounds* **15**(7):637–41.

27. Yildizeli B, Laçin T, Batirel HF, Yüksel M (2004). Complications and management of long-term central venous access catheters and ports. *J Vasc Access* **5**(4):174–8.

28. Zimmermann B (1945). Intravenous tubing for parenteral therapy. *Science* **101**:567–8.

Chapter 7

Anaesthesia for head and neck cancer surgery

Deanne Cheyne and Colm Irving

Incidence

The upper aerodigestive tract (UAT) consists of several connected structures including the lip, oral cavity, oropharynx, hypopharynx, larynx, nasopharynx, nasal cavity, sinuses, salivary glands, and thyroid. There were 10,323 new cases of head and neck cancer (including thyroid) reported in the UK in 2006, an incidence of 14.6/100,000 population.

Pathology and risk factors

Ninety per cent are squamous cell carcinomas of the head and neck (SCCHN). The remainder are thyroid, lymphoma, sarcoma, melanoma, and other skin cancers.
  Risk factors include:

◆ Tobacco—smoking or chewing

◆ Excessive alcohol consumption

◆ Human papillomavirus has been linked to an increased risk of oropharyngeal cancers

◆ Diet—the incidence of nasopharyngeal cancer (NPC) is higher in Asians, Eskimos, and Icelanders whose diets are rich in salt-cured fish and red meat

◆ There is a strong association between the development of NPC and Epstein–Barr virus

◆ UV light exposure (lip), previous radiation to head and neck

◆ Occupational exposure to nickel and wood dust

◆ Poor oral hygiene, ill-fitting dentures, chronic candidiasis.

Treatment

In 2004, the National Institute for Health and Clinical Excellence (NICE) published guidelines for improving services for head and neck cancer patients within the UK National Health Service. Key recommendations included centralization of services and treatment within multidisciplinary teams (MDT). The MDTs should treat a minimum of 100 new cases of UAT cancer per annum. Core members of the MDT include surgeons, oncologists, pathologists, radiologists, clinical nurse specialists, speech and language therapists, senior nursing staff, palliative care specialists, dieticians, and other supporting staff. An anaesthetist with a special interest in head and neck surgery is part of the extended MDT, and should make themselves available whenever their expertise is required.

Surgery and/or radiotherapy are the main forms of curative treatment, and offer equally good long-term results in early head and neck cancers. The choice of treatment modality depends on the site, stage, and resectability of the disease. For patients with non-metastatic, regionally advanced but resectable SCCHN (Stage III/IV, M0) the addition of concurrent chemotherapy to the adjuvant radiotherapy following surgical resection has resulted in significant improvement in survival. For those with unresectable, regionally advanced SCCHN, survival benefits have been observed with concurrent chemoradiotherapy compared with radiotherapy alone.

Survival

Despite the evidence that the majority of SCCHN are slow growing tumours, only around one-third of patients will present with early disease (stages I–II). The remaining two-thirds present with regionally advanced or metastatic SCCHN. The most common sites for metastases are lung, bone, and liver. With timely and appropriate treatment, 2-year crude survival for SCCHN can be as high as 95% for stage I, and up to 55% for stage IV.

Preoperative assessment

Head and neck cancer patients present the anaesthetist with a number of challenges relating to comorbidities, complications of the disease process, and complications arising from the treatment. Close cooperation among all members of the MDT is imperative to secure the best possible outcome for the individual patient.

Patient comorbidity

The vast majority of head and neck cancer patient are elderly. They may have significant cardiorespiratory disease and nutritional deficiencies, placing them in the intermediate-to high-risk category for perioperative pulmonary and cardiac complications. Their functional status should ideally be optimized prior to surgery. Unstable coronary syndromes, decompensated heart failure, significant arrhythmias, and severe valvular disease indicate a major clinical risk. These active coronary conditions need urgent management and may result in the delay of all but emergency surgery.

Patients with a history of alcohol abuse should be investigated for alcoholic liver disease and alcoholic cardiomyopathy. Early identification and treatment of alcohol withdrawal is essential in order to limit further complications.

Malnutrition and weight loss further increase the risk for postoperative complications. A systematic literature review for the American College of Physicians confirmed that a low serum albumin level (<35g/L) is an independent risk factor for postoperative pulmonary complications. However, routine total parenteral or enteral nutrition does not appear to reduce this risk.

Complications arising from tumour progression

Tumour invasion of the surrounding anatomical structures accounts for various symptoms with which the patient may present. Tumour encroachment into the airway may cause voice changes, dyspnoea, or stridor. A history of postural changes in these symptoms indicates impending obstruction. Airway compromise due to rapid progression or late presentation may limit the time available for preoperative optimization. Dysphagia and odynophagia further accelerates weight loss and nutritional deficiencies. Invasion of the carotid artery may present with a life-threatening haemorrhage, whilst fungating tumours may ulcerate and bleed leading to anaemia. Tumours may also invade cranial nerves around the base of the skull causing neuropathic pain. Unrelated to tumour size and invasion, patients may present with symptoms arising from paraneoplastic syndromes, e.g. hypercalcaemia and inappropriate antidiuretic hormone secretion.

Procedure-related risk

Head and neck surgery is a heterogeneous group of operations ranging from the relatively minor (e.g. endoscopy) to the complex (e.g. pharyngolaryngo-oesophagectomy with free flap reconstruction). The risk associated with any procedure depends on the degree of tissue trauma, the length of the operation, and any problems associated with a shared airway. These considerations will dictate the extent of preoperative investigation.

Complications arising from treatment

Radiotherapy-induced fibrosis of the irradiated tissues can cause trismus, decreased tongue mobility, limited neck movement, and lymphoedema. Therefore, a history of head and neck irradiation is a significant clinical predictor of both difficult intubation and difficult mask ventilation. These patients are often electively directed towards an awake fibreoptic intubation (see later section). Previous surgery causes scarring, induration, and distortion of the anatomy, further complicating airway management. The chemotherapeutic agents most commonly used are cisplatin, 5-flurouracil, taxanes, and cetuximab. The side effects of these agents include myelosuppression, nausea and vomiting, alopecia, nephrotoxicity (cisplatin), ototoxicity (cisplatin), peripheral neuropathy, myalgia, arrhythmias (taxanes), acneform rash, and hypersensitivity reactions (see Chapter 15). Chemotherapy may also exacerbate mucositis when used concurrently with radiotherapy.

Preoperative airway assessment

The preoperative airway assessment provides an opportunity for the anaesthetist to predict, plan, and prepare for the difficult airway. The assessment should include a history taking, clinical examination, and review of relevant radiological investigations. The assessment allows the anaesthetist, in conjunction with the surgeon, to formulate a plan specific to the individual patient and in particular to identify those patients where the predicted degree of difficulty is so great that they require an awake intubation or tracheostomy under local anaesthesia.

History and examination

A history of stridor, difficulty in breathing particularly on lying flat, snoring, previous irradiation, or surgery to the head and neck area should alert the clinician to potentially difficult airway management. The patient may volunteer information about a previous difficult intubation and may have medical correspondence providing details. Previous anaesthetic records can also provide valuable information bearing in mind intervening treatments or tumour progression.

Currently available bedside screening tests and physical characteristics that suggest difficult laryngoscopy include:

- Modified Mallampati class III/IV
- Interincisor distance <3cm
- Thyromental distance <6.5cm
- Sternomental distance <12.5cm
- Limited head and neck movement (atlantoaxial joint assessment)
- Immobile mandibular space due to tumour, previous surgery, or irradiation
- Protruding maxillary incisors (buck teeth)
- Receding mandible, limited jaw protrusion (grade C)
- High-arched/narrow palate
- Short, thick neck
- Obesity (body mass index >30).

The fallibility of these predictive tests is all too evident to anyone who has prepared for an anticipated difficult intubation, only to find direct laryngoscopy and intubation straightforward. While these tests can be highly sensitive (most difficult intubations are correctly predicted) there are a large number of false positives (many intubations predicted to be difficult are easy), i.e. positive predictive value is poor. In practice this is of little consequence as techniques employed for predicted difficulty are by definition associated with cardiovascular and respiratory stability and expose the patient to little additional risk.

Of greater concern are false negatives. Crucially, these tests are unable to predict the difficulty likely to be encountered with supraglottic and tongue base tumours that may obstruct the airway on induction of anaesthesia and impede laryngoscopy. The anaesthetist should study the findings of imaging and nasendoscopy to delineate the site and extent of these tumours and the degree to which they impede the view of the glottis.

Impossible mask ventilation is a rare occurrence in the general surgical population with an incidence of approximately 1 in 690 cases and one-quarter of patients who are impossible to mask ventilate are also difficult to intubate (1 in 2800 cases). Features found to be independent predictors of impossible mask ventilation include:

- Neck radiation changes
- Male sex
- History of sleep apnoea

◆ Mallampati class III or IV

◆ The presence of a beard.

Mouth opening limited to 20–25mm, is the only reliable test in predicting difficulty with the use of the laryngeal mask airway. Preoperative flexible nasendoscopy performed by the surgeon or experienced anaesthetist provide valuable information in particular regarding tongue base and supraglottic tumours.

Radiological investigations

The anaesthetist should examine the patient with computed tomography or magnetic resonance imaging to delineate the site and extent of the disease and discern whether there is any airway distortion or mediastinal disease. Flexion and extension cervical spine X-rays are indicated in patients with rheumatoid arthritis as exaggerated extension may be used during rigid bronchoscopy.

Anticipated difficult airway management

The American Society of Anesthesiologists, the Royal College of Anaesthetists, and Difficult Airway Society all stress the importance of a preplanned strategy for the management of the difficult airway. This systematic approach to airway management has led to the development of various airway management algorithms. These provide a framework around which the anaesthetist, in cooperation with the surgical team, can formulate an initial airway strategy and subsequent rescue strategies should the initial plan fail. Current algorithms focus on the unanticipated difficult airway that is likely to be encountered in general anaesthetic practice and awakening the patient is often recommended as a rescue strategy. Waking the patient is not an option where the airway is critically obstructed and is problematic in a patient who refused an awake technique at the outset. A simplified algorithm is described in Figure 7.1 which focuses on the predicted difficult airway and outlines strategies for dealing with the airway which is about to obstruct.

Airway management techniques to consider are:

◆ Awake intubation:
  • Awake fibreoptic intubation (FOI)
  • Primary tracheostomy
◆ Asleep techniques:
  • Inhalational induction of anaesthesia maintaining spontaneous respiration
  • Intravenous induction of anaesthesia with paralysis
  • Asleep FOI and the intubating laryngeal mask airway (ILMA)
◆ Prophylactic cricothyroid cannulation.

Awake fibreoptic intubation

This is a valuable tool in securing the airway of a patient with a high degree of predicted difficulty without critical airway obstruction. Absolute indications for awake FOI include

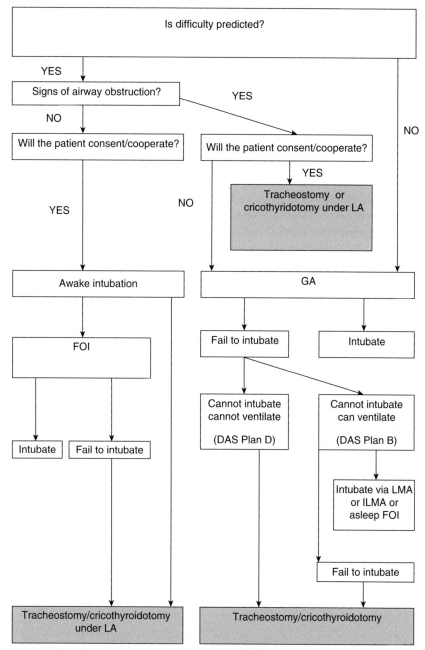

Fig. 7.1 Algorithm for management of the predicted difficult airway. DAS, Difficult Airway Society; FOI, fibreoptic intubation; GA, general anaesthetic; ILMA, intubating laryngeal mask airway; LA, local anaesthetic; LMA, laryngeal mask airway.

patients with trismus, an immobile mandibular space due to tumour, irradiation, or previous surgery, and those with supraglottic or tongue base tumours. It is contraindicated in those who refuse consent or are unable to cooperate. In patients with critical airway obstruction, awake FOI is contraindicated as it is all too easy to precipitate complete obstruction by causing bleeding, oedema, or dislodging friable tumour. In reality FOI is seldom carried out totally awake and it is common to administer conscious sedation during the procedure (Figure 7.2).

Primary tracheostomy

Tracheostomy under local anaesthesia (LA) is recommended for patients with a high degree of predicted difficulty with significant or imminent airway obstruction, and in whom less invasive techniques have failed or are likely to fail and who are not so hypoxaemic or hypercapnic that they are unable to consent or cooperate.

Asleep techniques

Conventional asleep intubation techniques can be used in those patients with no or lesser degrees of predicted difficulty and in those in whom awake techniques are contraindicated or refused. There is now good evidence to refute the classic teaching of inhalational induction and the avoidance of muscle relaxant in an obstructed airway. Uptake of inhalational agent is naturally slowed in this situation and it is difficult to get the patient deep enough

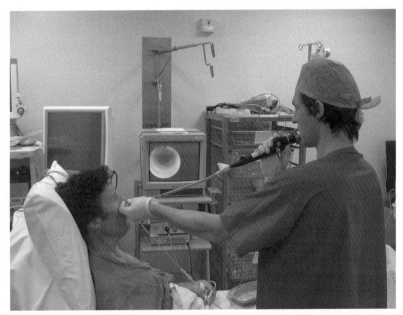

Fig. 7.2 Awake fibreoptic intubation under conscious sedation. Conscious sedation allows the patient to tolerate the procedure while maintaining a patent airway and spontaneous respiration.

using inhalational agent alone to permit bag/mask ventilation or to allow laryngoscopy. Using muscle relaxant will facilitate both bag/mask ventilation and laryngoscopy. Whatever technique is chosen for the obstructed airway the key is a planned rescue strategy which means having all the necessary equipment, personnel, and adjuncts immediately to hand. This means a prepared difficult airway trolley and a surgeon of appropriate experience ready to perform an emergency tracheostomy. Anaesthetizing the patient in the operating room means there is adequate space for equipment and expedites an emergency tracheostomy. Often it is easy to ventilate the asleep patient but difficult to intubate using direct laryngoscopy (can ventilate, can't intubate); in these circumstances an asleep FOI or the use of the ILMA will help to guide the endotracheal tube into the trachea.

Prophylactic cricothyroid cannulation

Elective insertion of a cannula (e.g. Ravussin) through the cricothyroid membrane under LA allows oxygenation of the patient prior to, and during, the planned intubation technique thus providing a further 'safety net' during the management of the anticipated difficult airway. Oxygenation can be provided by insufflation or transtracheal jet ventilation. The safety of this technique is dependent on it being tested prior to the planned intubation procedure, and ensuring that there is an adequate expiratory pathway.

Extubation

Tracheal extubation and the emergence and recovery from anaesthesia is a critical period and often neglected in the planning stage. If unplanned, the anaesthetist may find themselves stranded, dealing with a potentially threatened airway without the support of the key members of the surgical team.

The timing of extubation is critical. An awake extubation is indicated in patients whose airway was difficult and where the surgery has not improved it (e.g. endoscopy). An asleep extubation is indicated for easy airways where coughing or straining at extubation may precipitate bleeding or laryngospasm.

Staff recovering these patients in the postoperative period need to be vigilant in evaluating the patient for the potential complications arising from managing the difficult airway. These may include airway oedema, bleeding and obstruction, aspiration, tracheal or oesophageal perforation, pneumothorax, pneumomediastinum, and subcutaneous emphysema. The anaesthetist should provide clear documentation in the patient's medical notes, detailing the exact difficulty encountered, the various methods used, and how intubation was achieved.

The shared airway

Head and neck surgery forces the anaesthetist to share the airway with the surgeon and demands close cooperation. Both parties need to be aware of the condition of the patient, the anticipated surgical procedure, potential complications, and how best to achieve an unimpeded operative field whilst maintaining a safe, secure airway for oxygenation and ventilation.

Tracheal intubation

The majority of head and neck operations will be carried out with an endotracheal tube in place. For an endoscopy with or without a biopsy a small tube (e.g. a size 4 or 5 micro-laryngoscopy tube) will provide the surgeon with adequate access and allow adequate ventilation. They are not suitable for longer procedures due to a propensity to kink and obstruct due to their narrow diameter. For all other procedures a reinforced tube of size 6 or larger is indicated. Specialized tubes are required in laser surgery.

Tubeless techniques and jet ventilation

In certain circumstances an endotracheal tube will impede surgical access, especially with posterior vocal cord lesions, and oxygenation must be achieved by means of jet ventilation. A high pressure (1–2 bar) jet of oxygen-enriched air is delivered to the lungs at high frequency (100–200 breaths per minute) via a flexible or rigid cannula. This cannula can be placed above the cords (supraglottic), below the cords (subglottic), or externally through the cricothyroid membrane or tracheal rings (transtracheal). Anaesthesia must be maintained using a total intravenous technique.

Laser surgery

Laser surgery can be performed using a tubed or tubeless technique. When using a tube a specialized laser-resistant tube must be used which is constructed either of metal or has a covering of metal tape. It is important to remember that these tubes are laser resistant, not laser proof, and their non-metal components will ignite if sufficient laser energy is applied. Their cuffs are filled with saline which will partially absorb the energy of an inadvertent laser strike. Some tubes have a double cuff for added security.

Tracheostomy

Tracheostomy already in place

Many patients will come to theatre with a tracheostomy in place either as a result of previous elective surgery or an emergency procedure carried out to relieve airway obstruction. For all but the shortest of procedures it is common to replace this with a longer lower-profile cuffed tracheostomy tube (laryngectomy tube) which improves surgical access. If a tracheostomy is new always replace the tube over a bougie, if a false passage is created with a replacement tube in a patient who is likely to be a difficult endotracheal intubation the consequences can be dire.

Elective tracheostomy for postoperative airway protection

In most instances the decision whether to carry out an elective tracheostomy for postoperative airway protection is usually obvious or simple (e.g. following a total or partial laryngectomy). However, when the surgery is relatively distant from the airway it can be difficult to weigh the advantages of a tracheostomy against its rare but potentially lethal complications. In the latter circumstances the decisive factor should be ease or difficulty of intubation and grade of laryngoscopy at induction and at end of surgery. If intubation was difficult then it is likely to remain difficult, even if surgery has improved the airway there will be initial swelling and bleeding. For example, a good laryngoscopic view at induction may be degraded by a large tongue or buccal flap at the end of surgery. Predicted difficult intubation should therefore be added to the list of surgical indications for elective tracheostomy.

Conclusion

◆ Anaesthetists are not core members of the MDT but attendance at meetings will give early warning of difficult airways and the high risk patient. Early anaesthetic input can help decide between surgical and non-surgical therapy where neither offers a clear survival benefit.

◆ Encroachment on the airway may limit the time available for preoperative optimization in a population of patients likely to have multiple comorbidities.

◆ A thorough preoperative assessment of the airway is essential but be aware that classic bedside tests for the difficult airway will miss base of tongue and supraglottic tumours. The results of imaging and nasendoscopy will provide a more complete picture.

◆ Formulate a plan for managing the airway based on the degree of predicted difficulty and the patient's ability to consent or cooperate. Have rescue equipment and personnel immediately to hand.

◆ A shared airway demands close cooperation and team work between surgeon and anaesthetist.

◆ Predicted difficult intubation in the postoperative period is an indication for elective tracheostomy even where surgery is relatively remote from the airway.

Bibliography

1. American Society of Anesthesiologists Task Force on Management of the Difficult Airway (2003). *Practice Guidelines for Management of the Difficult Airway. An Updated Report by the American Society of Anesthesiologists Task Force on the Management of the Difficult Airway. Anesthesiology* **98**:1269–77.
2. Calder I, Yentis SM (2008). Could safe practice be compromising safe practice? Should anaesthetists have to demonstrate that face mask ventilation is possible before giving a neuromuscular blocker? *Anaesthesia* **63**:113–15.
3. Cancer Research UK. *Current information on incidence, mortality, aetiology, risk factors and treatment of oral, laryngeal and thyroid cancer.* Available at http://info.cancerresearchuk.org (accessed June 2010).
4. Evans KL, Keene MH, Bristow AS (1994). High-frequency jet ventilation – a review of its role in laryngology. *J Laryngol Otol* **108**(1):23–5.
5. Fleisher LA, Beckman BA, Brown KA, *et al.* (2007). ACC/AHA 2007 guidelines on Perioperative Cardiovascular Evaluation and Care for Noncardiac Surgery. A Report of the American College of Cardiology/American Heart Association Task Force on Practice Guidelines. *Circulation* **116**(17):418–500.

6. Henderson JJ, Popat MT, Latto IP, Pearce AC (2004). Difficult Airway Society guidelines for management of the unanticipated difficult intubation. *Anaesthesia* **59**:675–94.

7. Kheterpal S, Martin L, Shanks A, Tremper KK (2009). Prediction and outcomes of impossible mask ventilation. A review of 50 000 anesthetics. *Anesthesiology* **110**:891–7.

8. Mallampati SR, Gatt SP, Gugino LD, *et al.* (1985). A new sign for predicting difficult intubation. *Can Anaes Soc J* **32**:429–34.

9. Mingo OH, Ashpole KJ, Irving CJ, Rucklidge MWM (2008). Remifentanil sedation for awake fibreoptic intubation with limited application of local anaesthetic in patients for elective head and neck surgery. *Anaesthesia* **63**(10):1065–9.

10. National Institute for Health and Clinical Excellence (2004). *Improving Outcomes in Head and Neck Cancers. The Manual.* London: NICE.

11. Nouraei SAR, Giussani DA, Howard DJ, Sandhu GS, Ferguson C, Patel A (2008). Physiological comparison of spontaneous and positive-pressure ventilation in laryngotracheal stenosis. *Br J Anaesth* **101**(3):419–23.

12. Paes ML (1987). General anaesthesia for carbon dioxide laser surgery within the airway: a review. *Br J Anaesth* **59**:1610–20.

13. Rhys Evans PH, Montgomery PQ, Gullane PJ (2009). *Principles and Practice of Head and Neck Surgery and Oncology.* London: Informa Healthcare.

14. Robbie DS (1989). Anaesthesia for surgery in malignant disease of the head and neck. In Filshie J, Robbie DS (eds) *Anaesthesia and malignant disease*, pp.135–49 London: Edward Arnold.

15. The British Association of Otorhinolaryngology (2006). *Head and Neck Surgery. Pre-op tests – Guidelines for ENT 2006.* Available at http://entuk.org/publications.

16. Yentis SM (2002). Predicting difficult intubation–worthwhile exercise or pointless ritual? *Anaesthesia* **57**:105–9.

Chapter 8

Perioperative management for resection of upper gastrointestinal tract cancer

Matthew Hacking and Laurie Cohen

Introduction

Oesophagogastrectomy remains the only curative treatment option for cancer of the upper gastrointestinal (GI) tract. Surgery has historically involved the highest morbidity and mortality of all cancer resections. Recent Intensive Care National Audit & Research Centre (ICNARC) data confirms an intensive care unit mortality of 4.4% and in-hospital mortality of 11% although this has reduced over time. The incidence of surgically amenable disease is increasing due to earlier diagnosis and use of neoadjuvant therapies. Additional challenges are being faced with an increasing subpopulation of younger patients with significantly elevated body mass index (BMI) and treatable diagnoses in patients of advancing age with variable physiological reserves.

The surgical approach

The surgical approach is influenced by disease location, TNM (tumour, node, metastasis) stage, with consideration of comorbidities. Operable tumours are commonly adenocarcinoma or more rarely squamous cell carcinoma. Lower-third and oesophagogastric junctional tumours can be approached via a transhiatal approach. Mid-third tumours require a traditional Ivor Lewis right thoracoabdominal approach. Occasionally a third stage supramediastinal anastomosis needs to be made in the neck.

Minimally invasive approaches are in the ascendancy and may offer reduced early respiratory morbidity and mortality. However, the overall complication rates are not significantly different. Robotic technology affords the advantage of improved dexterity, manipulation, and stability control over 'straight-stick' laparoscopy although there are no current data on long-term advantage to outcome.

Preoperative assessment

Patient assessment prior to oesophagogastrectomy aims to identify mismatch between biological reserve and the physiological hurdle of proposed surgery. Anaesthetic review may influence several aspects of perioperative care (Table 8.1), with successful management

Table 8.1 The central role of preoperative assessment

Attribute	Example
Inform the consenting process	Describe the anticipated perioperative mortality risk
Inform MDT's decision to offer surgery, defer surgery, or recommend non-surgical interventions	Deferral for specific/non-specific organ dysfunction post neoadjuvant chemotherapy
Inform surgical decision on operative approach	Anticipate inability to tolerate OLV
Indicate specific preoperative interventions	Commencing beta blocker medication
Indicate specific perioperative interventions	Elective tracheostomy
Plan postoperative care location/duration	Recovery facility, ICU, or HDU

HDU, High Dependency Unit; ICU, Intensive Care Unit; OLV, one-lung ventilation.

often requiring several patient attendances and communication between many members of the multidisciplinary team.

The enhanced recovery programme for upper GI patients, part of the Quality Innovation, Productivity and Prevention (QIPP) programme, aims to optimize perioperative care, reduce morbidity and mortality, and reduce length of hospital stay. The focus is on patient education, particularly with respect to smoking, alcohol, exercise, and nutritional optimization.

Cardiorespiratory fitness

Major surgery significantly raises the body's demand for oxygen; an inability to meet this leads to organ dysfunction. Extent of existing comorbidity rather than age itself predicts postoperative complications. Assessment tools may indicate a broad risk-category or provide a more specific prediction. For upper GI surgery, the O-POSSUM (Physiological and Operative Severity Score for the enUmeration of Mortality and morbidity) model uses physiological and operative data to generate a mortality prediction. Other models use preoperative data alone and may predict organ-specific morbidity.

Mimicking the high postoperative metabolic demand, cardiopulmonary exercise testing (CPEX) documents functional response to ramped physical work performed during cycle ergometry. Electrocardiogram monitoring complements respiratory gas analysis, and the testing generating various parameters at submaximal and maximal work-rates. Landmark work in 548 patients having major abdominal surgery used CPEX findings plus surgery subtype to risk-stratify patients, assigning preoperative and postoperative care location accordingly. Nineteen of the 21 deaths were in the high-risk group, defined as either oesophageal or aortic surgery or an anaerobic threshold (AT) below 11ml/min/kg. Investigating oesophagectomy patients alone, studies have found that preoperative peak oxygen uptake (VO_2 peak), but not AT, is significantly lower in those developing cardiopulmonary complications. VO_2 peak correlates with distance walked during incremental shuttle walk test (SWT). One audit of 51 oesophagogastrectomy cases found that all five deaths occurred in patients achieving below 350m at SWT.

Preoperative inspiratory muscle training has produced a reduction in pulmonary complications following major surgery and respiratory exercises should be commenced preoperatively in patients considered at increased risk. Attention should also be placed upon extending preoperative exercise tolerance through the use of aerobic exercise regimes. Describing the postoperative mobilization schedule to the patient and their relatives helps to achieve enhanced recovery.

Preoperative beta blockade may have a roll in reducing cardiac complications in those at greatest risk. The POISE study confirms that this should be introduced cautiously since it found an increased stroke risk associated with high-dose day of surgery beta blockade. None of the randomized patients in this study underwent thoracic surgery. Additionally attempts to minimize positive fluid balance and optimize thoracic epidural sympathectomy may mitigate against beta blockade.

Nutrition

The degree and speed of preoperative weight loss may predict postoperative mortality. Hypoalbuminaemia from any cause is also an independent predictor of poor outcome. Patients with severe malnutrition (BMI $<18kg/m^2$) or those with weight-loss greater than 10% from baseline require preoperative supplemental nutrition. Evidence exists for improved outcome after parental nutrition up to 10 days prior to surgery in those that cannot be fed enterally. Meta-analysis suggests that oral supplementation with immune-enhancing nutrition including glutamine and perhaps omega-3 fatty acids and ribonucleic acids can reduce inflammatory cytokine levels, infection rates, and length of stay whilst increasing lymphocyte CD4 counts. Increasingly there is a trend towards administration of oral glucose loading the night before and the morning of surgery. It is proposed that this helps to reduce complications and improve GI recovery without increasing the risk of induction aspiration.

The route of early postoperative nutritional support should reflect the needs of the patient. There is evidence that early establishment of enteral intake in physiologically stable patients improves GI recovery, reduces translocation of bacteria, reduces stress ulcer rates, and possibly reduces cardiorespiratory complications without increasing risk of anastomotic breakdown. Enhanced recovery programme patients are encouraged to drink 30ml/h of water and commence low dose jejenostomy feed as early as day 2 postoperatively. Total parenteral nutrition is generally used to bridge the gap until full enteral nutrition is established.

Treatment goals for postoperative nutrition include avoiding excess catabolism, hypoalbuminaemia and hypo- or hypernatraemia, achieving glycaemic stability, and maintaining anastomotic integrity. Total fluid volume input should be scrutinized when establishing nutritional support and on transferring between routes of administration.

Airway considerations

Prior to transthoracic surgery, correct sizing of the double-lumen tube (DLT) should be established using chest X-ray or computed tomography scan. Smaller DLTs may reduce upper airway trauma, however less readily admit suction catheters, impair expiratory airflow, and may fail to achieve lung isolation. Endobronchial displacement risks obstruction and rupture, the risk of which may be minimized with a larger DLT. Wide variation in cuff-tip length (CTL) of left-sided DLTs increases the risk of upper lobe bronchus obstruction in patients with radiographic evidence of a short left main bronchus (LMB). A margin of safety (LMB length minus CTL) above 10mm is recommended.

Respiratory morbidity following oesophagogastrectomy is substantial, however accounts of elective tracheostomy are scarce. Patients with risk factors for postoperative ventilatory failure (including an FEV_1 below 65% predicted) should be considered for pre-emptive tracheostomy, as should patients with significantly elevated BMI.

Fluid management

How much fluid?

During major body cavity surgery, fluid management driven by empirical formulae is now considered to produce both an excessive fluid balance and complication rate. Deterioration in pulmonary function associated with fluid excess has been demonstrated in thoracotomy patients. Cumulative perioperative fluid balance is associated with morbidity and mortality following transthoracic oesophagectomy. Although a key element of a multimodal intervention programme for oesophagectomy, a restrictive fluid approach may still result in significant intraoperative fluid infusion. How best to avoid splanchnic and renal hypoperfusion during fluid restriction is not clear.

Goal-directed fluid management offers a more intuitive approach compared to formulaic or restrictive approaches. Although an oesophageal Doppler cannot be used, cardiac output (CO) measurement and optimization of stroke volume and oxygen delivery can improve outcome and length of stay without significantly altering the volume of infused fluids. Uncertainty remains with regard to optimum fluid management following oesophagogastrectomy. There may be a place for vasopressors and diuretics in limiting fluid accumulation.

What type of fluid?

Patients may present with varying degrees of dehydration prior to anaesthesia. Key factors include disease-related symptom severity, parenteral and oral nutritional supplementation, fasting duration, and bowel clearance preparations. Investigation of patients receiving the last factor has shown evidence of intravascular volume depletion without circulatory benefit from a preoperative crystalloid infusion. Evidence suggests that colloids are most suitable for intravascular volume expansion using goal-directed fluid management. However, salt-containing colloids risk iatrogenic hyperchloraemic metabolic acidosis and some colloids are associated with potentially deleterious effects on renal function and coagulation.

Ventilation

Evolution in ventilatory management has contributed to a downward trend in postoperative respiratory morbidity. However, complication rates of up to 28% are still reported in contemporary series. Even after procedures that avoid formal thoracotomy, such as gastrectomy and transhiatal oesophagectomy, significant pulmonary collapse and inflammatory changes still occur.

The effects of one-lung ventilation

Atelectasis occurs following induction of general anaesthesia, reducing total respiratory compliance. A correctly positioned DLT allows isolation of the two lungs; collapse occurs when one side is left non-ventilated. Pulmonary blood flow is diverted from the non-ventilated side in response to rising pulmonary vascular resistance (PVR) and the effect of hypoxic pulmonary vasoconstriction (HPV); this serves to limit the otherwise substantial ventilation/perfusion (V/Q) mismatch. These processes are not sufficient to prevent an interpulmonary shunt from developing. Decubitus positioning of the patient causes additional atelectasis in the dependent, ventilated lung. In the lung units most compressed by mediastinal and abdominal contents, intrapulmonary shunting will occur. Although PVR rises within these localities, there is little improvement in V/Q matching whilst in the lateral position, the overall effect is to promote interpulmonary shunting.

Modifying the impact of one-lung ventilation

Protective ventilation

In lung resection, trials of 'protective' strategies during one-lung ventilation (OLV) have generated inconsistent outcomes. Significantly, studies have used what would now be considered a harmful combination of high tidal volumes (TV) and zero positive end-expiratory pressure (PEEP) as their controls. One study of oesophagogastrectomy patients, open to similar criticism, found the protective group (5ml/kg tidal volume, 5cmH$_2$O PEEP) had significantly less deterioration in both perioperative oxygenation and inflammation profile, with reduced pneumonia, acute respiratory distress syndrome (ARDS), and intensive care length of stay. It is now established that insufficient PEEP and excessive TV are implicated in the pathogenesis of ARDS from any cause.

Optimizing lung compliance

PEEP applied during general anaesthesia enhances alveolar recruitment and improves oxygenation during both one- and two-lung ventilation. A pre-emptive approach uses pressure-controlled ventilation, PEEP, and dynamic compliance curves from the outset, aiming to avoid the need for hyperbaric recruitment manoeuvres. Adjustment of the PEEP to achieve optimal compliance should occur at all stages.

Anaesthetic agents

Volatile anaesthetic agents directly impair HPV, but this effect may be less substantial *in vivo*. For lung surgery with OLV, comparative studies of volatile anaesthetic agent versus propofol anaesthesia (without depth of anaesthesia monitoring) showed a clinical benefit with a reduced inflammatory profile using volatile. Investigations have focused on both the dependent and the non-dependent/operative lung, generating a hypothesis that volatile-impairment of HPV mitigates against hypoxia-induced lung injury. While this potentially protective role is explored, general anaesthesia with either volatile or propofol is acceptable, should have depth of anaesthesia monitoring to maintain optimal administration, and may be combined with intravenous opioids and regional anaesthesia.

Maintaining cardiac output

Low CO causes mixed venous oxygen saturation (SvO_2) to fall. By stimulating HPV, this may reduce interpulmonary shunt-associated hypoxaemia. However, tissue oxygen delivery may prove inadequate during low CO, the resulting metabolic acidosis further increasing PVR with the risk of progressive cardiopulmonary dysfunction. Increasing a low CO can improve oxygenation during OLV, while the same may not apply when elevating above a normal level of output. As prophylaxis against cardiac arrhythmia during mediastinal dissection, plasma electrolytes should be optimized and sustained rhythm disturbance should be treated promptly.

Fraction of inspired oxygen (FiO_2)

High FiO_2 is implicated in the aetiology of atelectasis and acute lung injury (ALI). When the interpulmonary shunt is greater than 30%, raising the FiO_2 to treat hypoxaemia may have little beneficial effect.

Managing desaturation

Confirmation of exact positioning of the DLT using fibreoptic bronchoscopy (FOB) is strongly recommended, both at initial placement and prior to commencing OLV. Parameters for initiating OLV include: FiO_2 below 0.6; TV approximately 6ml/kg; plateau pressure below 25cmH$_2$O. PEEP and respiratory rate should be optimized.

A period of desaturation is anticipated early during OLV, requiring assessment of CO and review of the spirometry. Sustained or substantial desaturation mandates rechecking of DLT position for which FOB is essential. Oxygenating the non-dependent lung by catheter insufflation or continuous positive airway pressure (CPAP) may rapidly improve interpulmonary shunt-related hypoxaemia and can be utilized prophylactically. Intermittent ventilation of the non-dependent lung may become necessary but must be coordinated with surgical activity.

The degree of cardiorespiratory instability during OLV has been associated with the subsequent development of ALI, the pathogenesis of which involves both pulmonary and circulating inflammatory elements. Additionally, duration of OLV has been associated with development of other pulmonary complications.

Extubation

Extubation on completing surgery has become routine in multimodal and fast-track management for oesophagogastrectomy. These strategies are associated with low mortality despite the prevalence of significant respiratory morbidity. A policy of extubating on the first postoperative day has achieved similar outcomes. Irrespective of the location of patient care in the initial postoperative period, access to facilities for managing respiratory failure is mandatory; non-invasive ventilatory support may be sufficient for this. High-risk patients selected for prophylactic tracheostomy will need ongoing multidisciplinary input while their respiratory support is weaned.

Analgesia

A balanced approach to analgesia is essential. Aims include high patient satisfaction, minimal cardiovascular and respiratory depression, with facilitation of physiotherapy and mobilization. Regional analgesia and regular review by a dedicated team are well-established elements of initial postoperative management. There is no consensus on which technique is most effective in preventing post-thoracotomy pain syndrome. Guidelines and clinical pathways favour thoracic epidural analgesia (TEA), however alternatives exist.

Thoracic epidural analgesia (TEA)

- Achieves significantly lower pain scores following major surgery compared to parenteral opioids. An association between lower pain scores and significant clinical benefit is less clear-cut and may be either delayed or absent.

- Is associated with fewer respiratory complications following oesophagectomy including significantly lower rates of pneumonia in patients receiving at least 2 days of TEA and lower ARDS rates in those receiving at least 3 days. Intensive care length of stay can be significantly shorter in TEA-treated groups.

- Bupivacaine bolus may significantly reduce gastric conduit perfusion during oesophagectomy. However, animal models and clinical studies demonstrate improved gastric conduit mucosal blood flow during TEA infusion. Moreover, TEA has been associated with a significantly reduced risk of anastomotic leak.

However, TEA significantly increases the risk of hypotension compared with intravenous opioid analgesia. Arterial hypotension reduces inferior mesenteric artery flow but an intravenous epinephrine infusion has been shown to mitigate this. While local anaesthetic (LA) with opioid and epinephrine is recommended for TEA following thoracotomy, such balanced solutions based around low concentration LA may also predispose to hypotension.

Paravertebral blockade (PVB) compared to TEA:

- Systematic reviews have shown PVB and TEA to be equianalgesic. However, one study showed PVB to be superior in terms of morphine consumption and pain scores.

- Measure of respiratory function is best preserved with PVB analgesia in patients undergoing transthoracic oesophageal surgery.

- Meta-analysis of pulmonary complications (pneumonia or atelectasis) following thoracotomy favours PVB over TEA. Bilateral intercostal motor block may be implicated in respiratory complications during TEA.

◆ Meta-analyses indicate that hypotension is more frequent during TEA than PVB, although high-concentration LA was used in the majority of these TEA infusions. Hypotension resulting from thoracic PVB is uncommon, irrespective of LA concentration.

◆ Paravertebral infusion catheter can be placed intraoperatively by the surgeon.

Other analgesic approaches

Interpleural infusion achieves similar analgesia to PVB while performing less well compared to TEA. Pulmonary function and hospital length of stay are both inferior. Systemic absorption of LA has been demonstrated during both interpleural and paravertebral infusion, toxicity occurring only with the former.

Intercostal nerve blockade by repeat injection or catheter-infusion reduces systemic opioid requirement following thoracotomy. Neither analgesia nor pulmonary function is superior to that during TEA or PVB.

Transversus abdominis plane (TAP) block can achieve abdominal wall sensory blockade without ventilatory or vasomotor impairment. A subcostal catheter technique has been reported in major upper abdominal surgery yet its contribution to analgesia following surgical incision for oesophagogastrectomy is unknown.

Bibliography

1. Allum WH, Griffin SM, Watson A, Colin-Jones D (2002). Guidelines for the management of oesophageal and gastric cancer. *Gut* **50**(Supplement):v1–v23.

2. Al-Rawi OY, Pennefather SH, Page RD, Dave I, Russell GN (2008). The effect of thoracic epidural bupivacaine and an intravenous adrenaline infusion on gastric tube blood flow during esophagectomy. *Anesth Analg* **106**(3):884–7.

3. Bussières JS (2009). Open or minimally invasive esophagectomy: are the outcomes different? *Curr Opin Anaesthesiol* **22**(1):56–60.

4. Cerfolio RJ, Bryant AS, Bass CS, Alexander JR, Bartolucci AA (2004). Fast tracking after Ivor Lewis esophagogastrectomy. *Chest* **126**(4):1187–94.

5. De Conno E, Steurer MP, Wittlinger M, *et al.* (2009). Anesthetic-induced improvement of the inflammatory response to one-lung ventilation. *Anesthesiology* **110**(6):1316–26.

6. Forshaw MJ, Strauss DC, Davies AR, *et al.* (2008). Is cardiopulmonary exercise testing a useful test before oesophagectomy? *Ann Thor Surg* **85**:294–9.

7. Internullo E, Moons J, Nafteux P, *et al.* (2008). Outcome after esophagectomy for cancer of the esophagus and GEJ in patients aged over 75 years. *Eur J Cardiothorac Surg* **33**:1096–104.

8. Joshi GP, Bonnet F, Shah R, *et al.* (2008). A systematic review of randomized trials evaluating regional techniques for postthoracotomy analgesia. *Anesth Analg* **107**:1026–40.

9. Juneja R, Hacking M, Wigmore T (2009). Peri-operative management of the oesphagectomy patient. *Curr Anaesth Crit Care* **20**(1):13–17.

10. Licker M, Fauconnet P, Villiger Y, Tschopp JM (2009). Acute lung injury and outcomes after thoracic surgery. *Curr Opin Anaesthesiol* **22**(1):61–7.

11. Low DE (2007). Evolution in perioperative management of patients undergoing oesophagectomy. *Br J Surg* **94**:655–6.

12. Low J, Johnston N, Morris C (2008). Epidural analgesia: first do no harm. *Anaesthesia* **63**:1–3.

13. Michelet P, D'Journo XB, Roch A, *et al.* (2005). Perioperative risk factors for anastomotic leakage after esophagectomy. *Chest* **128**(5):3461–6.

14. Michelet P, D'Journo XB, Roch A, *et al.* (2006). Protective ventilation influences systemic inflammation after esophagectomy: a randomized controlled study. *Anesthesiology* **105**(5):911–19.

15. Michelet P, D'Journo XB, Seinaye F, Forel JM, Papazian L, Thomas P (2009). Non-invasive ventilation for treatment of postoperative respiratory failure after oesophagectomy. *Br J Surg* **96**(1):54–60.

16. Murray P, Whiting P, Hutchinson SP, Ackroyd R, Stoddard CJ, Billings C (2007). Preoperative shuttle walking testing and outcome after oesophagogastrectomy. *Br J Anaesth* **99**:809–11.

17. Neal JM, Wilcox RT, Allen HW, Low DE (2003). Near-total esophagectomy: the influence of standardized multimodal management and intraoperative fluid restriction. *Reg Anesth Pain Med* **28**(4):328–34.

18. Park DP, Welch CA, Harrison DA, *et al.* (2009). Outcomes following oesophagectomy in patients with oesophageal cancer: a secondary analysis of the ICNARC Case Mix Programme Database. *Crit Care* **13**(Suppl 2):S1.

19. Partridge L, Russell WJ (2006). The margin of safety of a left double-lumen tracheobronchial tube depends on the length of the bronchial cuff and tip. *Anaesth Intensive Care* **34**:618–20.

20. PROSPECT: procedure specific postoperative pain management. *Thoracotomy recommendations algorithm.* Available at: http://www.postoppain.org/image.aspx?imgid=432.

21. Robertson SA, Skipworth RJE, Clarke DL *et al.* (2006). Ventilatory and intensive care requirements following oesophageal resection. *Ann R Coll Surg Engl* **88**(4):354–57.

22. Tekkis PP, McCulloch P, Poloniecki JD, Pryterch DR, Kessaris N, Steger AC (2004). Risk-adjusted prediction of operative mortality in oesophagogastric surgery with O-POSSUM. *Br J Surg* **91**:288–95.

Chapter 9

Anaesthesia for liver resection

Selena Haque, Richard Stümpfle, and Ravishankar
Rao Baikady

Introduction

Carl von Langenbuch performed the first successful liver resection in 1888 at the Lazarus
hospital in Berlin. In fact, the operation was first attempted 2 years prior to this, but the
patient did not survive the major perioperative haemorrhage associated with the procedure. Major intra- and postoperative haemorrhage precluded the widespread development of liver resection until the 1950s, when a standardized surgical technique was
devised based on the segmental anatomy of the liver. Mortality, however, remained high
(20–30%) until the late 1970s, when earlier diagnosis, better perioperative care, and technical advances led to improved patient survival. Currently the procedure has a mortality
rate of up to 2% where a well-practised multidisciplinary approach is taken.

Anatomy

For the anaesthetist, a sound understanding of liver anatomy and physiology is imperative for optimal perioperative management. The liver is the largest solid organ in the
body, weighing approximately 1.5kg in the average man. Based on surface features the
liver is traditionally divided into four lobes. From a surgical perspective, the liver is
divided into eight segments according to its venous drainage system (Figure 9.1).

The liver is unique in receiving blood from two different sources: the hepatic artery, a
branch of the coeliac trunk, and the portal vein, which carries venous blood from the
gastrointestinal tract. The hepatic artery provides only 30% of blood flow to the liver but
50–60% of the oxygen supply. The portal vein on the other hand provides 70% of blood
flow but only 40–50% of the oxygen supply. These structures enter the liver along with
the exiting bile duct at the porta hepatis. Major venous drainage is through the three
hepatic veins which attach the liver to the inferior vena cava (IVC). Liver blood flow
is dependent on splanchnic blood flow, hepatic arterial resistance, and portal venous
resistance.

The hepatic arterial buffer response is characterized by a one-way reciprocity between
hepatic arterial and portal venous flow. A reduction in portal venous flow results in an
increase in hepatic arterial flow. It is important to note that the reverse is not true; reductions
in hepatic arterial flow do not give rise to increased portal venous flow.

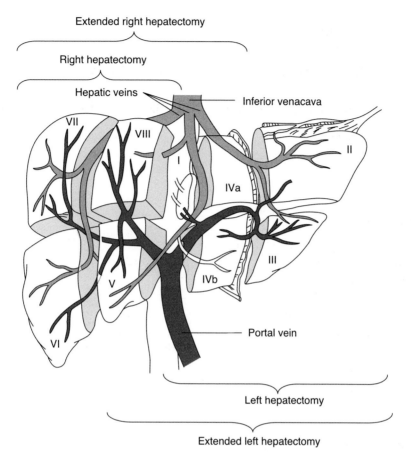

Fig. 9.1 Liver segments and definition of various resection types (reproduced with permission).

The basic functional unit of the liver is the lobule. The human liver contains 50,000–100,000 lobules. At the microscopic level, the bile ducts are found in the fibrous connective tissue separating adjacent lobules. Portal venules and hepatic arterioles, tiny branches of the portal vein and hepatic artery, are also found with the bile ducts together forming the portal triad. Blood flows from the triad to the central vein through the hepatic sinusoids. The central veins eventually join to form the hepatic veins. The portal system at the sinusoid has a low pressure (6mmHg) and high flow, whereas the hepatic arterial system has a higher pressure and relatively lower flow. In a non-cirrhotic liver, pressure within the sinusoid is only 2–4mmHg greater than vena caval pressure. Distortion of sinusoidal anatomy by nodular hyperplasia seen in liver cirrhosis can dramatically increase pressure within the system.

The liver is central to carbohydrate, lipid, urea, and haemoglobin metabolism, as well as protein and coagulation factor synthesis. It is also responsible for the breakdown of various hormones and toxin clearance.

Malignancies of the liver

Liver tumours may be benign or malignant. Benign lesions are largely asymptomatic, unless their size causes compression of adjacent structures. The commonest benign tumours are haemangiomata, hepatic adenoma, and focal nodular hyperplasia. Resection of these highly vascular lesions can prove challenging for the surgical and anaesthetic team as rapid major blood loss may occur.

Malignant liver lesions may be primary or secondary to metastatic disease. The most common primary malignancy, accounting for 80% of primary tumours is hepatocellular carcinoma (HCC).

Hepatocellular carcinoma

The incidence of HCC is increasing worldwide. Though a direct causal relationship has not been established, 75–80% of cases are associated with hepatitis B (HBV) and C (HCV) virus infection. The mechanism of development differs according to the underlying infection. HBV or HCV infection and subsequent development of liver fibrosis can cause rapid and deranged cellular turnover. This increases the formation of random DNA mutations which may lead to malignant proliferation. Chronic hepatitis B and C carriers have a 20–100-fold greater risk of developing HCC than non-infected individuals. Patients with HCC are often unsuitable candidates for surgery due to tumour characteristics such as invasion of major vessels, or degree of cirrhosis and liver failure. In addition, the tumour is largely unresponsive to systemic therapies.

Non-surgical treatments include percutaneous ethanol injection, percutaneous radio frequency ablation of tumour, and transarterial embolization. Partial hepatectomy or orthoptopic liver transplantation are the only curative treatment options. The postoperative mortality for tumour resection ranges from 0–21% depending on the age of the patient and the degree of cirrhosis.

Cholangiocarcinoma is the second most common type of primary liver cancer (15%). It usually arises from the bile duct, presenting with abdominal pain and progressive jaundice. Other rarer forms of primary liver malignancy include angiosarcoma.

Secondary liver cancers are metastatic tumours with primary lesions elsewhere, including large intestine, pancreas, stomach, skin, adrenal and neuroendocrine organs.

Approximately 90% of liver resections are for malignant disease of which 80% are metastatic lesions. The majority of liver resections in the UK are undertaken to treat metastatic colorectal cancer (CRC). In the UK more than 35,000 patients are diagnosed with CRC annually. Up to 25% of these will have liver metastases at the time of primary diagnosis while a further 20–25% will go on to develop metachronous liver lesions. Median survival for patients with untreated liver metastases is 6–13 months, while 5-year survival rates of up to 58% have been reported for those with treated disease with chemotherapy and surgery or either. Currently only 20–30% of patients with liver metastases are resectable (a potential 3000 liver resections per year). Advances in neoadjuvant chemotherapeutics, enhanced surgical techniques, and improved perioperative care may increase this number in the future.

Management of metastatic liver cancer

Metastatic disease is currently managed using a multidisciplinary approach encompassing chemotherapy, surgery, and ablative techniques.

Chemotherapy

The objectives of systemic chemotherapy in metastatic CRC were defined by the Central European Cooperative Oncology group:

1 Potential cure

    (a) Preoperative (neo adjuvant) chemotherapy for conversion to operable of initially inoperable lesions principally confined to the liver

    (b) Perioperative chemotherapy for the treatment of initially resectable disease

2 Palliation of symptoms

    Reducing tumour burden to improve quality of life

3 Prolongation of survival

    Control of disease progression.

Hepatic chemotherapy may be given systemically or as a hepatic arterial infusion. The former is the preferred method in Europe.

For nearly 40 years 5-fluorouracil (5FU) was the only first-line chemotherapeutic agent in advanced CRC. In the past decade three new cytotoxic agents have been developed— capecitabine (the prodrug of 5FU); irinotecan (a topoisomerase I inhibitor), and oxaliplatin (similar action to alkylating agents).

Common adjuvant chemotherapy regimens include:

♦ *FOLFOX:* 5FU, oxaliplatin, folinic acid (leucovorin)

♦ *FOLFIRI:* folinic acid, 5FU, irinotecan

♦ *Capecitabine:* alone or in combination.

Up to 12 cycles are administered with each cycle lasting 2 weeks.

Novel therapies are currently being developed including bevacizumab (Avastin), a vascular endothelial growth factor inhibitor. Cetuximab, an epidermal growth factor receptor (EGFR) inhibitor has been licensed for the treatment of EGFR expressing metastatic CRC.

While it is largely accepted that adjuvant chemotherapy is necessary for reducing the rate of recurrence and neoadjuvant chemotherapy is necessary to try and make inoperable disease operable, the use of neoadjuvant chemotherapy in initially resectable lesions remains contentious.

Sinusoidal obstruction syndrome which impairs regeneration and increases the risk of liver failure has been associated with the use of oxaliplatin. In addition, oxaliplatin has been shown to increase bleeding and biliary complications after resection. Irinotecan may cause a steatohepatitis, with a consequent increase in postoperative liver failure and mortality. Preoperative chemotherapy can make lesions extremely difficult to find where even the most detailed intraoperative ultrasound may fail to detect metastases still present.

The key to successful management of metastatic liver cancer is good communication between the various clinical specialties in order to optimize timing of treatment modalities. Recent studies have shown that simultaneous liver and colorectal resection is as efficient as staged resection in the treatment of metastatic disease. The outcome of combined procedures is largely determined by the extent of liver resection and patient age. Careful patient selection is required with anatomically difficult liver lobectomies and low anterior colorectal resections most often performed as staged procedures.

Surgical techniques

Surgical resection is standard treatment for metastatic disease confined to the liver. In assessing resectability, the first step is to determine anatomically:

- Whether the lesion may be safely resected in the context of its proximity to major vessels
- Whether sufficient liver parenchyma will remain post resection to allow normal hepatic function.

Up to 75% of liver parenchyma can be resected without adversely affecting postoperative liver function. Preoperative portal vein embolization may be considered in order to induce hypertrophy of the unaffected liver parenchyma. Theoretically this increases the functional reserve of the liver prior to surgery allowing it to better withstand the resection and possibly making lesions otherwise too large for resection operable. However there is little evidence for this.

Over recent years there have been significant advances in the surgical management of various liver pathologies assisted by major improvements in surgical technology. In the early 1990s the ultrasonic dissection device (CUSA, Tyco) was introduced. CUSA allows identification of small blood vessels during parenchymal transection, thus improving the accuracy of haemostatic measures. In the last decade the development of technologies such as pressurized jets of water (Hydrojet, Erbe), ultrasonic cutting and coagulation devices (Harmonic scalpel, Ethicon), the LigaSure vessel sealing system, dissecting sealer (Tissuelink), and radiofrequency-assisted liver transection, have transformed liver surgery. Endoscopic articulating linear staplers have simplified the division of large vascular structures during hepatic resection. These innovations in combination with low central venous pressure (CVP) anaesthesia have dramatically reduced blood loss during liver resection.

To further improve haemostasis of the transected liver parenchyma, various topical agents (Surgicel, Flo Seal Tachosil, Evicel spray) have been developed. When applied to the cut liver surface at the end of resection clot formation is improved and may reduce the bile leak from the surface postoperatively.

Recent advances have been made in the development of laparoscopic hepatectomy and robotic surgery reduces surgical stress response, postoperative pain and length of stay.

Radiofrequency ablative (RFA) therapies may be used as an alternative to surgery. RFA can be performed percutaneously, laparoscopically, or during open surgery for lesions smaller than 5cm. It remains unclear, however, whether long-term survival and progression-free survival rates are comparable to resection with chemotherapy. Morbidity is less than that with surgical resection and operative mortality is less than 1%. Complications include symptomatic pleural effusions, fever, shoulder tip pain, subcapsular haematomata, hepatic abscesses, and liver failure.

Preoperative assessment

All patients should be seen by the anaesthetic team well before surgery and have haematological, biochemical, and clotting profiles with the addition of liver function tests and a baseline electrocardiogram. The majority of liver resection patients however, are over the age of 50, and will have significant comorbidity.

In addition, any neoadjuvant chemotherapy administered to the patient can induce systemic side effects as well as the regional effects on the liver mentioned previously. These may manifest as malnutrition with reduced physiological reserve, increased susceptibility to infection, renal compromise, or, rarely, impaired cardiac function.

The presence of liver dysfunction will influence anaesthetic technique and the choice of analgesia with the avoidance of drugs that rely on hepatic metabolism. In addition, the presence of deranged liver function indicates extra risk of bleeding, by virtue not only of the potential derangement in clotting, but also the presence of abnormal liver architecture and consequent portal hypertension. Patients with decompensated liver failure are at very high risk of perioperative morbidity and mortality and are rarely considered for surgery.

Anaesthetic technique

General anaesthetic with endotracheal intubation is standard for all hepatic resections. Rapid sequence induction may be indicated where a large volume of ascites is present. Thoracic epidural is the analgesic modality of choice, the benefits of which may outweigh the postoperative risk of clotting derangement.

Effects of anaesthesia on liver blood flow

Many anaesthetic drugs are known to attenuate the hepatic arterial buffer response. This reduces the liver's ability to compensate for any fall in systemic blood pressure or cardiac output. Inhalational anaesthetic agents have significant effects on the hepatic arterial buffer response whilst intravenous anaesthetic agents such as propofol have minimal effect. Supporting systemic blood pressure with low-dose vasopressors or volume replacement will compensate for any reduction in liver blood flow.

Despite a demonstrable elevation in liver enzymes following prolonged administration of inhalational agents, no evidence exists to favour total intravenous anaesthesia (TIVA) over inhalational anaesthesia for liver resection surgery. There is a theoretical justification for avoiding hepatically metabolized neuromuscular blocking agents. However, in practice vecuronium and rocuronium are commonly used.

Major haemorrhage remains a significant risk during liver surgery and therefore wide-bore central venous access is recommended for major and complex liver resections. Invasive blood pressure monitoring is required to monitor the haemodynamic effects of vascular clamping and to allow early detection of haemorrhage. An oesophageal Doppler probe may be used to guide fluid replacement and optimize cardiac function during periods of vascular instability including IVC compression during liver resection. Caution should be exercised where there is any suggestion of portal hypertension with oesophageal varices.

Hepatic resection involves an extensive operative field and therefore causes significant patient exposure. Hypothermia will exacerbate any coagulopathy and should be avoided with heat conservation techniques. During RFA procedures the temperature may actually increase during the operation.

A nasogastric tube is recommended to decompress the stomach, aiding surgical access and providing the means for postoperative enteral nutrition.

The patient is typically supine for surgery, with or without 10–15 degree left lateral tilt. Antibiotic prophylaxis given in accordance with local guidelines is recommended, particularly in patients with evidence of ascites.

Central venous pressure and blood loss during major liver resection

Blood loss and transfusion requirements are major determinants of morbidity and mortality following liver resection. Minimizing blood loss is central to reducing operative mortality. Blood losses in excess of 2000ml are associated with a mortality of 43% as opposed to 8% for blood loss less than 500ml, in part, due to the immunomodulatory effect of blood transfusions. Blood transfusion is implicated in increased postoperative morbidity and a more rapid recurrence of primary or metastatic tumours. Shortage of blood products, risk of infection exposure, and increasing cost mean it is imperative to limit transfusion requirements.

The key to minimizing blood loss is maintaining a low CVP until hepatic vasculature is isolated and resected. A number of studies have demonstrated a clear correlation between CVP and haemorrhage during hepatic resection. Blood loss was reduced from 1000ml to 200ml when CVP was maintained below 6cmH$_2$O with a subsequent reduction in transfusion requirement from 48% to 5% of liver resections. Direct visualization of the IVC during surgery will help estimate the venous pressure. Methods of maintaining low venous filling pressures include:

- Preoperative bowel preparation
- Reverse Trendelenburg position
- Avoidance of PEEP
- Conservative fluid management
- Epidural anaesthesia (reduces systemic vascular resistance and CVP).

Pharmacological agents may be employed to further reduce CVP including glyceryl trinitrate (GTN) infusion or furosemide boluses. However these techniques have not shown clear benefit over non-pharmacological measures in reducing intraoperative blood loss. In reducing the CVP and inducing a state of hypovolaemia, normal compensatory mechanisms are severely compromised, and patients are vulnerable to any degree of blood loss. Potential organ hypoperfusion and air embolus are also significant concerns. Air embolus is a rare but serious complication of hepatic surgery and any sudden fall in end-tidal expired CO_2 should alert suspicion to its occurrence.

There is no evidence that a low CVP technique causes sustained detrimental effects on liver or renal function and its use has been shown to reduce hospital stay after surgery. Once the liver is resected, appropriate fluid boluses should be administered with the aid of invasive haemodynamic monitoring.

Haemorrhage may be massive and rapid. The complex anatomy and generous blood supply of the liver makes haemostasis more difficult to achieve. The effects of haemorrhage are compounded by a low CVP technique, which renders patients hypovolaemic and therefore less able to compensate for even minor blood loss. Transfusion requirements are higher if haemoconcentrated blood is lost during the low CVP intraoperative period. Bedside monitors of coagulation such as thromboelastography are increasingly used to guide clotting product administration.

Intraoperative cell salvage may be used in proven benign liver tumours. In malignancy the evidence is still unclear whether use of leucodepletion filters will prevent recirculation of malignant cells during resection of liver. Currently volume loss should be replaced with allogeneic blood and coagulation products.

Postoperative course and complications

At present mortality for elective resection of hepatic metastases is approx 3%, though the figure may be as low as 1–2% in high-volume centres. Around 20% of patients will experience complications after elective liver resection surgery. The commonest include respiratory infections and abdominal abscesses, both amenable to antibiotic therapy. More serious but less common are delayed haemorrhage, liver and renal failure. The extent of tissue resected and the presence of pre-existing liver dysfunction, determine the risk of developing postoperative liver failure.

The liver has an extraordinary capacity for regeneration. The residual parenchyma is able to double its volume within the first week of surgery. This rapid growth is fuelled by an increase in hepatic and splanchnic blood flow secondary to increased cardiac output. This hyperdynamic state is maintained for about 3 days. However, metabolic and synthetic capacity lags behind regeneration.

Diabetes and pre-existing liver dysfunction will impede recovery and the incidence of liver failure is greater in this population. Close monitoring of liver function and coagulation in the postoperative period is essential.

In some rare cases the imbalance between inflow and outflow of liver circulation after resection may lead to transudate formation and bile leak from the resected edges.

Management in such cases is conservative and involves replacement of lost volume with colloids until sufficient liver regeneration has taken place.

Most patients can be extubated at the end of the procedure and recovered within a high-dependency environment. Few will require intensive care and postoperative ventilation. Early enteral nutrition will facilitate postoperative recovery. Total parenteral nutrition (TPN) should be avoided to reduce the functional metabolic stress on the liver parenchyma.

Analgesia

There is significant pain associated with liver resection surgery. A functioning thoracic (T6–T9) epidural is the analgesic mode of choice. Coagulation parameters should be within normal limits prior to insertion and removal of the catheter. Good working epidural analgesia will facilitate early recovery. Although not evidence based, a paravertebral block is an alternative. Patient-controlled analgesia may be used with a local anaesthetic-only epidural, in particular with extensive right-sided liver surgery where the incidence of right-sided shoulder tip pain is high and will not be covered by an epidural alone. The incidence of shoulder tip pain is approximately 3%, but extreme retraction and longer operating times may increase its incidence in right-sided procedures. Intraperitoneal administration of local anaesthetic may be beneficial.

Paracetamol significantly reduces postoperative morphine requirement and is also useful for shoulder tip pain. It is safe to use in all but the most extensive liver resections, or those patients with pre-existing liver impairment. As a precaution, paracetamol should be administered after checking the liver function in the early postoperative period.

Non-steroidal anti-inflammatory drugs may worsen fluid retention associated with cirrhosis, and may precipitate renal failure. They are also avoided in patients with pre-existing impairment.

Conclusion

Management of liver malignancy has made significant progress in the last decade. Advances in perioperative care and surgical practice have significantly reduced morbidity and mortality. Most cases are managed uneventfully with minimal blood loss. Earlier diagnosis, technical advances in the practice of liver surgery, low CVP anaesthesia, and improved perioperative care have significantly reduced the mortality and morbidity associated with the procedure. Future directions will include greater numbers of patients being eligible for surgery with the development of neoadjuvant chemotherapeutics, greater numbers of patients presenting for repeat surgeries, and the further development of minimally invasive laparoscopic and robotic surgery.

Bibliography

1. Abbas SM, Hill AG (2008). Systematic review of the literature for the use of oesophageal Doppler monitor for fluid replacement in major abdominal surgery. *Anaesthesia* **63**(1):44–51.

2. Buggy DJ, Smith G (1999). Epidural anaesthesia and analgesia: better outcome after major surgery? *BMJ* **319**:530–1.

3. Chevalier A (2005). Anaesthesia and hepatic resection. *Anesthesiol Rounds* **4**(4).

4. Emond JC, Samstein, B, Renz JF (2005). A critical evaluation of hepatic resection in cirrhosis: Optimizing patient selection and outcomes. *World J Surg* **29**(2):124–30.

5. Garden OJ, Rees M, Poston GJ, *et al.* (2006). Guidelines for resection of colorectal cancer liver metastses. *Gut* **55**(suppl 3):iii1–iii8.

6. Gillams AR, Lees WR (2008). Five-year survival following radiofrequency ablation of small, solitary, hepatic colorectal metastases. *J Vasc Interv Radiol* **19**(5):712–17.

7. Hardy KJ (1990). Liver surgery: The past 2000 years. *ANZ J Surg* **60**(10):811–17.

8. Hawker F (1993). *The Liver*. Philadelphia, PA: Saunders.

9. Ho AMH, Karmakar MK, Cheung M, Lam GCS (2004). Right thoracic paravertebral analgesia for hepatectomy. *Br J Anaesth* **93**(3):458–61.

10. Kooby D, Stockman J, Ben-Porat L, *et al.* (2003). Influence of transfusions on perioperative and long term outcome in patients following hepatic resection for colorectal metastases. *Ann Surg* **237**:860–70.

11. Lentschener C, Ozier Y (2002). Anaesthesia for elective liver resections: some points should be revisited. *Eur J Anaesthesiol* **19**:780–8.

12. Malik HZ, Khan A (2008). Controversial topics in surgery; Adjuvant versus neo-adjuvant chemotherapy for colorectal liver metastases. *Ann R Coll Surg Engl* **90**:452–56.

13. McLoughlin JM, Jensen EH, Malafa M (2006). Resection of colorectal liver metastases: Current perspectives. *Cancer Control* **13**(1):32–41.

14. Melendez JA, Arslan V, Fischer ME, *et al.* (1998). Perioperative outcomes of major hepatic resections under low central venous pressure anesthesia: blood loss, blood transfusion, and the risk of postoperative renal dysfunction. *J Am Coll Surg* **187**(6):60–5.

15. Nakakura EK, Choti MA (2000). Management of hepatocellular carcinoma. *Oncology* **14**(7): 1085–100.

16. Pandya A, Jackson G, Wigmore T, Rao Baikady R (2008). Management of surgery-associated bleeding in cancer patients. *Current Anaesth Crit Care* **19**(2):59–69.

17. Rao Baikady R, Dinesh S, Hacking M, Wigmore T (2007). Cardiopulmonary exercise testing as a screeing test for perioperative management of major cancer surgery: a pilot study. *Critical Care* **11**(Suppl 2):P250.

18. Redai I, Emond J, Bretjens T (2004). Anesthetic considerations during liver surgery. *Surg Clin North Am* **84**:401–11.

19. Richter B, Schmandra TC, Golling M, Bechstein WO (2006). Nutritional support after open liver resection: A systematic review. *Dig Surg* **23**:139–45.

20. Soonawalla ZF, Stratopoulos C, Stoneham M, *et al.* (2008). Role of the reverse-Trendelenburg patient position in maintaining low-CVP anaesthesia during liver resections. *Langenbecks Arch Surg* **393**(2):195–8.

Chapter 10

Anaesthesia for plastic reconstructive and free flap surgery

Olivia Mingo

Introduction

Reconstruction after cancer surgery is required after a multitude of surgical procedures. The expertise of the plastic surgeon is called upon to fill defects exposed after tumour resection, restore functions such as speech and swallowing, and to provide an acceptable cosmetic result. Meticulous anaesthetic management is necessary as procedures are often prolonged. The anaesthetist may directly influence the viability of transferred tissue by control of haemodynamics and regional blood flow to the flap.

The surgery

Plastic surgery provides reconstructive options following cancer resection most commonly after breast and head and neck surgery but also after sarcoma, lower gastrointestinal, and gynaecological resection. Surgeons often work in tandem to allow resection of the tumour and reconstruction of the defect in one operation.

Surgical options for reconstruction include:

◆ Local flaps
◆ Pedicled flaps
◆ Free microvascular tissue transfer (free flaps).

A flap is a unit of tissue that is transferred from one site (donor site) to another (recipient site) while maintaining its own blood supply. Flaps can be composed of just one type of tissue including skin, fascia, muscle, bone, and viscera (e.g. colon, small intestine). Composite flaps include fasciocutaneous (e.g. radial forearm flap) and myocutaneous (e.g. transverse rectus abdominis muscle, TRAM) flaps. Distant flaps may be either pedicled, (transferred while still attached to their original blood supply, innervation, and lymphatics) or free. Free flaps are physically detached from their native blood supply and then reattached to vessels at the recipient site. This anastomosis is performed microsurgically.

Pedicled flaps

Pedicled myocutaneous flaps derived from pectoralis major, latissimus dorsi, and transversus abdominis can fill defects created in breast and head and neck surgery. Pedicle flaps are technically more straightforward and may be more suitable for higher-risk patients. However the use of these flaps is limited by the length of their vascular pedicle.

Free flaps

Free flaps can be raised from a variety of different sites, for example, the deep inferior epigastric perforator (DIEP) flap from the abdomen for breast reconstruction and the free fibula flap for bony mandibular reconstruction. These flaps can reconstruct soft and hard tissue defects. Their blood supply is divided to allow distant transfer of the flap before anastomosis to the recipient site. Free flaps suffer a period of primary ischaemia until blood flow is restored but are also prone to secondary ischaemia as flap blood flow frequently decreases by half during the first 6–12 hours post surgery. Dissection of the vessels also activates procoagulant processes leading to platelet sequestration which can cause stagnation of blood flow through the flap.

Free flaps are effectively denervated once dissected and lose their sympathetic tone, however the feeding artery and draining vein still respond to physical and chemical stimuli. Blood vessels can be put into spasm by cold, surgical handling, circulating catecholamines, and metabolites generated by ischaemia. Free flaps are also susceptible to oedema as their lymphatic drainage is disrupted. It can take weeks to months for lymphatic drainage to be restored.

Despite these physiological changes the success rates of free flap surgery are high. High success rates are due to meticulous surgical technique as well as rigorous peri- and postoperative management.

Physiological manipulation

Maintaining adequate regional blood flow is key to flap survival, particularly in free flaps where the flap is susceptible to secondary ischaemia.

The determinants of laminar flow are described by the Hagen–Poiseulle equation:

$$\text{Blood flow} = \frac{\Delta P \pi r^4}{8 \eta l}$$

where ΔP is pressure difference, r is radius, η is viscosity, and l is length.

Blood flow is directly dependent on a driving pressure across the flap and greatly influenced by the radius of the vessel. During microsurgery, vessels (usually with diameters from 1–4mm) are anastomosed thus optimization of flow is crucial.

The anaesthetist can manipulate the variables in the equation above to ameliorate flow.

◆ Perfusion pressure: flow is dependent on an adequate mean arterial pressure (MAP) maintained by optimal fluid loading and occasionally vasopressor support.

◆ Calibre of the vessel: vasodilatation is favourable and achieved via adequate fluid loading and active warming. External pressure on the vessel from oedema, tight dressings, and haematoma should be avoided.

◆ Viscosity: there is a non-linear relationship between blood viscosity and haematocrit with viscosity rising steeply when the haematocrit reaches 40%. Low viscosity favours flow but the concomitant haemodilution decreases oxygen carrying capacity. The optimal haematocrit is not known but a value of 27–30% is frequently aimed for. Viscosity is also increased by cold.

The practical implications for optimal anaesthetic management include maintenance of an adequate MAP, normothermia, and a relatively low blood viscosity.

Preoperative assessment

All patients undergoing reconstructive surgery should be preassessed paying particular attention to the site and local effects of the tumour and the effects of radiotherapy and chemotherapy. Flap failure was thought to be more common after radiotherapy, yet a recent review could not demonstrate a significant difference in flap success rate due to the overall high success rate of flaps. However operative complications increase as the time between radiotherapy and surgery increase.

The only independent risk factor associated with increased flap loss is obesity (Table 10.1).

Patients with head and neck cancers often have comorbidity related to a history of smoking and alcohol consumption. Nutritional status should be assessed as weight loss and difficulty with oral intake are likely. Consideration should be made to inserting a percutaneous endoscopic gastrostomy (PEG) preoperatively. Airway anatomy can be distorted by tumour, previous surgery, and radiotherapy and tissue fibrosis. The anaesthetist should assess and be prepared to manage a difficult airway.

Conduct of anaesthesia

Anaesthesia should ensure optimal perfusion of the transplanted tissue whilst minimizing morbidity associated with prolonged surgical time.

Positioning

Careful positioning is vital to prevent neuropraxias and pressure necrosis or pressure sores. Soft gel pads and cotton wool based dressing pads are used to protect vulnerable areas. Eyes should also be protected. Arm boards are often required for breast reconstruction

Table 10.1 Risk factors in free flap surgery

Risk factor	Postoperative complications/flap failure
Increasing age	No effect on complication rate or flap failure
Smoker	Higher rates of skin flap necrosis, infection and delayed wound healing. Smoking cessation 4 weeks prior to surgery decreases complications
Obesity	Increased complication rate and flap loss if body mass index >30
Diabetes	Increased rate of postoperative infection

and care must be taken with positioning to avoid hyperextension of the brachial plexus. Arms should rest in a pronated position with slight flexion at the elbow. In head and neck surgery the table should be tilted 30° head up to minimize blood loss. A head ring is often used to provide extension of the neck for surgical access in head and neck surgery but is avoided in breast procedures as it is unnecessary and can cause areas of pressure necrosis. Endotracheal tubes should be taped rather than tied to avoid venous congestion.

Intraoperative access and monitoring

The level of intravenous access and invasive monitoring required depends on the expected blood loss which mainly arises from the tumour resection.

Essential:

◆ Large-bore intravenous access.

Consideration of:

◆ Central venous access if major blood loss anticipated or difficult peripheral access (use subclavian or femoral lines for head and neck surgery away from the surgical field)

◆ Invasive blood pressure monitoring for prolonged surgery to monitor gas exchange, pH and haematocrit

◆ Urinary catheter to avoid bladder distension and monitor fluid balance.

Maintenance

Anaesthesia can be maintained with a combination of volatile agent and remifentanil or a target-controlled infusion of propofol and remifentanil used in conjunction with cerebral cortex monitoring. Isoflurane has been shown to maintain microcirculatory flow in free flaps in animal models. Newer agents such as sevoflurane and desflurane have not been investigated although have favourable properties of cardiovascular stability and quick offset time.

A remifentanil infusion is ideal for these procedures as it provides analgesia which is titratable to the changing surgical stimulus. A long-acting opioid needs to be given well before the end of the procedure to ensure postoperative analgesia after the remifentanil is stopped.

Vasoactive agents

There is some controversy over the use of vasopressors in flap surgery. The anaesthetist may use a vasopressor to increase a low MAP thus increase flow to vital organs and provide a driving pressure across the flap. However, vasoconstriction will potentially reduce flap blood flow. To maintain an adequate MAP the first aim should be optimal fluid management, however once the patient is adequately filled a vasopressor may still be required.

There is limited evidence to indicate which agent offers the ideal combination of increasing MAP as well as flap flow. Pedicle flaps have intact innervation while free flaps are denervated and it is difficult to predict the action of vasoactive agents on free flaps. However, their vasculature will respond to local physical and chemical factors and their feeding artery and draining vein still have intact innervation.

Vasodilators

Vasodilators increase vessel diameter and should theoretically increase flow to the flap. However, infusing milrinone, a phosphodiesterase inhibitor with the actions of arterial dilatation and increased cardiac output, does not improve flap survival and can require vasopressor support to maintain MAP. Topically applied vasodilators (verapamil, lignocaine) are often used by surgeons to prevent vasospasm and there is some evidence to indicate they may be effective.

Vasopressors

Effect on pedicle flaps

In animal studies adrenaline increased flow across all dose ranges given (0.5–2mcg/kg/min) in contrast to phenylephrine which decreased flow in the pedicle artery and decreased microvascular perfusion. For pedicled TRAM flaps both dobutamine and dopamine raised MAP and cardiac output, however only dobutamine increased blood flow in the recipient and donor blood vessels.

Effect on free flaps

A recent study investigated the effect of dobutamine infusion after completion of the microsurgical anastomosis for head and neck reconstruction. Dobutamine infusions of 4 and 6mcg/kg/min increased blood flow as well as increasing cardiac output which putatively could improve free flap perfusion.

Phenylephrine (1mcg/kg/min) has been shown to increase MAP and systemic vascular resistance (SVR) whilst having no deleterious effect on free flap blood flow in normovolaemic and hypovolaemic pigs. A human study comparing phenylephrine to sodium nitroprusside again showed an increase in MAP with no effect on flap blood flow with phenylephrine whilst sodium nitroprusside caused a severe reduction in flow linked with a drop in SVR and MAP.

Ephedrine or metaraminol may be used as an intraoperative vasopressor in free flap surgery. Metaraminol and phenylephrine should probably be avoided in pedicle flap surgery based on the above evidence. Consideration should be given to dobutamine due to its favourable effect on regional blood flow and cardiac output.

Fluid management

Traditionally in reconstructive surgery liberal fluid administration (hypervolaemic haemodilution) was utilized to decrease haematocrit and viscosity with the aim of increasing flap blood flow. However, excessive fluid loading can lead to flap oedema, venous congestion, and flap failure. One retrospective study investigating free flap loss in latissimus dorsi transfer to the lower leg found higher intraoperative crystalloid administration in the flaps that failed.

Fluid management should aim to maintain adequate cardiac output without vaso-pressors if possible. There are few data to compare crystalloid with colloid or on the effect of goal-directed fluid therapy for reconstructive surgery. It is reasonable to guide fluid administration aiming for a urine output of greater than 0.5–1.0ml/kg/h. Blood transfusion is rarely required for reconstruction alone, and indeed haemodilution decreases viscosity and may ameliorate flap blood flow. A liberal transfusion policy has been found to be associated with increased morbidity and mortality. In animal models normovolaemic haemodilution (Hb 9g/dl) has been shown to improve microcirculation in ischaemic flaps.

Temperature

Maintaining normothermia avoids the deleterious effects of hypothermia: increased blood viscosity, vasoconstriction, and vasospasm. In an animal model of skin free flaps, blood flow varied directly with temperature between 22°C and 38°C (increase in flow of 3.4% per degree). Active management of perioperative temperature may improve flap survival compared to no active warming. One must not only maintain normothermia but aim for a narrow core–peripheral temperature gradient (<2°C).

Coagulation and antithrombotic prophylaxis

All patients without contraindications should have compression stockings and pneumatic boot calf compression applied. Prophylactic subcutaneous heparin is routinely given and a large case series of free flap surgery associated its use with improved flap survival. In this series no other antithrombotic regime was shown to influence flap survival.

Other agents used

- Aspirin given postoperatively gives equivalent outcomes to subcutaneous heparin
- Clopidogrel reduces the rate of venous thrombosis in animal models
- Intravenous heparin has not been shown to influence thrombosis rate
- Low-molecular-weight dextran (known antiplatelet and antifibrin effects) does not improve flap survival and risks complications, such as congestive cardiac failure
- Thrombolytic agents (e.g. streptokinase) can be infused into vessels in cases of flap thrombosis although evidence for efficacy is scant.

Pain management

Effective analgesia is essential for patient comfort and to prevent systemic sympathetic stimulation leading to vasoconstriction. Epidurals may decrease rate of microvascular complications and flap loss, but benefit may be outweighed by the theoretical 'steal' phenomenon, by which blood flow is diverted from a denervated flap to intact vessels vasodilated by the epidural. Some studies have shown a 20–30% decrease in blood flow to the free flap as well as a marked drop in MAP, exacerbated in the presence of hypovolaemia. Epidurals are not contraindicated in flap surgery but care should be taken to avoid hypovolaemia and vasopressors may be required to maintain an adequate MAP.

Effective analgesia can be provided by opioids given perioperatively and continued as patient-controlled analgesia postoperatively. Regional techniques such as paravertebral and rectus sheath blocks can be opioid sparing. Continuous local anaesthesia catheters can also be placed in the wound and under the rectus sheath to decrease opioid consumption.

Extubation

The majority of patients can be extubated at the end of the procedure despite long anaesthetic times. A period of elective ventilation may be advocated in head and neck patients to avoid head movement and in anticipation of postoperative airway swelling, but sedation and ventilation may require vasopressors to maintain MAP. An elective tracheostomy may be required to protect the airway and flap which may negate the need for sedation and thus vasopressors postoperatively.

Postoperative care

Intensive postoperative care is required to continue the intraoperative measures taken to ensure good tissue perfusion and to monitor the flap for signs of failure. The patient should ideally be nursed on a high dependency unit.

The aims of postoperative management are to maintain normothermia, MAP, and an adequate fluid status. Fluids should be given to maintain a urine output of 0.5–1ml/kg/h and vasopressors only used to maintain MAP once the patient is fluid resuscitated.

Regular flap observations are crucial as the salvage of compromised flaps depends on early detection and re-exploration. Simple manoeuvres such as repositioning the patient to avoid vessel kinkage and removal of tight dressings can prove vital in flap management. A recent large study of free flaps showed 6% incidence of re-exploration with a third of these occurring in the first 24 hours. The most common finding was microvascular occlusion (53%) followed by flap haematoma (30%). Venous thrombosis was more common than arterial and was associated with a higher salvage rate. Flap failure may also be due in part to trauma from flap handling and long surgical ischaemic time, although only if prolonged over 3 hours.

A flap should be warm, pink, and have a capillary refill time (CRT) of 2–3 seconds. Problems with venous drainage result in a dusky, congested flap with a brisk CRT whereas arterial occlusion is marked by a pale and cool flap that does not bleed on pin prick testing. Both are indications for re exploration. Clinical observation is of limited use in monitoring buried flaps, and Doppler flowmetry is a reliable non-invasive monitor. Implantable Doppler probes and microdialysis, which allows continuous monitoring of flap metabolism, have been employed although these techniques are less widely used.

Conclusion

Outcomes after reconstructive surgery are excellent due to honed surgical technique and intensive perioperative care. The role of the anaesthetist is diverse and challenging particularly in flap surgery where they are central to presenting a patient in the optimum physiological state to ensure best surgical results.

Bibliography

1. Banic A, Krejci V, Erni D, Petersen-Felix S, Sigurdsson GH (1997). Effects of extradural anesthesia on microcirculatory blood flow in free latissimus dorsi musculocutaneous flaps in pigs. *Plast Reconstr Surg* **100**(4):945–55.

2. Bui DT, Cordeiro PG, Hu QY, Disa JJ, Pusic A, Mehrara BJ (2007). Free flap reexploration: indications, treatment, and outcomes in 1193 free flaps. *Plast Reconstr Surg* **119**(7):2092–100.

3. Chang DW, Wang B, Robb GL, *et al.* (2000a). Effect of obesity on flap and donor-site complications in free transverse rectus abdominis myocutaneous flap breast reconstruction. *Plast Reconstr Surg* **105**(5):1640–8.

4. Chang DW, Reece GP, Wang B, *et al.* (2000b). Effect of smoking on complications in patients undergoing free TRAM flap breast reconstruction. *Plast Reconstr Surg* **105**(7):2374–80.

5. Chien W, Varvares MA, Hadlock T, Cheney M, Deschler DG (2005). Effects of aspirin and low-dose heparin in head and neck reconstruction using microvascular free flaps. *Laryngoscope* **115**(6):973–6.

6. Evans GR, Gherardini G, Gürlek A, *et al.* (1997). Drug-induced vasodilation in an in vitro and in vivo study: the effects of nicardipine, papaverine, and lidocaine on the rabbit carotid artery. *Plast Reconstr Surg* **100**(6):1475–81.

7. Gurlek A, Kroll S (1997). Ischaemic time and free flap success. *Annals of Plastic Surgery* **38**:503–5.

8. Heller L, Kowalski AM, Wei C, Butler CE (2008). Prospective randomized double-blind local anaesthetic infusion and intravenous narcotic patient controlled anaesthesia pump for pain management after free TRAM flap breast reconstruction. *Plast Reconstr Surg* **122**(4):1010–18.

9. Jones SJ, Scott DA, Watson R, Morrison WA (2007). Milrinone does not improve free flap survival in microvascular surgery. *Anaesth Intensive Care* **35**(5):720–5.

10. Massey MF, Gupta DK (2007). The effects of systemic phenylephrine and epinephrine on pedicle artery and microvascular perfusion in a pig model of myoadipocutaneous rotational flaps. *Plast Reconstr Surg* **120**(5):1289–99.

11. Nataranjan SK, Clarke S, Mitchell V, Kalavrezos N, Ramasamy P (2008). Anaesthesia for reconstruction of head and neck defects using microvascular tissue transfer. *CPD Anaesthesia* **10**(1):17–23.

12. Panchapakesan V, Addison P, Beausang E, Lipa JE, Gilbert RW, Neligan PC (2003). Role of thrombolysis in free-flap salvage. *J Reconstr Microsurg* **19**(8):523–30.

13. Scholtz A, Pugh S, Fardy Shafik M, Hall JE (2009). The effect of dobutamine on blood flow of free tissue transfer flaps during head and neck reconstructive surgery. *Anaesthesia* **64**:1089–93.

14. Schramm S, Wettstein R, Wessendorf R, *et al.* (2002). Acute normovolemic hemodilution improves oxygenation in ischemic flap tissue. *Anesthesiology* **96**:1478–84.

15. Scott GR, Rothkopf DM, Walton RL (1993). Efficacy of epidural anesthesia in free flaps to the lower extremity. *Plast Reconstr Surg* **91**(4):673–7.

16. Serletti JM, Higgins JP, Moran S, Orlando GS (2000). Factors affecting outcome in free-tissue transfer in the elderly. *Plast Reconstr Surg* **106**(1):66–70.

17. Sigurdsson GH (1995). Perioperative fluid management in microvascular surgery. *J Reconstr Microsurg* **11**(1):57–65.

18. Sigurdsson GH, Thomson D (1995). Anaesthesia and microvascular surgery: clinical practice and research. *Eur J Anaesthesiol* **12**:101–22.

19. Smit J, Acosta R, Zeebregts C, *et al.* (2007). Early reintervention of compromised flaps improves success rates. *Microsurgery* **27**:612–616.

20. Spear SL, Ducic I, Cuoco F, Hannan C (2005). The effect of smoking on flap and donor-site complications in pedicled TRAM breast reconstruction. *Plast Reconstr Surg* **116**(7):1873–80.

21. Thankappan K (2010). Microvascular free tissue transfer after prior radiotherapy in head and neck reconstruction–A review. *Surg Oncol* **19**(4):227–34.

22. Xu H, Luo J, Huang F (2007). Clinical study on effect of keeping perioperative normal body temperature on skin flap survival. *Chin J Reparative & Reconstructive Surg* **21**(7):718–21.

23. Yi N, Evans G, Miller MJ, *et al.* (2001). Thrombolytic therapy: What is its role in free flap salvage? *Ann Plast Surg* **46**:601–4.

Chapter 11

Anaesthesia for gynaecological oncology surgery

Andrew McLeod, Joanna Moore, and
Desmond P.J. Barton

Introduction

Gynaecological cancers are relatively uncommon, with the incidence of cervical cancer, for example, being fifteen times less than that of breast cancer. Management in the UK is therefore increasingly concentrated in specialist centres, where outcomes have been improved by specifically trained gynaecological oncologists working with experienced anaesthetists and nursing colleagues. This chapter will describe the main types of gynaecological cancer (except trophoblastic disease), and their current management. These patients are surgically challenging, and also require careful evaluation and postoperative care, as they are at risk of significant postoperative morbidity especially after visceral resection and prolonged laparotomies.

Ovarian cancer

Ovarian cancer has a deservedly notorious reputation characterized by a late stage of presentation and low overall survival rates. The classic presentation is of a 50–70-year-old woman with complaints of altered bowel habit or abdominal distension. These patients are often misdiagnosed with irritable bowel syndrome and may initially have been referred to colorectal units. At first presentation, 75% will have malignant disease spread to the peritoneal cavity (classified as stage 3 disease, FIGO (International Federation of Gynecology and Obstetrics)), or to the liver parenchyma (stage 4). The majority of patients with stage 3 ovarian cancer will have ascites, sometimes incapacitating. Not infrequently, patients will also have a symptomatic unilateral or bilateral pleural effusion. Women who have stage 3 or 4 disease can only expect a 20–30% chance of survival at 5 years. The surgical goals depend on the tumour type, patient characteristics, and stage of disease. Four groups of patients can broadly be considered:

- Healthy women predisposed to ovarian cancer (e.g. carriers of BRCA gene mutations) are increasingly being offered prophylactic salpingo-oophorectomy.
- Young patients with presumed early-stage cancer—many of these patients will have germ cell cancers, which can behave aggressively and are very chemosensitive. The surgical goal is to resect the disease while preserving fertility, i.e. the uterus and

one fallopian tube and ovary are conserved. Pelvic and para-aortic lymph nodes are sampled.

♦ Postmenopausal patients with evidence of abdominal disease but who are well—surgical treatment aims at optimal 'de-bulking', i.e. maximal reduction of tumour volume. The degree to which this can be achieved correlates well with disease-free interval and overall survival. Outcomes are most improved when all visible disease has been removed. To achieve this requires multiple surgical procedures, both pelvic and abdominal.

♦ Unwell postmenopausal patients with evidence of abdominal disease—these patients are typically malnourished, with significant ascites, low serum albumin, and a poor performance status. In such cases, the perioperative risks are increased, and in the absence of a significant palliative benefit from surgery (e.g. a painful mass) the usual initial management is neoadjuvant platinum-based chemotherapy. These patients typically have a laparotomy ('delayed primary surgery') after three cycles of chemotherapy and then receive a further three cycles after surgery. Second laparotomy may be required for resection of recurrent disease, or where optimal tumour debulking could not be achieved initially. A common scenario with recurrent disease is subacute bowel obstruction and these cases when managed surgically have the highest morbidity and mortality of any gynaecological oncology procedure.

Cervical cancer

Cervical cancer is broadly distributed across all age groups over 25 years (Table 11.1), but advanced disease is more common in older women. Cervical smear testing can provide early diagnosis, but most patients are symptomatic, presenting with irregular vaginal bleeding and/or discharge. The cancer usually spreads local–regionally before metastasizing beyond the pelvis, and this local spread may result in constipation, or affect the urological system causing haematuria, hydronephrosis, and renal impairment. Early disease can be treated with cone biopsy, but radical hysterectomy is employed for stage

Table 11.1 Cancer incidence, age of presentation, and treatment modes

Type of cancer	Incidence (UK) per 100,000 standardized population[a]	Age of presentation	Treatment modes
Ovarian cancer	17.0	50–70 years	Surgery Chemotherapy
Cervical cancer	8.4	25–80 years	Radiotherapy + chemotherapy Surgery
Uterine cancer	18.1	50–70	Surgery Radiotherapy
Vulval cancer	2.4	>65 years	Surgery Radiotherapy ± chemotherapy

[a]Source: Cancer Research UK CancerStats reports 2006/2007 data. http://info.cancerresearchuk.org/cancerstats/reports/index.htm.

Ib1, Ib2, and less often, stage IIa. Pelvic exenteration is considered more rarely for advanced primary malignancy. Adjuvant brachytherapy and pelvic radiotherapy are also used, sometimes with chemotherapy. Recurrent disease is treated with radiotherapy but if the patient has had this treatment already, the only potential salvage is an exenterative operation (see below).

Endometrial carcinoma

There are many cancers of the uterine body but the vast majority arise in the endometrium as endometrial endometrioid adenocarcinomas. Unlike ovarian cancer, 75% of patients present with early disease. Although this cancer is considered to have a lower mortality, stage for stage it is in fact as lethal as cervical or ovarian cancer. Endometrial cancer is associated with hypertension, heart disease, and diabetes, but the main underlying risk factor is obesity (two to three times increased risk). Operative management ranges from simple hysterectomy and oophorectomy without lymph node sampling, to radical hysterectomy with extensive lymph node dissection. Increasingly surgery is performed laparoscopically and there is evidence that obese patients are better managed this way. Patients at increased anaesthetic risk can also be treated by a vaginal hysterectomy (with or without bilateral salpingo-oophorectomy) and without node dissection. Pelvic radiotherapy and brachytherapy are commonly employed as adjuvant treatments (Table 11.1).

Vulval and vaginal carcinoma

Vulval cancer is rare, and mainly affects women over 65 years of age, with older patients presenting with later stages of disease. Surgical strategies range from radical wide local excision to (modified) radical vulvectomy with unilateral or bilateral groin node dissection. Vaginal cancer is even rarer, and usually arises from metastatic spread from another primary site. The mainstay of treatment of primary vaginal cancer is radiotherapy or chemo-radiotherapy (Table 11.1).

General management considerations

Preoperative assessment

Women with gynaecological cancer need good information about the likely outcomes and potential complications of surgery, as well as possible alternatives of chemoradiotherapy or palliative treatment. Preoperative assessment and preparation must therefore define perioperative risks as far as possible, and improve them as far as practicable. Assessment should be as for any major surgical procedure, but should also focus on the systemic effects of these malignancies, and the consequences of previous chemoradiotherapy:

◆ A careful history and examination should be undertaken to identify any symptoms or signs of cardiorespiratory disease, and an electrocardiogram and chest X-ray should be routine before major surgery. Cardiac impairment may also result from prior chemotherapy. Initial evaluation with echocardiography or MUGA (multi-gated acquisition) scan is useful, and a cardiologist may be able to help to optimize cardiac function. Cardiorespiratory function may also be impaired by large pleural effusions or tense abdominal ascites, detected on clinical examination or computed tomography. Thoracocentesis is indicated for significant pleural effusions. Predicting overall cardiac fitness for surgery remains difficult, but cardiopulmonary exercise testing shows promise in assessing functional status, establishing statistical risks for morbidity and mortality (which can assist patients to make informed choices) and allowing appropriate postoperative care to be planned.

◆ Several investigations are recommended (Table 11.2).

◆ Carboplatin and paclitaxel are the principal drugs used in the treatment of ovarian cancer. Carboplatin is nephrotoxic, and can cause thrombocytopenia. Cardiac impairment is unusual but can occur. Paclitaxel causes peripheral neuropathy and sometimes neutropenia. Twenty-five per cent of patients relapse early on this regimen and second-line agents are then considered. Although these patients are less likely to be operative candidates, they may present for surgery to relieve bowel obstruction. Doxorubicin can cause cardiomyopathy in 7.5% of patients, and this may be irreversible. Etoposide and topotecan are also used, and are both associated with blood count abnormalities.

◆ Patients may have received previous radiotherapy, which causes progressive fibrosis of pelvic tissues, making surgery more difficult and increasing the likelihood of blood loss.

Table 11.2 Investigations for gynaecological preoperative assessment

Blood test	Significance in gynaecological malignancy
Full blood count	Anaemia (from bleeding, radiotherapy, or bone marrow suppression) may require preoperative iron therapy or transfusion
	Low white cell count (from chemotherapy)[a]
	Thrombocytopenia (from platinum chemotherapy)
Urea and electrolytes	Renal impairment (from ureteric obstruction or chemotherapy)
Calcium	Biochemical derangement due to paraneoplastic syndromes
Glucose/HbA$_{1C}$	If diabetes or poor diabetic control is suspected due to obesity
Serum albumin	Hypoalbuminaemia is common and a proven risk factor for delayed wound healing, anastomotic breakdown, and poor overall outcome. It may also indicate malnourishment
CA125	CA (cancer antigen) 125 levels contribute to the diagnosis and monitoring of ovarian cancer, but do not predict the extent of surgery
Pregnancy test	May be indicated. 1% patients diagnosed with cervical carcinoma are pregnant, which can alter their management. Some treatments may also have a second aim of fertility preservation

[a]Source: (Cancer Research UK cancer registry data 2007). A neutrophil count $<1.0 \times 10^9.l^{-1}$ is an indication to postpone surgery.

♦ Massive intra-abdominal tumours can occasionally compromise breathing, and may also cause a supine hypotensive syndrome if venous return is affected. Pelvic masses can cause neurological symptoms in the legs due to nerve compression. Any symptoms or signs should be documented preoperatively, particularly if epidural anaesthesia is being considered, and patients should also be warned that their symptoms may be worsened by surgery.

♦ Significant ascites is common in ovarian cancer, and drainage can alleviate distension and dyspnoea. However, excessively rapid removal of a large ascitic volume can cause hypotension, fatally so in some cases. Fluid resuscitation is indicated to maintain circulating volume, but there are limited data to guide this procedure. Ascitic drainage should always be accompanied by cardiovascular monitoring, and withdrawal of volumes greater than 5L may require intravenous fluid replacement.

♦ Some patients, particularly with ovarian cancer, are malnourished due to direct disease effects, chemotherapy-induced vomiting, or poor appetite. Weight loss may not be a reliable indicator, however, as it can be confounded by ascitic fluid mass or tumour bulk. Bowel obstruction (with aspiration risk) should always be considered.

♦ A number of varied paraneoplastic syndromes have been reported, mainly in association with ovarian malignancy which is more immunogenic. These are rare overall, but can cause:

  • Hypercalcaemia
  • Cushing's syndrome
  • Nephrotic syndrome
  • Cerebellar degeneration
  • Stroke secondary to microembolization
  • Osteoarticular disorders causing rheumatoid-like symptoms.

  It is wise to be wary of unexplained clinical findings, and investigate them further. Some syndromes will resolve with treatment of malignancy, but neurological effects can be irreversible.

♦ Venous thromboembolism (VTE) affects 15% of all women with cancer, and this incidence is likely to be much greater where pelvic masses are compressing major blood vessels. Where VTE is detected, surgery can be deferred to allow treatment, but this delay may be unacceptable in progressive disease. Alternatively, an inferior vena cava filter (IVCF) can be placed by an interventional radiologist, ideally 24–48 hours before surgery. Patients with IVCFs continue to require thomboprophylaxis with low-molecular-weight heparin (LMWH). Current NICE (National Institute of Health and Clinical Excellence) guidance would classify all women undergoing major gynaecological surgery as at high risk of VTE. Patients should receive information about VTE risk and prophylaxis, compression stockings, and prophylactic LMWH (or unfractionated heparin in renal failure) on the night before surgery.

Intraoperative management

◆ Surgery for gynaecological malignancy is performed supine or more usually in a modified lithotomy position which can sometimes be for prolonged periods leading to risks of peripheral nerve injury or compartment syndrome in the legs. Meticulous positioning and padding of all pressure points is essential. Head-down tilt may also cause facial or airway oedema. Normothermia can be difficult to maintain where there is significant peritoneal exposure. Postoperative bowel dysfunction is common after major surgery, and a nasogastric tube is routinely placed after induction. Fluid and heat loss from the exposed bowel can be reduced by the use of a bowel bag during major abdominal procedures.

◆ Significant blood loss should be anticipated, particularly in exenteration surgery, or if pelvic side wall tumours involve major blood vessels. Circulating volume must also be maintained in spite of ongoing ascitic production, or fluid loss from prolonged peritoneal exposure. Direct monitoring of arterial and central venous pressure is routine for major procedures, and some form of cardiac output monitoring, e.g. oesophageal Doppler, can be useful in patients with poor cardiac function.

◆ Electrolyte and acid–base balance abnormalities are also common during major procedures. Hypokalaemia and hypomagnesaemia can result from gastrointestinal losses, while metabolic acidosis may be due to inadequate tissue perfusion, or iatrogenic hyperchloraemia.

◆ Massive blood transfusion may become necessary, requiring adequate venous access, fluid warming devices and maintenance of normal body temperature, and correction of coagulopathy and/or thrombocytopenia. Although there have been concerns that allogenic blood transfusion may modify tumour recurrence, this should not delay treatment of significant anaemia. Intraoperative cell salvage (ICS) is currently believed to be contraindicated in most gynaecological cancer surgery, based on concerns of spreading malignancy. However, in certain situations (e.g. a Jehovah's Witness patient), ICS may be justified following expert consultation, and full discussion with the patient.

◆ Epidural analgesia can provide good postoperative pain relief, but has yet to be shown conclusively to alter outcome overall. Morphine delivered by a patient-controlled analgesia device provides acceptable analgesia, and thus informed patient choice should be the overriding factor. If an epidural technique is chosen, the block should be developed carefully during surgery in case significant blood loss occurs. An alternative strategy is to use a remifentanil infusion during surgery, and then establish the epidural block before closure. Where epidural analgesia is contraindicated or declined, an ultrasound-guided transversus abdominis plane (TAP) block may also contribute to analgesia for midline or Pfannenstiel incisions.

◆ Surgical site infection precautions are supported by some evidence, but precise choice of agent(s) should be guided by local policy. Broad-spectrum antibiotics such as a cephalosporin and metronidazole are usually given on induction, and continued postoperatively following prolonged surgery, major blood loss, or contamination by bowel contents.

◆ Intraoperative measures to prevent VTE should be in place, including compression stockings and use of active calf compression devices.

Considerations specific to individual procedures

Ovarian cancer surgery

Surgery for ovarian cancer routinely includes excision of the uterus, ovaries, and adnexa, together with omentectomy and sampling of peritoneal deposits and lymph nodes. However, further spread of disease may require bowel resection including partial gastrectomy and/or splenectomy, and prolonged surgery. Anaesthetic considerations are;

◆ The midline incision is routinely full-length and a thoracic epidural placement is required to achieve reliable postoperative analgesia.

◆ Intraoperative blood loss and fluid balance may be difficult to estimate, particularly when it is accompanied by significant ascites or fluid loss from the peritoneal surface.

◆ Formal haemoglobin estimation is indicated, either using a point of care monitor such as Haemocue, or laboratory-based full blood count.

Radical hysterectomy

Radical hysterectomy includes the removal of uterus and cervix, paracervical tissue and upper vagina, and variably pelvic and para-aortic lymph nodes, ovaries, and fallopian tubes, either via a low transverse or midline incision. An initial lymph node dissection is performed and the procedure may not be continued if nodes are found to be positive on frozen section analysis. This procedure can sometimes be performed vaginally and also laparoscopically or robotically.

Anaesthetic considerations include:

◆ Patients may have a range of comorbidities due to the broad age group affected by cervical cancer and also its association with smoking.

◆ Duration of surgery is typically 3–6 hours.

◆ Expected blood losses 500–1500ml.

◆ Fluid balance requires care, particularly in the case of lymph node dissection, which can increase third-space losses.

◆ Ureteric injury can occur, and patients should be observed for haematuria and oliguria.

Pelvic exenteration

Pelvic exenteration has an appreciable mortality but is indicated as a curative procedure usually for recurrent cervical carcinoma, or rarely for locally advanced primary malignancy. It may also be employed for some recurrent endometrial, vulval, ovarian, vaginal, and other tumours. Occasionally it may be carried out as a palliative procedure, but this is the subject of some debate. Exenteration involves en bloc resection of all or some of the internal reproductive organs, bladder, pelvic ureters, rectum and sigmoid colon, pelvic peritoneum, and lymph nodes. This is followed by reconstruction including bowel anastomosis or stoma formation, urinary diversion, and vaginal and pelvic reconstruction using an omental flap and myocutaneous grafts. It is carried out via abdominal midline, and perineal incisions. Anterior and posterior exenterations may be performed to preserve either bowel or bladder function in some cases. Pelvic exenteration is contraindicated by distant or peritoneal metastases, and metastases to the bowel.

Anaesthetic considerations are:

- Most patients have recurrent disease and have either received chemoradiotherapy or have undergone previous surgery.
- Surgery is prolonged (8–12 hours), and involves at least two surgical teams.
- Large blood losses (1500–4000ml) should be expected and a rapid fluid infusion device must be prepared.
- Patients will require critical care postoperatively.
- Operative mortality is around 5% and morbidity is also high. The incidence of major perioperative complications is 45–60%, and common problems include postoperative infections, fistula formation, ileus and anastomotic leakage.

Radical vulvectomy

Radical vulvectomy is the primary management for invasive vulval carcinoma, and includes excision of the vulva, sometimes with bilateral dissection of the inguinal and femoral lymph nodes via a 'butterfly' or three separate incisions. Skin or myocutaneous grafting may be necessary to achieve wound closure. The procedure is associated with considerable perioperative morbidity and mortality, and there has been a move away from radical surgery. Hemivulvectomy with unilateral groin node dissection or wide local excision may be utilized. The use of sentinel node technology is being evaluated and may allow selective lymphadenectomy in future.

Anaesthetic considerations are:

- These patients are older (average 70 years), and may suffer from age-related comorbidities. There is an association between vulval carcinoma and smoking.
- Duration of surgery is typically 3–4 hours.
- Injury to femoral vessels can cause significant blood loss.

Laparoscopy

Laparoscopic techniques have a well-established range of applications in gynaecological cancer surgery, including staging laparoscopy, lymphadenectomy, sentinel node sampling, and hysterectomy. Radical hysterectomy and even exenterations may now be performed in this way. Improved visualization, lower blood loss, shorter hospital stay, and reduced analgesic requirements make these techniques attractive alternatives. The introduction of robotically-assisted procedures increases the range of applications still further. Anaesthetic considerations are similar to those of any laparoscopic surgery, but the potential for conversion to an open procedure must always be considered.

Brachytherapy

Brachytherapy is a technique of local radiotherapy used in the management of cervical, endometrial, and vulval cancers and recurrent pelvic malignancies. A radioactive source is placed close to the tumour either via a body cavity (e.g. uterus or vagina) or interstitially. It may be used either as an adjuvant therapy or as an alternative treatment in those patients unfit for surgery, and may involve the siting of an applicator with repeated attendances for short fractions of radiotherapy or a single application with a source that remains *in situ* for several days. Laparoscopy or even laparotomy is occasionally necessary to allow placement of interstitial sources.

Anaesthetic issues are:

- Many patients are elderly or unfit for major surgery and comorbidities are common.
- Procedures typically last 1.5–3 hours but may be prolonged further.
- Sedation may not deliver adequate immobility.
- Regional techniques may be employed, but some procedures may be too long to allow use of spinal or single-bolus epidural techniques. Epidural catheter techniques may be useful, particularly in unfit patients, and give continued analgesia postoperatively.
- It may be necessary to transport anaesthetized patients between theatre and radiotherapy departments.
- Pain can be problematic, and if not addressed may result in patients terminating therapy early.
- Postoperative radioactivity can preclude the use of the recovery room and may result in a patient with comorbidities being nursed in an isolated environment.
- Postoperative immobility may be necessary but increases the risk of VTE, and prophylaxis should be considered.
- Intraoperative radiotherapy is the subject of current investigation and may become more commonplace in the future.

Postoperative care

- Patients will require high dependency care following major procedures, and may need positive pressure ventilation after very extensive surgery. Longer stays in critical care facilities are more likely in patients over 65 years old, in those who are malnourished, and where intraoperative fluid replacement has been significant. Extensive surgery may also lead to a systemic inflammatory response syndrome, requiring vasopressor drug infusions and continued fluid administration.

◆ Electrolyte derangement, coagulopathy, and ongoing fluid loss may all need to be addressed where necessary. Fluid requirements are likely to remain increased due to continued ascites formation and other third-space losses, while a urinary diversion can also contribute to metabolic acidosis and electrolyte disturbance.

◆ Bowel complications are common after major procedures (2–30%), and must be considered if enteric nutrition fails, or signs of peritonitis occur. Total parenteral nutrition is indicated if bowel dysfunction is prolonged. Late complications such as wound breakdown and ureteric obstruction may also occur.

◆ Epidural analgesia may also contribute to postoperative hypotension, requiring correction with vasopressors. Parental opioids may be given if epidural analgesia has been unsuccessful, or has not been used. Women may also have pre-existing pain conditions due to their primary disease or pelvic nerve compression. Pain specialists and palliative care teams may provide valuable advice in these cases.

◆ VTE prophylaxis should be maintained, except where a significant coagulopathy or bleeding risk persists. LMWH dosages will need to be coordinated with epidural catheter removal, but must be continued at least until the patient is fully ambulant, and any IVCF device has been removed. The ongoing risk of VTE after discharge from hospital remains high, and has probably been underestimated in the past. Current guidance from NICE advises continuing pharmacological prophylaxis for 28 days after major surgery.

Bibliography

1. Abbas SM, Hill AG (2008). Systematic review of the literature for the use of oesophageal Doppler monitor for fluid replacement in major abdominal surgery. *Anaesthesia* **63**(1):44–51.
2. Adib T, Belli A, McCall J, *et al.* (2008). The use of inferior vena caval filters prior to major surgery in women with gynaecological cancer. *Br J Obstet Gynaecol* **115**(7):902–7.
3. Amant F, Moerman P, Neven P, Timmerman D, Van Limbergen E, Vergote I (2007). Treatment modalities in endometrial cancer. *Curr Opin Oncol* **19**(5):479–85.
4. American College of Obstetricians and Gynecologists (1997). Educational bulletin. Antibiotics and gynecologic infections. *Int J Gynecol Obstet* **58**(3):333–40.
5. Becker G, Galandi D, Blum HE (2006). Malignant ascites: systematic review and guideline for treatment. *Eur J Cancer* **42**(5):589–97.
6. Cannistra SA (2004). Cancer of the ovary. *N Engl J Med* **351**(24):2519–29.
7. Carney J, McDonnell JG, Ochana A, Bhinder R, Laffey JG (2008). The transversus abdominis plane block provides effective postoperative analgesia in patients undergoing total abdominal hysterectomy. *Anesth Analg* **107**:2056–60.
8. Cho JE, Liu C, Gossner G, Nezhat FR (2009). Laparoscopy and gynecologic oncology. *Clin Obstet Gynecol* **52**(3):313–26.
9. Crosbie EJ, Slade RJ, Ahmed AS (2009). The management of vulval cancer. *Cancer Treat Rev* **35**(7):533–9.
10. del Carmen MG, Eisner B, Willet CG, Fuller AF (2003). Intraoperative radiation therapy in the management of gynecologic and genitourinary malignancies. *Surg Oncol Clin N Am* **12**(4):1031–42.
11. Díaz-Montes TP, Zahurak ML, Bristow RE (2007). Predictors of extended intensive care unit resource utilization following surgery for ovarian cancer. *Gynecol Oncol* **107**(3):464–8.

12. Elit LM, Thomas H, Trim K, Mazurka J, Moens F (2004). Evaluation of postoperative pain control for women undergoing surgery for gynaecological malignancies. *J Obstet Gynaecol Can* **26**:1051–8.

13. Fader AN, Rose PG (2007). Role of surgery in ovarian carcinoma. *J Clin Oncol* **25**:2873–83.

14. Hudson CN, Curling M, Potsides P, Lowe DG (1993). Paraneoplastic syndromes in patients with ovarian neoplasia. *J Roy Soc Med* **86**:202–4.

15. Laky B, Janda M, Bauer J, Vavra C, Cleghorn G, Obermair A (2007). Malnutrition among gynaecological cancer patients. *Eur J Clin Nutr* **61**:642–6.

16. National Institute for Health and Clinical Excellence (2010). *Venous thromboembolism: reducing the risk*. London: NICE.

17. Ng R, Better N, Green MD (2006). Anticancer agents and cardiotoxicity. *Semin Oncol* **33**:2–14.

18. Riley J, Ross J, Bates C (2004). Management of difficult pain in patients with carcinoma of the ovary. In Kehoe S, Gore M, Miles A (eds) *The effective management of ovarian cancer*, 3rd edn, pp. 135–47. London: Aesculapius Medical Press.

19. Roessler B, Six LM, Gustorff B (2008). Anaesthesia for brachytherapy. *Curr Opin Anaesthesiol* **21**:514–18.

20. Schneider A, Köhler C, Erdemolgu E (2009). Current developments for pelvic exenteration in gynecologic oncology. *Curr Opin Obstet Gynecol* **21**(1):4–9.

21. Sweetland S, Green J, Liu B, *et al.* (2009). Duration and magnitude of the postoperative risk of venous thromboembolism in middle aged women: prospective cohort study. *BMJ* **339**:b4583.

22. Yap OW, Husain A, Kapp DS, Teng NN, Carroll I, Rosenthal MH (2004). Gynecologic oncology. In Jaffe RA, Samuels S (eds) *Anesthesiologists' manual of surgical procedures,* 3rd edn, pp. 591–629. Philadelphia, PA: Lippincott Williams & Wilkins.

Chapter 12

Anaesthesia for urological cancer surgery

James Burrows, Charlotte Moss, and Tim Wigmore

Introduction

Increases in prevalence, improvements in medical treatment, and advances in minimal access surgical techniques are resulting in increasing numbers of patients of all ages and comorbidities presenting for surgical management of their urological tumour.

In this chapter we consider different types of urological cancers that are encountered, potential management strategies for these, and the anaesthetic approach. We include preoperative considerations, intraoperative approach, and also focus on specific surgery that has particular anaesthetic requirements, and postoperative care.

Preoperative management

General considerations

With the exception of testicular cancer most are over 50 and have significant comorbidities. A comprehensive preoperative assessment is required. Of particular interest are the cardio-vascular and respiratory systems. Smoking is a risk factor for many urological cancers.

Tumour-specific considerations

Renal function

It is common for malignancies affecting the urogenital tract to adversely affect renal function either as a direct result of diseased renal tissue itself or due to tumour obstructing the renal tract.

Consequences may include:

- Deranged electrolytes
- Uraemia
- Acidaemia
- Fluid overload
- Impaired drug clearance and metabolism (including anaesthetic agents)
- Anaemia due to decreased erythropoietin production.

Renal function may improve postoperatively (e.g. post removal of an obstructing tumour) but recovery is likely to be delayed. Nephrectomy may result in the patient becoming dialysis-dependent postoperatively if the remaining kidney cannot compensate for the lost function. Therefore it is important to assess function in both kidneys prior to nephrectomy.

Paraneoplastic syndromes

Ten to 40% of patients with renal cell carcinoma may suffer from paraneoplastic syndromes, with a variety of symptoms and signs from constitutional symptoms (malaise, fever, cachexia, and weight loss) to metabolic and biochemical abnormality from ectopic hormone production (see Table 12.1). Non-metastatic hepatic dysfunction, amyloidosis, dermatological manifestations such as pemphigoid, and neurological problems have also been described.

These effects can be wide-ranging and include hypertension, polycythaemia, hepatic dysfunction, amyloidosis, and many endocrine abnormalities (e.g. Cushing's syndrome, hyper/hypoglycaemia, galactorrhoea, elevated human chorionic gonadotropin or adrenocorticotropic hormone).

Malnutrition

Cancer patients are commonly malnourished due to disease, treatment, and consequent anorexia. The malnourished patient lacks fat and muscle mass, which reduces the volume of distribution of most intravenous anaesthetic agents. They are also at greater risk from hypothermia, hypoglycaemia, pressure sores, and refeeding syndrome.

Hypoalbuminaemia

Albumin is one of the principal proteins to which drugs bind and hypoalbuminaemia has significant effects on the pharmacokinetics of many drugs. Hypoalbuminaemia is an independent risk factor for poor outcome.

Prior radiotherapy and chemotherapy

Radiotherapy may have been administered externally or, with prostate cancer, internally as brachytherapy. Long-term systemic side effects are minimal but radiotherapy causes localized fibrosis resulting in a more challenging and lengthy surgery with increased blood loss.

Table 12.1 Paraneoplastic syndromes arising from ectopic hormone production in renal cell carcinoma

Hormone produced	Physiological derangement
Erythropoietin	Polycythaemia
Parathyroid hormone-related peptide	Hypercalcaemia
Adrenocorticotrophic hormone	Cushing's syndrome
Renin	Hypertension
Glucose	Diabetes
Insulin	Hypoglycaemia

Table 12.2 Side effects of chemotherapeutic agents commonly administered against urological tumours

Drug	Significant adverse effects
Gemcitabine	Haemolytic uraemic syndrome, hepatic/renal impairment, pulmonary toxicity
5-Fluorouracil	Hepatic impairment, mucositis, myelosuppression
Vinblastine	Hepatic impairment, myelosuppression, neuropathy
Paclitaxel	Arrhythmias and cardiac conduction defects, myelosuppression, peripheral neuropathy
Carboplatin/cisplatin	Neurotoxicity, ototoxicity, renal impairment
Ifosfamide	Haemorrhagic cystitis, myelosuppression, renal impairment
Doxorubicin (anthracycline)	Cardiomyopathy and heart failure, hepatic impairment, supraventricular tachycardia
Mitoxantrone	Cardiotoxicity, myelosuppression
Etoposide	Myelosuppression, renal impairment
Methotrexate	Mucositis, myelosuppression, pneumonitis, pulmonary fibrosis
Bleomycin	Pulmonary fibrosis

A variety of chemotherapeutic agents may have been employed prior to surgery either as a primary therapy or as neoadjuvant therapy—an attempt to reduce the tumour size or extent in order to facilitate surgery. Many of the drugs commonly used against urological cancers have long-term systemic side effects of significance to the anaesthetist (see Table 12.2 and Chapter 15).

Individual tumour-specific issues

Renal cancer

Most commonly renal cell carcinoma (renal adenocarcinoma or hypernephroma), accounts for over 80% of renal cancer. Transitional cell carcinoma makes up the majority of the remainder together with Wilm's nephroblastoma in children.

Anaesthetic preassessment issues:

♦ Renal cell carcinoma is also associated with early onset of constitutional symptoms of weight loss, fever, and lethargy, which may be the only apparent symptoms both at initial presentation and upon disease recurrence. Weight loss may be compounded by a lack of appetite and by chemotherapy-induced nausea and vomiting.

♦ Paraneoplastic syndromes as above.

♦ Invasion of local structures including liver, colon, and spleen.

♦ Tumour extension can occur into the inferior vena cava, which can extend up to the right atrium in 4–10%.

♦ Metastasis to the brain, bone, and lungs.

♦ Standard surgical treatment for localized renal cell carcinoma involves radical nephrectomy (5-year survival rate over 80%). Surgery extending into the inferior vena cava may require cardiothoracic and vascular surgeons, and is occasionally performed under cardiopulmonary bypass.

- For small, solitary tumours, nephron-sparing surgery involving local removal of a small tumour can have equivalent success rates to radical nephrectomy, and is associated with a lower long-term risk of chronic renal failure.

Bladder cancer

Most commonly transitional cell carcinoma.
  Anaesthetic preassessment issues:

- Patients usually older and as risk factors include smoking often have associated cardiopulmonary morbidity.
- Disease is usually limited to the mucosa and submucosa and is managed by cystoscopic resections, and close surveillance.
- For more invasive tumours involving the muscle wall a radical cystectomy is preferred. Radical cystectomy is also used for recurrent superficial tumours, and extensive papillary disease not controlled by transurethral resection and intravesical therapy.

Prostate cancer

Most are adenocarcinomas arising in the peripheral prostate and the majority of malignant foci remain dormant.
  Anaesthetic preassessment issues:

- Spread may occur locally to structures including seminal vesicles, bladder, and rectum, or metastasize to lymph nodes, bone, or lung.
- Primary curative surgical treatment is radical prostatectomy, usually reserved for low-grade, localized cancers in men with a life expectancy exceeding 10 years.
- Other treatment options include active surveillance, external bean radiation, brachytherapy, high-intensity focused ultrasound (HIFU), and cryotherapy.
- Brachytherapy involves implantation of radioactive sources directly into the prostate under ultrasound guidance in the form of small seeds that emit low-dose radiation locally for several weeks, or high-dose implants which are removed after several hours.
- HIFU and cryotherapy involve heating or cooling the tissues respectively to remove cancerous tissue.

Testicular cancer

One to 2% are bilateral. Ninety to 95% are germ cell tumours, peak incidence occurring in the third decade for non-seminoma (60% of total and includes teratoma, intratubular germ cell neoplasia, spermatocytic seminoma, embryonal carcinoma, yolk sac tumour, choriocarcinoma and those with more than one type) and the fourth decade for seminoma. Seventy-five per cent of seminomatous tumours are stage 1 (localized) at diagnosis and are highly radiosensitive. Chemotherapy (bleomycin, etoposide, and cisplatin) is useful for stage 2 (regional lymph node spread) and stage 3 (spread to distant nodes and viscera) disease.

Anaesthetic preassessment issues:

- Non-seminomatous germ cell tumours tend to spread via the lymphatics from the spermatic cord into the retroperitoneal lymph chain.

- Embryonal carcinomas and choriocarcinomas are more aggressive, spreading haematogenously to the brain, lungs, and liver particularly. They are less radiosensitive than seminomatous tumours and treated with orchidectomy followed by cisplatin-based chemotherapy or retroperitoneal lymph node dissection for removal of lymph nodes lying in the anatomical chain draining the spermatic cord.

- Patients may have received bleomycin, which can cause pulmonary fibrosis, especially in the presence of high oxygen concentrations which should be avoided if at all possible.

Intraoperative management

Anaesthesia—general principles

Surgery for urological malignancy is often lengthy and typically involves the abdominal and/or pelvic body cavities. These features make general anaesthesia with tracheal intubation frequently necessary.

Patient temperature should be monitored and intraoperative hypothermia should be avoided with the use of a range of warming devices (e.g. mattresses, hot air blankets and intravenous fluid warmers).

Thromboprophylaxis should be undertaken with graduated compression stockings and intermittent pneumatic calf compression devices.

Analgesia

Pain experienced following open procedures is usually severe. There remains controversy over the use of epidural analgesia. Several studies demonstrate reduced postoperative respiratory failure, in addition to reduction in other postoperative complications including myocardial infarction, venous thromboembolism, and improved pain scores when compared to an opioid-based technique. In addition, studies have demonstrated a reduction in long-term development of metastatic disease in those receiving regional analgesia, avoiding the use of opiates which may reduce tumour immunosurveillance. Nevertheless, problems with failure (10–30%) of epidural analgesia necessitate the addition of supplemental systemic opioids. Epidural infusion can increase requirements for additional fluid boluses and vasopressor treatment. Rarely, neurological complications may occur. Regional nerve blocks can be used as an alternative in certain circumstances (see below), and supplemented by the use of opioids where necessary. An opiate patient-controlled analgesia (PCA) system is an alternative. Non-steroidals should be avoided in patients where renal function is of concern.

Haemorrhage

Urological tumour resections have the potential for major haemorrhage. Large-bore intravenous access as well as central venous catheterization and invasive blood pressure monitoring is often required to optimally manage the haemodynamic changes. For high-risk patients undergoing major surgery intraoperative cardiac output monitoring by oesophageal Doppler has been shown to improve outcomes.

Blood and blood products should be readily available for transfusion via rapid infusion devices as blood loss can be extremely swift. Transfusion should be guided, where possible, by timely analysis of blood samples either in the laboratory or with point of care testing (e.g. thromboelastography). In 2008, the National Institute for Health and Clinical Excellence (NICE) approved the use of intraoperative cell salvage during radical prostatectomy and radical cystectomy. The report notes concern over the potential for reinfusion of viable malignant cells causing metastases, but concludes that there is no reported evidence that this occurred and that the known benefits would outweigh this theoretical risk.

Laparoscopic surgery

Laparoscopic techniques are becoming increasingly prevalent because they are associated with faster recovery, and generally avoid the need for high dependency postoperative care. However, the surgical time tends to be longer and there are significant effects and potential complications in addition to those of the Trendelenburg position. Carbon dioxide is used to achieve pneumoperitoneum because it has a low toxicity and high solubility. Insufflation of gas for pneumoperitoneum can cause vagal stimulation and associated bradycardia. Caval compression by the gas causes a reduction in venous return and cardiac output. The carbon dioxide itself is absorbed, further contributing to cerebral hyperaemia from the Trendelenburg position. Ventilation may need to be increased to offset this. There is a reduction in functional residual capacity and lung compliance and an increase in intragastric pressure which compounds that caused by Trendelenburg.

Other complications of laparoscopic surgery that the anaesthetist must be aware of are:

◆ Vessel injury resulting in sudden and severe haemorrhage
◆ Pneumomediastinum
◆ Pneumothorax
◆ Subcutaneous emphysema
◆ Sympathetic response
◆ Injury to abdominal organs, e.g. bowel perforation
◆ Venous gas embolism.

Anaesthesia—specific tumours

Renal cell carcinoma

Simple nephrectomy and partial nephrectomy can be performed laparoscopically but many are still performed open. The surgical incision may be abdominal, flank, or thoracoabdominal depending upon the location and extent of the tumour. All these approaches cause significant intra- and post-operative pain, particularly if rib resection is required. Appropriate analgesic techniques include epidural, or paravertebral block, opiate PCA, field or transversus abdominis plane block, and catheters for local anaesthetic infusion placed in the surgical wound or intercostal space.

The patient is positioned in the lateral decubitus position such that the upper body is at an angle of about 45 degrees pronation. Careful positioning and padding of the arms is required to avoid brachial plexus and ulnar nerve injuries. The dependent leg is flexed at the hip whilst the other leg remains extended and padding is placed between them. The table is broken to raise the flank in relation to the head and feet. This causes pooling of blood in the dependent zones, which combined with potential compression of the vena cavae, may significantly reduce venous return and thus cardiac output. Major haemorrhage and haemodynamic instability must be anticipated and invasive monitoring, large-bore IV access, and the availability of fluid-warming rapid infusion devices is generally indicated.

If removal of high vena caval thrombus is planned then facilities for cardiopulmonary bypass should be available and intraoperative transoesophageal echocardiography is desirable to detect tumour thrombus embolization or migration.

Bladder cancer

Transurethral resection (TUR) is performed under general or regional anaesthesia. The patient is placed in the lithotomy position. This reduces pulmonary compliance and increases ventilation/perfusion mismatch and increases venous return leading to increased stretch and myocardial oxygen demand. The lithotomy position also risks compression to the saphenous and common peroneal nerves, compartment syndrome, as well as back and hip injuries.

Tumours that are more invasive at presentation or which have progressed despite TUR (43%) will require cystectomy. Cystectomy may also be performed as a palliative procedure for very advanced tumours causing distressing symptoms, e.g. bleeding, pain, dysuria, or bowel obstruction. Radical cystectomy involves removal of the bladder, lymph nodes, and adjacent structures (prostate and seminal vesicles in men, and uterus and adnexa uteri in women). This is an extensive operation with the potential for large-scale blood loss, significant fluid shifts, and hypothermia. Patients receive bowel preparation preoperatively and urine output is often impossible to measure throughout surgery. Therefore fluid and electrolyte balance pose a significant challenge to the anaesthetist and invasive pressure monitoring is indicated and cardiac output/preload monitoring should be considered.

Robust analgesia is required and can be provided as opiates with or without an epidural bearing in mind that the level of block would need to cover any stoma as well as the pelvic drains.

Following cystectomy a new pathway for urine to exit the body needs to be provided. This can take the form of an ureterosigmoidostomy (ureters anastomosed to sigmoid colon) or, more commonly, a diversion to an abdominal wall stoma utilizing some ileum as a conduit. It is also possible to fashion a neobladder from some stomach or ileum which acts as reservoir for urine. This can be connected to the urethra which enables micturition to take place via abdominal straining or may require the formation of a continent stoma (the Mitrofanoff) through which intermittent self-catheterization is performed.

Postoperatively these patients need close attention to fluid balance, analgesia, thromboprophylaxis, and nutrition. In addition there may metabolic disturbances as described below. A high dependency environment is desirable.

Prostate cancer

Open prostatectomy

The prostate can be approached through the perineum with the patient in an extended lithotomy position where the feet are elevated and the hips flexed such that the thighs are all but parallel to the trunk. This position exacerbates the physiological challenges and pressure area hazards of the standard lithotomy position.

More commonly a retropubic approach to the prostate is taken—this requires a supine patient with a hyperextension at the iliac crests to facilitate access. Again, for these open procedures opiates and/or central or regional blocks are appropriate.

Laparoscopic prostatectomy

Laparoscopic and, more recently, robotically-assisted laparoscopic prostatectomy are increasingly becoming the preferred option. Although these less invasive techniques do pose significant intraoperative challenges for patients, surgeons, and, anaesthetists there are benefits for appropriately selected patients in terms of reduced blood loss, pain, enhanced recovery (from 4–6 to 2–3 weeks) and nerve-sparing surgery increasing the likelihood of preserved sexual function.

Both the laparoscopic and particularly the robotic prostatectomy require a steep Trendelenburg. The tilt is such that the patient is at risk of sliding on the operating table and needs careful supporting to avoid this, as any extraneous movement whilst the laparoscopic instruments are positioned in the abdomen could be catastrophic. Shoulder braces have been used but run the risk of brachial plexus injury. Steep head-down results in splinting of the diaphragm and reduces pulmonary compliance and ventilation leading to an increase in $PaCO_2$ whilst increased shunt from ventilation–perfusion mismatching can lead to hypoxia. Increased venous return increases myocardial stretch and oxygen demand. The head-down position also promotes cerebral blood inflow whilst impeding venous drainage; this can lead to raised intracranial pressure (exacerbated by higher $PaCO_2$) and raised intraocular pressure. This circulatory congestion leads to a generalized oedema of the head and neck, which may result in facial and periorbital swelling, retinal detachment, and laryngeal oedema with stridor. In an attempt to ameliorate this situation, the patient's head should be kept in neutral alignment and the endotracheal tube should be taped rather than tied in position. Regurgitation is also more likely in this position.

Postoperatively a period of careful monitoring is prudent and analgesic requirements may be significant if an open approach is used. The robotic prostatectomy is considerably less painful and often a PCA is not required.

Testicular cancer

Orchidectomy

Commonly a day case procedure and anaesthesia can be effectively achieved with either general or spinal/epidural anaesthetic and may be complemented with an inguinal field block.

Retroperitoneal lymph node dissection

Retroperitoneal lymph node dissection has both a diagnostic and therapeutic role. In low-grade cases it may be offered in addition to orchidectomy to assess disease spread and potentially eradicate the cancer without chemotherapy. In higher-grade cases it may be offered to those who have residual retroperitoneal masses following chemotherapy (usually a combination chemotherapy including bleomycin and cisplatin).

Bleomycin can cause pulmonary fibrosis particularly in the presence of high oxygen concentrations, which should be avoided intraoperatively.

The complexity or otherwise of retroperitoneal lymph node dissection depends almost entirely upon the location and extent of the nodes to be removed. The principal anaesthetic concerns are major haemorrhage and pain. Analgesia may include thoracic epidural/other blocks as appropriate and/or opioid PCA. These patients are generally otherwise well and can usually be managed on a surgical ward postoperatively.

Postoperative care

The nature and extent of the operation performed as well as the pre-existing physical status of the patient will largely determine the level of postoperative care required. In most cases this is predictable from the information gained during the preoperative work-up.

Postoperative analgesia is multimodal. Simple analgesics, including non-steroidal anti-inflammatory drugs only where renal function is not a concern, are supplemented with opioids as required taking into consideration any preoperative opiate exposure that will have resulted in a degree of tolerance. Local anaesthetic techniques employed include nerve blocks such as the transversus abdominis plane block as well as catheters placed at the time of surgery at the wound site or in the intercostal or pleural space through which local anaesthetic is infused.

Perioperative fluid shifts may be significant. Surgery is often lengthy and involves an open abdomen from which significant heat and moisture may be lost. Add to this potentially large blood losses and high third space losses (particularly where bowel is involved in the surgery) and it is clear that large fluid deficits and acid–base disturbances may occur. Urine output coupled with clinical examination for markers of adequate filling (warmth of extremities, capillary refill time, and jugular venous pressure) is often enough to give a good indication of fluid balance status although for more complex clinical scenarios invasive measures including central venous pressure and cardiac output monitoring will be required. Renal function is at risk after urological surgery and adequate filling is a mainstay of supportive management, however, a balance needs to be achieved such that cardiac failure and oedema to delicate suture lines are avoided. A low-dose vasopressor infusion may support the blood pressure and renal perfusion particularly in cases where overtransfusion is a concern or to counteract epidural sympathetic blockade. Choice of replacement fluid should reflect the nature of the fluid deficits being addressed. It should be noted that even with optimum management a number of patients will require postoperative renal replacement therapy in the short or long term.

Patients having urinary diversion can experience specific metabolic problems. Where the colon or ileum has been used as a conduit, absorption of chloride, with concomitant secretion of bicarbonate can cause a normal anion gap hyperchloraemic acidosis. Urinary ammonium is absorbed and converted to ammonia and hydrogen ions in the liver which can contribute to the acidosis. This occurs less often where ileal conduits are used as the urine drains rapidly into a bag, limiting contact time. There is higher risk with use of ileum as a neobladder as contact time is increased. If the acidosis is severe, bicarbonate supplementation may be required.

If resumption of normal dietary intake is delayed, consideration must be given to ongoing nutrition especially those previously malnourished. Depending upon the type of surgery and the expected duration of starvation total parenteral nutrition or nasogastric or nasojejunal feeding may be considered worthwhile.

Antibiotic prophylaxis is usually continued to complete 24 hours of therapy in uncomplicated surgery, guided by local microbiological policies.

Thromboembolic disease remains a significant cause of perioperative morbidity and mortality. Postoperatively, patients should continue to wear thromboembolic deterrent stockings and pneumatic sequential compression devices and the timely introduction of prophylactic low-molecular-weight heparin will mitigate this risk. Early mobilization should be encouraged. In cases where haemorrhage is a concern, unfractionated heparin may be used instead as this can be antagonized with protamine should bleeding occur.

Conclusion

Rigorous preoperative assessment and preparation are important when it comes to planning and delivering optimum care. The perioperative demands of major urological surgery include uncompromising patient positioning, major haemorrhage, fluid balance, and analgesia and require a robust but careful and precise approach.

Bibliography

1. Cancer Research UK (2007). *Cancer incidence – UK statistics*. Available at: http://info.cancerresearchuk.org/cancerstats/incidence/.
2. Danic MJ, Chow M, Alexander G, Bhandari A, Menon M, Brown M (2007). Anesthesia considerations for robotic-assisted laparoscopic prostatectomy: a review of 1,500 cases. *J Robotic Surg* 1(2):119–23.
3. European Association of Urology (2004a). *Guidelines on Bladder Cancer*. Arnhem: European Association of Urology.
4. European Association of Urology (2004b). *Guidelines on Testicular Cancer*. Arnhem: European Association of Urology.

5. Johnston N, Morris C, Low J (2008). Epidural analgesia: first do no harm. *Anaesthesia* **63**:1–3.

6. National Institute for Health and Clinical Excellence (2008). *Intraoperative red blood cell salvage during radical prostatectomy or radical cystectomy.* Available at http://www.nice.org.uk/nicemedia/pdf/IPG258Guidance.pdf (accessed 15 December 2009).

7. Older P, Hall A, Hader R (1999). Cardiopulmonary exercise testing as a screening test for perioperative management of major surgery in the elderly. *Chest* **116**:355–62.

8. Pahernik S, Roos F, Wiesner C, Thüroff JW (2004). Nephron sparing surgery for renal cell carcinoma in a solitary kidney. *World J Urol* **25**:513–17.

9. Palapattu GS, Kristo B, Rajfer J (2002). Paraneoplastic syndromes in urologic malignancy: the many faces of renal cell carcinoma. *Rev Urol* **4**(4):163–70.

10. Rhodes A (2010). Anaesthesia for cancer patients: The prognostic implications of anaesthetic technique. *Anaesth News* **274**:24–6.

11. Sessler DI, Buggy DJ, Biki B, Mascha E, Moriarty DC, Fitzpatrick JM (2008). Anesthetic technique for radical prostatectomy surgery affects cancer recurrence: A retrospective analysis. *Anesthesiol* **109**:180–7.

12. Shenoy S, Ward P, Wigmore T (2009). Surgical management of urological malignancy: Anaesthetic and critical care considerations. *Curr Anaesth & Crit Care* **20**(1):22–7.

13. Stainsby D, MacLennan S, Thomas D, Isaac J, Hamilton PJ (2006). Guidelines on the management of massive blood loss. *Br J Haematol* **135**(5):634–41.

14. Sterrett S, Mammen T, Nazemi T, *et al.* (2007). Major urological oncological surgeries can be performed using minimally invasive robotic or laparoscopic methods with similar early perioperative outcomes compared to conventional open methods. *World J Urol* **25**(2):193–8.

15. Williams SK, Hoenig DM, Ghavamian R, Soloway M (2010). Intravesical therapy for bladder cancer. *Expert Opin Pharmacother* **1**(6):947–58.

16. Wong KK, Harris JR (2005). Parathyroid adenoma presenting as paraneoplastic syndrome secondary to renal cell carcinoma. *J Otolaryngol* **34**(4):280–1.

17. Zacharias M, Gilmore IC, Herbison GP, Sivalingam P, Walker RJ (2005). Interventions for protecting renal function in the peri-operative period. *Cochrane Database Syst Rev* **3**:CD003590.

Part 3

Malignant disease and critical care

Chapter 13

Stem cell transplantation and the implications for critical care

Rachel Harrison and Tim Wigmore

Introduction

Haematopoietic stem cell transplantation (HSCT) is increasingly used to treat many life-threatening malignant and non-malignant diseases and up to 40% of stem cell transplant patients require intensive care unit (ICU) treatment.

Types of transplantation

HSCT is defined as 'any procedure where haemopoietic stem cells of any donor type and any source are given to a recipient with the intention of repopulating and replacing the haemopoietic system in total or in part'. Stem cells are harvested from bone marrow, peripheral blood, or umbilical cord blood. The donor may be the patient themselves (autologous) or another individual (allogeneic).

Autologous transplantation

Autografts use the patient's own stem cells. They are removed when the cancer is in remission and can be reinfused within days of harvest or years later after relapse. The patient is treated with chemotherapy with or without radiotherapy to eliminate the marrow immediately prior to transplantation. There follows a period of profound myelosuppression (up to 25 days) followed by engraftment.

Oncological indications for autologous transplantation include:

- Non-Hodgkin's lymphoma (NHL)
- Hodgkin's lymphoma
- Acute myeloid leukaemia (AML)
- Acute lymphoblastic leukaemia (ALL)
- Multiple myeloma (MM)
- Relapsed germ cell tumours
- Ewing's sarcoma
- Neuroblastoma.

Allogeneic transplantation

Allografts involve the infusion of a donor's (either sibling or matched unrelated donor, 'MUD') stem cells. Donor and recipient need to be a full or near human leukocyte antigen (HLA) match with siblings having an approximately one in four chance of being a complete match. In addition, cytomegalovirus (CMV) seronegative donors should be used for CMV seronegative patients due to the risk of CMV transmission. Indications for allografts include;

- AML
- ALL
- Chronic myeloid leukaemia (CML)
- Chronic lymphocytic leukaemia (CLL)
- NHL
- Hodgkin's lymphoma
- MM
- Myelodysplastic syndromes.

In myeloablative regimes, the patient receives high-dose chemotherapy and/or total body irradiation to eliminate the host marrow. The period of severe myelosuppression before engraftment is generally 7–21 days. Long-term immunosuppression is required post infusion to prevent graft-versus-host disease (GvHD) and graft rejection. This predisposes to infection although the allogenicity of the transplant does result in a graft versus disease effect as well as GvHD.

Autologous versus allogeneic transplantation

The major advantage of autografts is that the patient acts as their own donor, eliminating the subsequent risk of incompatibility, GvHD, and the requirement for immunosuppression. There is a low early treatment mortality (2–5%) and morbidity, making it particularly attractive for older patients (younger than 70 years). The trade-off is the risk of reinfusing tumour cells and of increased recurrence later.

Allogeneic transplant has a high associated morbidity and mortality (20–40% early treatment-related) but may offer the only hope of cure (notably for CML). It requires more intensive conditioning regimes (either total body irradiation or intensive chemotherapy) and immunosuppression post transplant to prevent GvHD and graft rejection. It is generally reserved for younger patients with fewer comorbidities and a higher chance of cure. 'Mini' or 'reduced intensity' allografts with less intensive conditioning that is strongly immunosuppressive but not myeloablative are increasingly used in either older patients or those with pre-existing comorbidities.

Stem cell sources

Stem cells can be isolated from bone marrow, peripheral blood (with granulocyte colony-stimulating factor (GCSF) stem cell mobilization), or umbilical cord blood (cord blood stem cell CBST) from a donated cord and placenta.

Most transplant centres use peripheral sources for autologous transplants following work showing them to be faster to engraft and to be associated with lower morbidity. There is no conclusive evidence as to which is better for allogeneic transplants. Meta-analysis suggests engraftment is faster using peripheral sources but associated GvHD may be more severe.

CBST are largely limited to children and adolescents due to limitations imposed by the relatively small number of cells collected.

Complications

Early complications occur either as a result of the conditioning regime (e.g. widespread mucosal damage causing mucositis, oesphagitis, gastritis and diarrhoea, or nausea and vomiting) or from infection due to myelosuppression. Allografts are, in addition, associated with GvHD.

Multiorgan system complications

Graft-versus-host disease

GvHD occurs in up to 50% of patients post allograft and arises when immunocompetent cells in the donor marrow recognize host tissue as foreign and mount an immune response. T-cell mediated activation leads to inflammation followed by apoptosis of the host cells and typically affects the eyes, skin, intestines, liver, and lungs. The reaction may be acute (less than 100 days post transplant) or chronic (more than 100).

Risk factors:

- Degree of HLA matching of the transplant (the less the match, the greater the risk)
- Older age of donor or recipient
- Males receiving female transplants (particularly if the female was previously pregnant).

Acute GvHD classically exhibits a triad of:

- Dermatitis—ranges from mild with a maculopapular rash affecting the hands and feet to complete desquamation
- Hepatitis—typically causes intrahepatic cholestasis
- Enteritis—abdominal pain with nausea, vomiting, copious secretory diarrhoea, ileus, and haemorrhage.

Diagnosis is through skin biopsy, rectal biopsy (to distinguish from *Clostridium difficile* colitis), and (as a last resort) liver biopsy.

Management of acute GvHD lies initially in prophylaxis with immunosuppressants such as methotrexate, cyclosporine, steroids, or antithymocyte globulin. Another approach is removal of T lymphocytes from the donor graft, although this may be associated with increases in graft failure or disease relapse due to a decrease in graft versus disease effect.

If prophylaxis fails, treatment is with further immunosuppression, typically with methylprednisolone in the first instance. Other agents may be used for symptom control, e.g. octreotide for secretory diarrhoea and patients may need to be parenterally fed.

Mortality is typically from sepsis associated with immunosuppression. Manifestations of chronic GvHD and its implications for organ systems are discussed in the relevant sections later in this chapter.

Infection

Infections are common post transplant and if the patient is sufficiently unwell to be referred to ICU tend to present as septic shock with either respiratory failure or abdominal pain that can be mistaken for an acute abdomen. The patterns of infection are determined by post-transplant progress.

- Pre-engraftment period (up to 30 days): recipients are neutropenic and have breaks in mucocutaneous barriers, with consequent bacterial, candidal, and *Aspergillus* infections.

- Early post-engraftment period (first 3 months): a deficiency in cell-mediated immunity in particular with viral and fungal infection predominating.

- Later, allogenic recipients suffer from impaired cell-mediated and humoral immunity due to ongoing immunosuppression, with viral, mycobacterial, and encapsulated bacterial infections.

Bacterial

Bacterial infection usually occurs either in the 3 weeks prior to engraftment or in the late post-transplant phase (>3 months). Pre-engraftment infection tends to be with Gram-positive cocci rather than Gram-negative organisms due to the routine use of antibiotics active against Gram-negatives and of selective gut decontamination.

Late infection is generally only a problem in allogeneic transplants and is often secondary to encapsulated bacteria (*Pneumococcus, Haemophilus,* or *Neisseria meningitidis*), *Staphylococcus,* and *Pseudomonas.*

Pneumocystis jirovecii (PCP) infections have become rare through the routine use of co-trimoxazole (Septrin) prophylaxis. Nevertheless, the diagnosis should always be considered in patients on immunosuppressive therapy or using less potent prophylaxis due to intolerance particularly as symptoms may be relatively non-specific.

Treatment and investigation are similar to that of the non-transplant patient, although the use of antibiotic prophylaxis may make identification of a specific organism more difficult. Cultures should include bronchoalveolar lavage (BAL) with real-time polymerase chain reaction (PCR) and a high-resolution chest computed tomography (CT) scan may show infection specific diagnostic features. Broad-spectrum antibiotics should be commenced as soon as possible after cultures have been taken and treatment modified to directive therapy once bacterial sensitivities and specificities are established.

Viral

Viral infections predominate from day 31–100 post transplant.

- Up to 70% of patients, particularly allogeneic recipients, develop CMV infections, 40% of whom go on to develop pneumonitis. Infection is typically secondary to latent virus reactivation in the immunocompromised (particularly if the host T cells have been eliminated), but may also be caused by transmission from CMV-positive donor to a negative recipient through stem cells or blood products. Patients who are CMV seronegative with CMV-seronegative donors should only receive CMV-negative blood products.

◆ Pneumonitis usually presents 6–8 weeks post transplant with fever, dyspnoea, hypox-aemia, and a non-productive cough, eventually progressing to respiratory failure. Chest X-ray demonstrates non-specific bilateral interstitial shadowing, and high-resolution CT shows bilateral asymmetrical ground-glass opacities and small centri-lobular nodules predominantly in the mid and lower zones.

◆ CMV can also cause hepatitis, oesphagitis, encephalitis, retinitis, and bone marrow suppression.

◆ Diagnosis is usually with PCR for early antigens or for CMV DNA polymerase.

◆ Management is primarily through the prevention of *de novo* or reactivated infection. CMV-negative donors and blood products and antiviral prophylaxis (aciclovir or ganciclovir) are used. Treatment is with ganciclovir (itself immunosuppressive) with or without foscarnet and CMV intravenous immunoglobulin (IVIG). The combina-tion of ganciclovir and IVIG has reduced the mortality of pneumonitis from around 90% to 50%.

Other viral infections are less prevalent. The most common early viral infection is gingi-vostomatitis from herpes simplex virus (HSV). HSV is also a rare cause of severe pneumonia. Human herpesvirus-6 (HHV6) infection is increasingly recognized.

Seasonal viruses such as respiratory syncytial virus (RSV) and influenza that affect the respiratory system tend to be seen in the first month post transplantation. Presenting with mild coryzal symptoms they can progress to severe pneumonia with mortality rates approaching 80% in RSV. Treatment is with aerosolized ribavarin and intravenous immunoglobulin.

Fungal

Fungal infections are increasingly common in post transplant patients. *Candida* and *Aspergillus* are the most common although other opportunistic fungal infections (e.g. fusarium and zygomycetes) are becoming more frequent. Diagnostic tests tend to be poorly sensitive, as reflected by the disparity between the rates infection diagnosed pre- and postmortem.

Risk factors include:

◆ Allogenic transplants (due to the use of immunosuppression)

◆ Prolonged neutropenia

◆ Colonization

◆ Intensive conditioning

◆ Regimen-related mucositis

+ Premorbid diabetes
+ Central venous catheters
+ Prolonged use of broad-spectrum antibiotics
+ Renal replacement therapy.

Aspergillosis Approximately 10% will develop an *Aspergillus* infection. It primarily affects lung, presenting with non-specific symptoms; fever, dry cough, dyspnoea, pleuritic chest pain, and occasionally haemoptysis although it can also disseminate to brain, kidney, liver, and skin. *Aspergillus* may be angioinvasive, leading to haemorrhagic infarction, and/ or airway invasive, leading to bronchiectasis, pneumonia, or tracheobronchitis.

Early diagnosis and treatment are key to outcome. Diagnosis depends on:

+ Culture—often falsely negative.

+ Serum galactomannan—a constituent of *Aspergillus* cell wall. False positives may occur if the patient is receiving a fungal derived antibiotic (e.g. Tazocin).

+ Lung CT—early angioinvasive aspergillosis may appear as a nodule surrounded by a 'halo' of ground glass, representing the infection surrounded by haemorrhagic infarction. This is non-specific, also being seen in other infections, inflammatory conditions, and neoplasms. The 'air-crescent sign' is seen on CT during the recovery phase of infection with resolution of neutropenia and indicates cavitation within nodules.

Whilst prevention of pulmonary aspergillosis is vital, no anti-fungal agent has yet been identified that reduces the risk of infection, so practical measures such as laminar-airflow systems and high efficiency particulate (HEPA) air filters are used. GCSF is often used to reduce the neutropenic phase, reducing the period of highest risk. In established infection voriconazole is first line with caspofungin and liposomal amphotericin B alternatives. Mortality from invasive pulmonary aspergillosis is extremely high (up to 90%).

Candida Invasive candidal infection is less common than previously due to the use of azole prophylaxis, although this is simultaneously leading to the more common isolation fluconazole resistant species such as *C. glabrata* and *C. kruseii*. Infections produce non-specific symptoms and signs, and the diagnosis is often made late from blood culture. Fluconazole is first line for treatment but resistance or evidence of endophthalmitis (which should always be looked for) requires use of an echinocandin (e.g. caspofungin) liposomal amphotericin B, voriconazole, or itraconazole.

Tumour lysis syndrome

Patients undergoing HSCT (particularly for AML and ALL) are at risk of tumour lysis syndrome, which comprises of a range of metabolic abnormalities that result from the rapid death of large numbers of tumour cells. Specifically it results in:

+ Hyperuricaemia (and subsequent uric acid nephropathy)
+ Hyperkalaemia

- Hyperphosphataemia

- Hypocalcaemia (due to the precipitation of calcium phosphate).

Prophylaxis is traditionally with allopurinol (a xanthine oxidase inhibitor) and fluid hydration, although more recently rasburicase (recombinant urate oxidase) has been used. Alkalinization of urine is controversial (as it risks increased precipitation of calcium phosphate in the renal tubules).

Keys to treatment are the management of the hyperkalaemia and hyperphosphataemia (which may require haemofiltration). Hypocalcaemia should not be treated unless symptomatic again because of the risk of calcium phosphate deposition in the kidneys.

Pulmonary system

Respiratory complications remain a major limitation to HSCT. It is vital to differentiate the infective and non-infective complications, since the former may respond to antibiotics and the latter to steroids. Most early complications are infective and occur in up to 50% of patients. Non-infective are detailed chronologically below with the exception of the pulmonary manifestations of systemic phenomena, such as veno-occlusive disease (VOD) and GvHD.

Engraftment syndrome

Engraftment syndrome, also known as capillary leak syndrome or pulmonary alveolar proteinosis develops within 96 hours of HSCT.

It has a complex pathophysiology involving the production and release of pro-inflammatory cytokines and rapid neutrophilia. A neutrophil-mediated endothelial injury similar to that observed in acute respiratory distress syndrome is a possible cause.

Presentation:

- Pyrexia

- Erythematous rash

- Non-cardiogenic pulmonary oedema

- Hepatic dysfunction

- Transient encephalopathy

- Haemodynamic compromise, multiorgan failure, and death in severe cases.

Investigation includes high-resolution CT and BAL revealing a milky aspirate due to the high protein content.

Management is supportive. GCSF should be discontinued and antimicrobial therapy used if appropriate. Corticosteroids effectively reduce the duration of the syndrome, particularly the pulmonary complications.

Diffuse alveolar haemorrhage (DAH)

Typically occurring within 30 days of HSCT, DAH occurs in up to 15% of patients. Pathogenesis is unclear but involves injury to small vessel endothelium.

Presentation:

◆ Deteriorating respiratory function or multiorgan failure/sepsis

◆ Dyspnoea

◆ Cough

◆ Pyrexia

◆ Hypoxaemia

◆ Haemoptysis is rarely seen.

The key to diagnosis is via BAL which reveals fresh blood progressing to haemosiderin-laden macrophages.

Treatment is supportive. Some retrospective studies have shown an association between high-dose corticosteroids and improved outcome. Prognosis is poor with a mortality rate approaching 70%.

Cryptogenic organizing pneumonia (COP)

COP, previously known as bronchiolitis obliterans organizing pneumonia (BOOP), is an acute lung injury linked to GvHD. It develops in approximately 1% of HSCT patients within 1–3 months.

Biopsies show intraluminal granulation with fibroblasts throughout small airways, alveolar ducts and alveoli.

Presentation may be suggestive of pneumonia with pyrexia, dyspnoea, and dry cough, but no organism is cultured. Progression to hypoxaemia and acute respiratory failure requiring mechanical ventilation follows. The diagnostic gold standard is lung biopsy while HRCT typically reveals patchy consolidation with ground glass appearance. There is typically a good response to long-term corticosteroid treatment, but the mortality rate is still around 20%.

Bronchiolitis obliterans (BO)

In 10% of chronic GvHD, BO produces severe obstructive airway disease at 3–18 months post transplantation. Prognosis is poor with deterioration over months or years and progressive inflammation of the small airways leading to irreversible airway obstruction, respiratory failure, and death. Diagnosis is by lung biopsy. Little response is seen to immunosuppressants, although azithromycin (via an immunomodulatory effect) may limit progression.

Graft-versus-host disease

Pulmonary manifestations of GvHD include bronchiolitis, bronchiectasis, and associated infections.

Idiopathic pneumonia syndrome (IPS)

IPS is widespread alveolar injury in the absence of infection (ruled out by sequential BAL or lung biopsy). Generally occurring within 6 months of transplantation, it is seen in 10%

of patients. Pathogenesis is unclear, but it probably represents a heterogenous group of conditions with varying aetiologies (e.g. intensive chemotherapy regimes and GvHD) but a common final pathway of lung damage. Treatment is supportive and mortality rates are high (>70%).

Cardiac and circulatory systems

Cardiac failure

Cardiac failure with consequent pulmonary oedema is a common complication. Risks include premorbid dysfunction, cardiotoxic drugs (e.g. ciclosporin and anthracyclines), fluid overload from medications and dimethyl sulfoxide (used in cryopreservation of marrow). Management is similar to non-transplanted patients.

Pericardial effusion

Effusions secondary to cardiotoxic chemotherapy, chronic GvHD, renal failure, or from infection occasionally occur. Of infective syndromes, viruses such as Epstein–Barr virus or CMV are most commonly implicated, but cases linked to bacterial infection or aspergillosis have been reported.

Endocarditis

Endocarditis seen in the post-transplant phase may be non-infective or infective in origin, and is seen in approximately 1% of patients post HSCT. Clinical infection may be inconspicuous with only 25% identified before death. Causative organisms are typically gram-positive bacteria (*Staphylococcus aureus* or *S. viridans*) or fungi (*Candida* and *Aspergillus* species). Risk factors include venous cannulation (central lines in particular), breached mucosal barriers or skin attenuation (GvHD and high-dose chemotherapy), and immunosuppressants. Treatment centres on aggressive targeted antimicrobial therapy as patients are frequently unfit for surgery.

Hepatic system

A common site for GvHD and infections, particularly fungal and viral, the hepatic system may also sustain insults from VOD and splenic rupture.

Veno-occlusive disease

- VOD occurs within the first 21 days post transplant and is a result of endothelial cell damage from high-dose preconditioning chemotherapy (particularly busulphan and melphelan). The incidence used to be 20–50% with a similar mortality, but is decreasing with the use of defibrotide (an antithrombotic and fibrinolytic agent, used both prophylactically and as treatment).
- Typically thrombosis develops in the small central hepatic venules leading initially to weight gain and (often painful) hepatomegaly, ascites, and hyperbilirubinaemia. The clinical course ranges from a mild, self-terminating liver enzyme derangement to a

devastating, rapid disease with associated multiorgan failure. VOD is also seen in other organs, such as the kidney where it causes acute renal failure.

◆ Diagnosis is usually made with Doppler ultrasound showing reduced or reversed portal blood flow in hepatic vessels. Hepatic vein catheterization is rarely used but enables direct measurement of portal pressures; A hepatic venous pressure gradient greater than 10mmHg is diagnostic. Liver biopsy is also diagnostic, although associated with a high risk of haemorrhage.

Splenic rupture

GCSF is commonly used in patients to improve granulocyte counts after chemotherapy or HSCT. Its use is associated with generalized symptoms such as fatigue and nausea, but more serious complications such as splenic rupture have been described.

Neurological system

Patients admitted to ICU are at risk from general complications such as critical illness polyneuropathy and myopathy, encephalopathy, and cerebrovascular accidents together with specific complications of therapy.

Cerebrovascular accident

Post-transplant patients are at increased risk of haemorrhage, embolism, and thrombosis. Haemorrhage is typically secondary to thrombocytopenia, whilst thrombosis may occur either due to the prothrombotic state or disseminated intravascular coagulation. Emboli may be due to infection (typically aspergillosis) or non-bacterial endocarditis.

Management is similar to that of non-HSCT patients although they are unlikely to be candidates for thrombolysis.

Metabolic encephalopathy

Presents as confusion, decreased level of consciousness, agitation or seizures. The aetiology is diverse including hypoxaemia, electrolyte disturbance, hepatic failure, sepsis, and drugs (analgesics and sedatives in particular). Wernicke's may also develop secondary to GvHD of the gut with subsequent malabsorption and thiamine deficiency.

Central nervous system infections

This can be secondary to a number of different pathogens including bacterial, viral (CMV, herpes zoster), fungal (*Aspergillus, Candida, Crypotococcus*) and protozoal (toxoplasma) infection.

Neurological complications of therapeutic agents

Several commonly used agents have the potential to produce serious neurological side effects:

◆ Ciclosporin can lead to oedema of the posterior cerebral white matter causing posterior reversible encephalopathy (PRES). This produces headache, visual changes, reduced Glasgow Coma Scale score, confusion, seizures, and hypertension. Treatment is blood pressure and symptom control.

◆ OKT3 (muromonab), a murine monoclonal antibody used as an immunosuppressant can lead to aseptic meningitis 24–72 hours after injection. The use of corticosteroids prior to administration may reduce or prevent its occurrence.

◆ Corticosteroids have well documented neurological effects including myopathy, psychosis, and withdrawal complications.

Chronic graft-versus-host disease

Polyneuropathy, polymyositis, and myasthenia gravis may result from GvHD of the central nervous system. Increased immunosuppression is the mainstay of treatment.

Gastrointestinal tract

All critically ill patients are at increased risk of gastrointestinal (GI) complications, including peptic ulcer disease, pancreatitis, and cholecystitis. After HSCT, pancreatitis is particularly prevalent and at autopsy pancreatitic inflammation is found in 20%, although clinical disease is diagnosed far less often. This propensity is probably due to the use of drugs such as steroids and ciclosporin, infections (adenovirus and CMV), GvHD, and biliary sludge. Other GI complications include

◆ Enteritis—either infectious (following *Clostridium difficile* or viral infection with CMV, adenovirus and rotavirus) or related to GvHD.

◆ Neutropenic colitis (typhlitis).

◆ Ileus—mulitfactorial, including sepsis, opioid analgesia, GvHD and electrolyte imbalance.

◆ Perforation due to ulceration secondary to GvHD, infections (e.g. CMV) and long-term steroid use.

◆ GI haemorrhage—common post transplant. May be secondary to GvHD (the majority of cases), peptic ulcer disease, infective mucosal ulceration (CMV, adenovirus) and mucosal injury due to chemotherapy. Coexisting thrombocytopenia increases risk.

Treatment options are limited as diffuse involvement of the GI tract is typical in these conditions with the exception of peptic ulcer disease, haemorrhage from which may be managed endoscopically. GvHD is treated with additional immunosuppression.

Renal tract

Acute renal failure (ARF)

ARF is common with some degree of impairment affecting up to 80% of patients within the first month. Aetiologies include sepsis, drug nephrotoxicity (particularly from myeloablative chemotherapy, and antibiotics such as aminoglycosides, amphotericin, and aciclovir) and hypotension with additional patient group-specific causes.

ARF due to tumour lysis syndrome (previously discussed) and the toxicity of the infused stem cells is seen within the first 5 days (marrow infusion-associated toxicity). Stem cells are stored in dimethyl sulfoxide which may precipitate haemolysis of the cells and lead to acute tubular necrosis (ATN) and ARF on infusion. The effect is potentiated by other risk factors for ATN such as hypovolaemia and acidosis.

Hepatorenal syndrome secondary to VOD is another frequent cause of early ARF. Later causes include HSCT nephropathy, ciclosporin toxicity and thrombotic microangiopathy (all > 4weeks post transplant).

Haemorrhagic cystitis

Haemorrhagic cystitis is seen in around 25% of patients post HSCT. The cause is damage to the bladder urothelium resulting from either from metabolites of chemotherapeutic agents (especially cyclophosphamide and busulfan), radiotherapy, or infection (adenovirus, BK virus, and CMV). Subsequent bleeding leads to obstructive uropathy. Prevention is with superhydration and furosemide, and additionally with mesna following administration of cyclophosphamide or ifosfamide.

Haematological system

The main complications after a transplant will be those relating to pancytopenia. Other specific complications are discussed below.

Thrombotic thrombocytopenic purpura (TTP)

TTP is a disorder of coagulation in which platelets are consumed in microvascular occlusive platelet plugs. Idiopathic TTP is related to an inhibition or deficiency of ADAMTS13 (a metalloproteinase that cleaves von Willibrand factor). Secondary TTP, as occurs in these patients, is thought to be due to an unrelated process, possibly involving chemotherapy-related endothelial damage.

Classically, TTP presents with a pentad of renal failure, fever, thrombocytopenia, fluctuating neurological signs, and microangiopathic haemolytic anaemia (MAHA). Neurological signs and renal failure may however be absent in the post-transplant patient.

Differential diagnoses include ciclosporin toxicity (renal failure, MAHA, and neurological signs) and haemolytic uraemic syndrome (but renal impairment is more pronounced).

Unfortunately the response to traditional therapy with plasma exchange is highly variable when compared to idiopathic TTP (25% versus 90%).

Conclusion

HSCT has revolutionized the treatment of many conditions and is seen by many patients as a miracle cure. Whilst a transplant may induce remission of their disease, the common and potentially life-threatening complications show that it is not without significant risk. It is important to counsel patients and families before such a procedure to reduce the psychological difficulty that may result from a death or debilitating condition, often requiring significant hospital and ITU stay, which may be a direct complication of the transplant and not their original disease.

Bibliography

1. Afessa B, Tefferi A, Hoagland HC, *et al.* (1992). Outcome of recipients of bone marrow transplants who require intensive-care unit support. *Mayo Clin Proc* **67**:117–22.
2. Ho VT, Weller E, Lee SJ, Alyea EP, Antin JH, Soiffer RJ (2001). Prognostic factors for early severe pulmonary complications after haemopoietic stem cell transplantation. *Biol Blood Marrow Transplant* **7**:223–9.
3. Kotloff RM, Ahya VN, Crawford SW (2004). Pulmonary complcations of solid organ and hematopoietic stem cell transplantation. *Am J Respir Crit Care Med* **170**:22–48.
4. Leung AN, Gosselin MV, Napper CH, *et al.* (1999). Pulmonary infections after bone marrow transplantation: clinical and radiographic findings. *Radiology* **210**:699–710.
5. Ljungman P, Urbano-Ispizua A, Cavazzana-Calvo M, *et al.* (2006). Allogeneic and autologous transplantation for haematological diseases, solid tumours and immune disorders: definitions and current practice in Europe. *Bone Marrow Transplant* **37**:439–49.
6. Nichols WG (2003). Management of infectious complications in the haematopoietic stem cell transplant recipient. *J Intensive Care Med* **18**:295–312.
7. Pawson H, Jayawera A, Wigmore T (2008). Intensive care management of patients following haematopoietic stem cell transplantation. *Curr Anaesth Crit Care* **19**:80–90.
8. Raman T, Marak PE (2006). Fungal infections in bone marrow transplant recipients. *Expert Opin Pharmacother* **184**:350–4.
9. Sable BA, Donowitz GR (1994). Infections in bone marrow transplant recipients. *Clin Infect Dis* **29**:273–81.
10. Soubani AO (2006). Critical care considerations of haematopoietic stem cell transplantation. *Crit Care Med* **34**:251–67.
11. Soubani AO, Miller KB, Hassoun PM (1996). Pulmonary complications of bone marrow transplantation. *Chest* **109**:1066–77.
12. Soubani AO, Kseibi E, Bander JJ, *et al.* (2004). Outcome and prognostic factors of haemopoietic stem cell transplantation recipients admitted to a medical ICU. *Chest* **126**:1604–11.
13. Wah TM, Moss HA, Robertson RJ, Barnard DL (2003). Pulmonary complications following bone marrow transplantation. *Br J Radiol* **76**:373–9.
14. Winston DJ (1993). Prophylaxis and treatment of infection in the bone marrow transplant recipient. *Curr Clin Topics Infect Dis* **13**:293–321.

Chapter 14

Outcomes for cancer in intensive care

Katie Blightman and Tim Wigmore

Introduction

Intensive care provides advanced support for patients with a reasonable prospect of recovery from a reversible disease process and is an expensive and scarce resource. This poses the dilemma of whether admission should be available, or indeed appropriate, for those patients with significant or terminal underlying disease. Cancer is one such disease and is present in 15% of patients admitted to European intensive care units (ICUs). They are heavy consumers of resources and are presenting in greater numbers to critical care due to longer survival times and increasing incidence.

Traditionally there has been a reluctance to escalate levels of care in cancer patients due to the perception of high short-term mortality. The presence of cancer is frequently employed as a reason to refuse admission to ICU and patients with other significant chronic illnesses are still more likely to be admitted. However, in reality, mortality rates for patients with cancer who are admitted to ICU vary widely, reflecting the heterogeneous nature of both the disease and the cause of clinical deterioration, and actually show a steadily improving trend. The evidence is evolving towards the need for a less blanket admission or refusal policy and to identify those in whom ICU admission is likely to prove beneficial.

Overall trends in mortality

Over the last 40 years there have been huge improvements in 5-year survival for most cancer types as shown in Table 14.1. This reflects the growth in new targeted therapies and improvements in the management of treatment and disease-related complications.

This has been matched by improvements in survival of patients with a primary diagnosis of cancer admitted to critical care, with studies over the last 25 years showing a progressive decrease in mortality for cancer as a whole (Table 14.2) and more specifically for those with haematological malignancies (see Table 14.3).

Specific prognostic factors

Cancer type and progression

Many studies have evaluated cancer as an independent risk factor for poor outcome in ICU and shown that the degree of acute physiological disturbance is far more predictive than the presence of cancer itself. That said, cancer can affect any organ system and

Table 14.1 Mortality trends in cancer

Cancer type	5-year survival, early 2000s	5-year survival, early 1970s
Breast	80%	52%
Bowel	50%	25%
Hodgkin's lymphoma	80%	25%
Non-Hodgkin's lymphoma	50%	30%
Leukaemia	40%	10%

manifests a wide range of behaviours. The fundamental difference in prognosis is between solid and haematological tumours.

Solid tumours

Patients with solid tumours (such as renal, lung, or ovarian cancer) are more likely to be admitted to ICU following surgery than for a medical complication. They have similar severity scores and general profiles to the non-cancer population, and generally have comparable hospital and intensive care mortality rates.

Haematological tumours

Patients with hematological malignancies have historically had higher mortality and longer-term survival was often low. Patients tend to be more severely unwell at presentation to critical care than those with solid tumours, but although overall mortality remains higher than for the general ICU population (43% vs. 21%, Intensive Care National Audit & Research Centre (ICNARC) 2010) prognosis has improved over the last 20 years (Table 14.3). Contrary to popular belief, ICU mortality of these patients is not predicted by the long-term prognosis of the underlying haematological malignancy and its premorbid severity (although they are obviously linked to long-term survival).

This improvement probably reflects the use of marrow growth factors (e.g. granulocyte colony-stimulating factor, GCSF) that shorten periods of neutropenia, the development of novel antibiotics and antifungals, together with a general changes in ICU care (such as goal-directed treatment of sepsis, and strategies to limit ventilator-associated lung injury).

Haemopoietic stem cell transplantation (HSCT)

Those patients requiring HSCT represent a separate subgroup. They are made more vulnerable to systemic illness from infection due to treatment-related marrow suppression and up to 40% of all HSCT recipients may require ICU following their transplant, most often within the first 100 days.

Table 14.2 Hospital mortality of patients with a primary diagnosis of cancer admitted to intensive care

Year	Hospital mortality	Study
1982	55%	Hauser et al. (1982)
1998	42%	Groeger et al. (1998)
2009	30%	Soares et al. (2010)

Table 14.3 Hospital mortality of patients with a primary diagnosis of haematological malignancy admitted to intensive care

	Hospital mortality (%)	Study
1986	82	Lloyd Thomas et al. (1988)
1990	85	Brunet et al. (1990)
2002	54	Benoit et al. (2003)
2009	58	ICNARC[a] Case Mix Programme (2009)

[a]Intensive Care National Audit & Research Centre.

Allogenic transplants pose an additional risk as recipients require the use of post-engraftment immunosuppression to prevent or ameliorate graft-versus-host disease. They tend to present more often to intensive care than autografts and to be higher acuity on presentation.

Generally the mortality in patients receiving HSCT has trended downwards and reasons for this are likely to be multifactorial, including the use of newer treatments involving the use of non-myeloablative transplants which require less aggressive conditioning regimens. However, morbidity and mortality remain high, particularly in those requiring mechanical ventilation, where it is quoted at 70–90%, double that of those not requiring it.

Cancer progression

The progression of cancer is usually associated with a longer-term worsened outcome. With specific cancers such as lung cancer the extent of chest involvement due to disease progression is an obvious influencing factor on requirements for respiratory support and in turn survival to ICU discharge.

Metastatic disease

The presence of metastases usually suggests advanced disease which is less modifiable. Generally this will herald a new stage in the disease process and may alter treatment goals. Significant physiological impairment may arise from the presence of lung and liver involvement. Whilst the presence of metastases has been shown to be an adverse prognostic indicator for hospital survival for patients with solid tumours, there has been contesting evidence to suggest that neither progression of solid tumour disease nor the presence of metastases are associated with increased shorter-term mortality in ICU.

Specific ICU factors

As a broad diagnosis, cancer does not necessarily mean a worse outcome from intensive care and although consideration of the type and progression of the cancer may help in overall prognostication, we need to look elsewhere for ICU-specific factors.

Age

Cancer is a prevalent disease in the elderly, a group making up an increasing percentage of the population. Whilst age should not be a preclusion to intensive care treatment, a recent study showed that patients older than 60 admitted to ICU with cancer had a higher mortality than their younger counterparts The difference seemed to result from those patients with severe comorbidity; elderly patients with a good performance status and lacking severe comorbidities had similar outcomes to their younger counterparts.

Length of stay

A prolonged stay on ICU increases the risk of adverse events. Very long-stay patients in the general adult population have been shown to have a worse outcome if ventilated for greater than 90 days, required inotrope support or renal replacement therapy after day 30, or were immunosuppressed. However, within the cancer population only a minority (15%) have a prolonged length of stay (>21 days). In a recently published study, the recorded hospital and 6-month mortality in this long-stay group were similar to those of patients spending shorter periods on ICU (50% and 60% respectively). In addition, longer-term prognosis was also reasonable with a reported hospital discharge mortality of 18%, suggesting that prolonged ICU admission in isolation should not be used as the decider in continuance of treatment.

Specific treatments

Chemotherapy regimens have been expanded and refined over the years but still cause many adverse side effects including severe end-organ damage. Careful monitoring should be maintained but simply being in ICU does not preclude administration of ongoing chemotherapy treatment regimens, and with acute presentations of certain cancers may represent the only chance of survival. Similarly, the recent administration of chemotherapy does not preclude admission to ICU and some studies have actually found this to be a good prognostic indicator.

Radiotherapy, either curative or palliative, is widely incorporated in certain cancer treatment programmes for both solid tumour and haematological cancer types. Acute complications (particularly bone marrow suppression) within the first few weeks following therapy may require ICU support. Longer-term problems include mucositis, gut disturbances, pneumonitis, and tissue fibrosis. Improving understanding and increasingly targeted therapy may translate into a lesser risk of end-organ damage.

Need for mechanical ventilation

Respiratory failure is a common reason for admission to ICU. It is usually secondary to sepsis, an inflammatory reaction, cardiac failure, or localized tumour involvement. The institution or recommencing of mechanical ventilation for respiratory failure in cancer sufferers is associated with a poorer outcome, although recent ICNARC case-mix data for haemato-oncological admissions to ICU showed that mechanical ventilation within 24 hours was not linked to increased ICU mortality once other prognostic factors had been taken into account. Instituting non-invasive ventilation (NIV) has been shown to reduce the need for intubation and ventilation although it must be recognized that as many as 50% of patients may fail NIV which in itself may worsen their overall outcome by delaying appropriate aggressive treatment. Prompt referral and review of patients with deteriorating respiratory function is paramount. In common with all critically ill patients, the use of lung protective ventilatory strategies has resulted in overall improvement in survival for patients with acute lung injury and respiratory distress in recent years.

Acute kidney injury

Acute renal failure poses particular problems as it may continue as a persistent pathology which limits treatment options. It may be secondary to a wide variety of insults including sepsis, nephrotoxic pharmaceuticals, tumour lysis syndrome, and tumour-related obstruction. Whilst isolated renal failure is not predictive of poor outcome, the need for renal replacement therapy (RRT) is associated with a higher predicted mortality than in the non-cancer population, and as a contributing organ failure it is been shown as an independent risk factor for mortality. In the context of sepsis, the outcome for cancer patients requiring RRT has improved but the occurrence with other organ failures or the development of renal failure whilst in critical care are bad prognostic indicators.

Multiorgan failure

In common with other groups of patients the key to predicting ICU outcome for cancer patients is the degree and progress of physiological derangement. Multiorgan failure is a strong predictor of poor outcome and both ICU and hospital mortality increase with number of organ failures present on admission. In those with greater than two organ failures, mortality may exceed 75%, higher than in the non-cancer population. This is especially true for haematological malignancies (Table 14.4).

Moreover, progression of organ failure has been shown to be closely correlated with survival. Deterioration in organ failure scores or the development of new organ failures by 72 hours following admission to ICU predicts a poor outcome.

Sepsis and neutropenia

It is estimated that 8.5% of all cancer deaths are attributable to sepsis. The mortality associated with severe sepsis in general ICU patients is still around 30–50% although

Table 14.4 Hospital mortality rates for patients admitted to ICU with haematological malignancy, ICNARC Case Mix Programme 2009

Number of organ failures	Hospital mortality (%)
0	33.8
1	50.3
2	68.3
3	83.9
4	92.3
5	98.8

most recent studies have reported a significant improvement probably due to prompt and aggressive resuscitation and early appropriate antibiotic use. The Sepsis Occurrence in Acutely ill Patients (SOAP) study demonstrated that cancer patients are more frequently hospitalized and admitted to intensive care with sepsis when compared with the general population and that overall the outcome in those with solid tumours was similar to non-cancer patients, although those with haematological cancers had a far greater relative risk.

Neutropenic sepsis occurs particularly in the haemato-oncological population or those who have undergone stem cell transplantation. Interestingly, neutropenia per se may have little influence on outcome. Neutropenia is far less important as a predictor of mortality, even within specific diseases such as leukaemia, lymphoma, and lung cancer, than the number of organ failures contributing to physiological disturbance. In patients admitted to intensive care for support with septic shock there is often no difference in mortality between neutropenic and non-neutropenic groups. Evidence also suggests neither the severity nor duration of neutropenia has a great impact on mortality, although recovery from neutropenia is a good prognostic sign.

Intercurrent acute illness

Patients with cancer are vulnerable to the same pathological insults that might lead to ICU admission as the general population. Whilst there has been little interest to date in examining outcome in cancer patients admitted to ICU for supportive therapy following unrelated life-threatening events such as myocardial infarction, pulmonary embolus, exacerbations of airways disease, or polytrauma, the diagnosis of cancer may impact on whether full treatment is offered due to a perception of a likely poor outcome. However, the fact that large multicentre studies such as the SOAP study report similar mortality outcomes for cancer and non-cancer patients presenting to ICU would seem to mitigate in their favour.

Predictive scoring models

Scoring models have been developed to help quantify severity of illness and predict outcome in populations of patients. Most models are derived from large databases of general ICU patients and unsurprisingly fit these populations best. Cancer is a catch-all term that encompasses numerous disease processes and most established ICU outcome models are less accurate in this group.

The majority of ICUs currently use the familiar systems of acute physiology and chronic health evaluation (APACHE), simplified acute physiology score (SAPS), mortality probability model (MPM), or the ICNARC Case Mix Programme model. Versions of these well-established traditional scoring systems have tended to underestimate mortality in the cancer population requiring intensive care although they still adequately identify those patients at very high risk of dying.

Cancer-focused mortality models have been designed to include specific disease-related factors to help more accurately predict outcome. The cancer mortality model (CMM) includes HSCT, intracranial mass effect, disease progression and relapse, as well as evaluation of severity of illness with physiological data. This has been extensively compared against traditional models but unfortunately has not been found to be prognostically more useful (in this case tending to overestimate mortality). It may be that subgroups of cancer patients (e.g. haematological malignancies versus solid tumours) are simply too disparate to be suitable for analysis with one scoring system.

Whilst scoring systems may provide some indication of the likely outcome of a patient they cannot be used for triage decisions. They do, however, highlight the importance of the degree of acute physiological derangement and organ failures as being the major influencing factors of outcome.

Resuscitation and palliation

Whilst it is fair to argue that outcome from intensive care in cancer patients has become more positive, a realistic approach must still be adopted towards dealing with end-of-life decisions or limitations on therapy. Cardiopulmonary resuscitation (CPR) overall offers limited recovery and cancer patients are likely to fair worse. As with other groups of patients, CPR is generally most effective and appropriate in patients who suffer a cardiac arrest due to an acute insult. Those with metastatic disease are least likely to regain spontaneous circulation and survive to discharge. There is a notable difference between solid and haematological cancers with outcome less favourable in the latter group.

Death is still an emotive and difficult subject within this particular patient group. Many institutions have established care protocols (such as the Liverpool Care Pathway) to assist healthcare professionals dealing with palliation. Once a decision has been made to discontinue aggressive therapy there should be emphasis on the alleviation of ongoing suffering. It is still appropriate that this care takes place in the ICU environment providing suitable arrangements can be made.

Re-admission to ICU

Follow-up studies have shown that whilst survival outcome from ICU in the cancer population is improving, malignant disease is still the most frequent cause of death following ICU discharge while in hospital and at 1-year discharge. The requirement for re-admission predicts a poor outcome in the absence of an acutely remediable cause and palliation may be appropriate.

Conclusion

Despite historic reticence to admit patients with cancer to intensive care, there is now good evidence that this is unwarranted. Traditional markers of mortality have lost much of their value. The characteristics of the malignancy (including source and metastasis) are often not associated with likelihood of survival in ICU and scoring systems are also of little help in prediction. Solid tumours in particular should be treated as with any other chronic disease. The key to prognosis is in the degree of acute physiological derangement that leads to critical care admission. In all but the most extreme cases, a reasonable approach should be a trial of organ support and aggressive management with frequent and repeated reassessment of the degree of organ dysfunction.

Bibliography

1. Benoit DD, Vanderwoude KH, Decruyenaere JM, Hoste EA, Colardyn FA (2003). Outcome and early prognostic indicators in patients with a hematological malignancy admitted to the intensive care unit for a life threatening complication. *Crit Care Med* **31**(1):320–1.

2. Brunet F, Lanore JJ, Dhainaut JF, *et al.* (1990). Is intensive care justified for patients with haematological malignancies. *Intensive Care Med* **16**(5):291–7.

3. Cancer Research UK (2007). *Trends in cancer mortality - UK statistics.* Available at:http://info. cancerresearchuk.org/cancerstats/mortality/timetrends/ (accessed 15 October 2009).

4. den Boer S, Keizer N, de Jonge E (2005). Performance of prognostic models in critically ill cancer patients: a review. *Critical Care* **9**(4), R458–463 doi.10.1186/cc3765.

5. Depuydt PO, Benoit DD, Vanderwoude KH, Decruyenacre JM, Colardyn FA (2004). Outcome in non-invasively and invasively ventilated haematologic patients with respiratory failure. *Crit Care Med* **36**(10):2766–72.

6. Groeger JS, Lemeshow S, Price K, *et al.* (1998). Multicentre outcome study of cancer patients admitted to the intensive care unit: a probability of mortality model. *J Clin Oncol* **16**(2):761–70.

7. Hampshire PA, Welch CA, McCrossan LA, Francis K, Harrison DA (2009). Admission factors associated with hospital mortality in patients with haematological malignancy admitted to UK adult general critical care units: a secondary analysis of the ICNARC Case Mix Programme Database. *Critical Care* **13**(4):R137 doi.10.1186/cc8016.

8. Hauser MJ, Tabak J, Baier H (1982). Survival of patients with cancer in a medical critical care unit. *Arch Intern Med* **142**(3):527–9.

9. Lecuyer L, Chevret S, Theiery G, Darmon M, Schlemmer B, Azoulay E (2007). The ICU Trail: A new admission policy for cancer patients requiring mechanical ventilation. *Crit Care Med* **35**(3):808–14.

10. Lloyd Thomas AR, Wright I, Lister TA, Hinds CJ (1988). Prognosis of patients receiving intensive care for life-threatening medical complications of haematological malignancy. *BMJ* **290**:1025–9.

11. Pene F, Aubron C, Azoulay E, *et al.* (2006). Outcome of critically ill allogenic HSCT patients: A reappraisal of indications for organ failure supports *J Clin Oncol* **24**(4):643–9.

12. Reisfield GM, Wallace SK, Munsell MF, Webb FJ, Alvarez ER, Wilson G (2006). Survival in cancer patients undergoing in-hospital cardiopulmonary resuscitation: a meta-analysis. *Resuscitation* **71**(2):152–60.

13. Soares M, Fontes F, Dantas J, *et al.* (2004). Performance of six severity-of-illness scores in cancer patients requiring admission to the intensive care unit: A prospective observational study *Critical Care,* **8**(4):R194–203 doi.10.1186/cc2870.

14. Soares M, Salluh JI, Torres VB, Leale JV, Spector N (2008). Short-and long-term outcomes of critically ill patients with cancer and prolonged ICU length of stay. *Chest* **134**(3):520–6.

15. Soares M, Caruso P, Silva E, *et al.* (2010). Characteristics and outcomes of patients with cancer requiring admission to intensive care units: A prospective multicentre study. *Crit Care Med* **38**(1):9–15.

16. Taccone ST, Artigas AA, Sprung CL, Moreno R, Sakr Y, Vincent JL (2009). Characteristics and outcomes of cancer patients in European ICUs. *Crit Care* **13**(1):R15 doi.10.1186/cc7713.

Chapter 15

Chemotherapy and radiotherapy: considerations for the intensivist and anaesthetist

Craig Carr

Introduction

Whilst anaesthetists and intensivists frequently enjoy a sound grasp of the implications of surgery and its sequelae, there is generally less awareness of the implications of chemotherapy and radiotherapy. However, with an increasing number of patients presenting post- or pericancer treatment, an awareness of the risks of anaesthesia and critical care to patients who have received chemotherapy and radiotherapy as well of the risks presented by the chemotherapy and radiotherapy to the patients' health is crucial.

With over 200 chemotherapeutic agents and multiple different radiotherapy regimens in use, this chapter will provide a rudimentary overview of the types of treatments in common use and outline the spectrum of the common toxicities of anticancer therapies.

Chemotherapy

Cancer treatment may be intended to be:

- *Cytostatic* preventing proliferation of malignant cells
- *Cytotoxic* resulting in the death of tumour cells or both cytostatic and cytotoxic.

Cytostatic therapies such as anti-oestrogen therapies for breast tumours or anti-androgen therapies for prostate tumours are targeted therapies blocking receptors in hormone-sensitive tumours. As these hormone receptors have limited distribution about the body these treatments tend to have fewer systemic side effects. However, adverse effects can occur (e.g. thrombosis with tamoxifen).

Most cytotoxic treatments used affect normal as well as malignant cell replication processes. Death of some healthy cells is inevitable during chemotherapy and radiotherapy; the guiding principle of treatment is that higher death rates are expected in the malignant cell population owing to their higher rate of cell division.

Anticancer therapies may be described as:

- Adjuvant
- Neoadjuvant
- Concomitant

- Induction
- Consolidation
- Intensification
- First-line, second-line, etc.
- Palliative.

1 *Adjuvant therapy* is additional treatment to reduce the risk of relapse or recurrence after the primary curative therapy (usually surgery or radiotherapy) has been completed. Occasionally, but less correctly, adjuvant therapy is also used to describe treatments in non-curative treatment programmes, aimed at prolonging survival if not achieving cure. Examples include:

  - Radiotherapy to reduce the risk of recurrence of a breast tumour following complete surgical excision of the tumour.

  - Hormonal control of a metastatic prostatic cancer not cured by the main treatment modality. However, in the strictest sense this is not adjuvant but maintenance treatment.

2 *Neoadjuvant therapy* is non-curative treatment given to reduce the disease mass prior to the main intended potentially curative therapy, e.g. administration of chemotherapy to shrink a tumour before surgery. This may convert an irresectable tumour into a resectable one or allow the preservation of important structures at the time of surgery to minimize patient disability afterwards. Not all neoadjuvant therapies have a proven survival benefit and many studies are ongoing to work out who best benefits from this approach.

3 *Induction therapy* is treatment given with the aim of inducing a remission or cure of the cancer and is usually applied to haemato-oncological conditions.

4 *Consolidation* or *intensification* therapy is treatment given once remission has been achieved and aims to sustain or prolong the remission. It is most commonly applied to treatment of leukaemias.

5 *Concomitant treatments* run at the same time as one another, e.g. the administration of multiple chemotherapy agents in a treatment regimen or in combination with radiotherapy. Where several chemotherapeutic agents are used in combination as part of a single regimen, an acronym is often applied (Table 15.1).

6 *First-line chemotherapy* is the standard treatment regimen given to treat an individual tumour on the basis of it having the highest likelihood of achieving a cure or disease control.

7 *Second-line chemotherapy* is given if the tumour fails to respond to first-line treatment, becomes resistant to first-line therapy, or if following remission achieved with first-line chemotherapy, there is later relapse.

8 *Palliative therapy* is given to reduce the symptoms caused by the tumour rather than to prolong life. This may include radiotherapy to treat bony metastases and pain.

Table 15.1 Commonly used acronyms for chemotherapy regimes in the UK. Many other acronyms exist. The use of letters in acronyms is inconsistent; sometimes the same letter is used to represent a generic name and sometimes a brand name for a different generic drug, e.g. V = vincristine, etoposide (VP-16), and vinblastine

Chemotherapy regimen acronym	Drugs associated with acronym
AC—breast cancer	Adriamycin (doxorubicin), cyclophosphamide
BEACOPP—Hodgkin's disease	Bleomycin, etoposide, Adriamycin (doxorubicin), cyclophosphamide, Oncovin (vincristine), procarbazine, prednisone
BEP—germ cell tumours	Bleomycin, etoposide, platinum agent (cisplatin)
CBV—lymphoma	Cyclophosphamide, BCNU (carmustine), etoposide
CHOP—non-Hodgkin's	Cyclophosphamide, hydroxydoxorubicin (doxorubicin), vincristine (Oncovin), prednisone
R-CHOP—B-cell non-Hodgkin's	CHOP + rituximab
FEC—breast	Fluorouracil (5-FU), epirubicin, cyclophosphamide
FLAG-Ida—leukaemia	Fludarabine, Ara-C (cytarabine), G-CSF, Idarubicn
FOLFOX—colorectal tumours	Fluorouracil (5-FU), leucovorin (folinic acid), oxaliplatin
ICE—lymphoma	ifosfamide, carboplatin, etoposide
VAD—myeloma	Vincristine, Adriamycin (doxorubicin), dexamethasone
VIP—germ cell tumours	Etoposide, ifosfamide, platinum agent cisplatin

Classification of chemotherapeutic agents

Investigation of cellular physiology, biochemistry, and genetics has seen an explosion in the understanding of tumour cell behaviour and resulted in targeted therapies to control this. Different drugs are often used in combination to achieve better outcomes (Table 15.1). Individual drugs can generally be classified into broad categories based on their mode of action or chemical composition, yet many drugs have several different actions and to classify them to one category only is inaccurate. For example, etoposide is both a topoisomerase II inhibitor and an alkylating agent. For the sake of simplicity, we shall list only 40 or so commonly used drugs and categorize each only once (Table 15.2).

Radiotherapy

Irradiation of malignant tissues induces tumour cell death by irreparably damaging the malignant cells' DNA. The radiation causes direct ionization of water molecules within the cells generating oxygen free radical species that damage cellular DNA. The involvement of reactive oxygen species in this process means hypoxic cells are several times more resistant to radiotherapy than well oxygenated ones. Therefore, haemoglobin values should be maintained at higher than 10g/dl in patients receiving radiation therapies.

◆ *External beam radiotherapy* with X-rays primarily damages replicating cells and so the total dose of radiation is usually divided into several fractions to ensure that all tumour cells are in division at some point during the treatment. By contrast, gamma irradiation

Table 15.2 Chemotherapeutic agents, their mechanisms of action, and common side effects

Category	Mode of action	Examples	Main toxicities
Alkylating agents	Highly chemically reactive and form covalent bonds with DNA inducing breaks and formation of new cross-links. This induces cell death and apoptosis	Busulfan Chlorambucil cyclophosphamide Ifosfamide Mitomycin	Myelosuppression Thrombosis Mucositis Diarrhoea Neuropathy Electrolyte disturbance
Platinum-based agents	Enter cells and form chemically reactive compounds that form covalent bonds with DNA inducing breakage and new cross-link formation. Similar mechanism of action to alkylating agents	Carboplatin, Cisplatin Oxaliplatin	Myelosuppression Nephrotoxicity Neurotoxicity Peripheral neuropathy Cardiac arrhythmias
Antimetabolites	Act as inhibitors of enzymes processing the naturally occurring purines and pyrimidines in the nucleic acid synthesis pathway. Furthermore, they can be incorporated into the DNA and RNA resulting in aberrant synthesis resulting in cell death. In addition, anti-folate drugs can be used to reduce the regeneration of reduced folate necessary for thymidine synthesis	Antipyrimidines antimetabolites Cytarabine Gemcitabine Capecitabine (a 5-FU precursor) 5-fluorouracil Antipurine antimetabolites 5mercapto-purine 6-thioguanine Fludarabine Pentostatin Antifolate antimetabolite: methotrexate	Myelosuppression (For methotrexate only, folinic acid 'rescue therapy' may be administered following treatment to reduce the severity of myelosuppression. However, once established there is no advantage to be gained from administration) Diarrhoea Cardiac arrhythmias Pneumonitis

(Continued)

Table 15.2 (*continued*)

Category	Mode of action	Examples	Main toxicities
Cytotoxic antibiotics—anthracyclines and anthraquinolones	Multiple concurrent cytotoxic effects with inhibition of DNA and RNA polymerization, generation of oxygen free radicals, induction of DNA breakage, disruption of cell and mitochondrial membranes, and cell death	Daunorubicin, Doxorubicin, Epirubicin, Idarubicin Bleomycin	Cardiomyopathy Pulmonary fibrosis colitis
Microtubule poisons	Taxanes increase tubulin assembly but inhibit microtubule disassembly leading to cell death	Docetaxel Paclitaxel	Pneumonitis Bronchospasm Ischaemic colitis Conduction defects
	Vinca alkaloids bind to tubulin and prevent it incorporating into microtubules also leading to cell death	Vincristine Vinblastine	Thrombosis Paralytic ileus Nausea Urinary retention Myelosuppression
Topoisomerase inhibitors	Interfere with the control process for unwinding of super-coiled DNA and with controlled breakage of DNA strands and thus interfere with cell function and replication	Topoisomerase I inhibitors Irinotecan Topotecan Topoisomerase II inhibitors Etoposide Some anthracyclines	Acute cholinergic syndrome Hypotension Myelosuppression Myelosuppression Ovarian failure Diarrhoea Nausea
Tyrosine kinase inhibitors	Inhibit tyrosine kinase directly or via antagonism of tyrosine kinase linked membrane receptors thereby reducing mitogenesis	Imatinib Erlotinib Sunitinib Gefitinib Cetuximab Traztuzumab (Herceptin)	Cardiac failure Pneumonitis Diarrhoea Bowel perforation

Category	Description	Agents	Side effects
Hormone therapies	Some tumours (primarily breast and prostate) express oestrogen or androgen receptors whose stimulation by these hormones induces or accelerates tumour cell growth. Blockage of these receptors by antagonists or reduction of hormone production by prevention of the conversion of hormone precursors to the active hormone can result in tumour cell stasis and shrinkage	Oestrogen receptor antagonists Tamoxifen	Thrombosis Endometrial ca
		Aromatase inhibitors block the conversion of androgens to oestrogen and can be used as second-line treatments if there is a failure of receptor antagonist therapy Letrozole Exemestane Anastrozole	Oedema Hypertension Dyspnoea Headache Arthralgia Hot flushes Constipation
		Luteinizing hormone releasing hormone (LHRH) analogues induce anergy in the pituitary with downregulation of release of LH and FSH, reduction in ovarian oestrogen/progesterone and testicular androgen synthesis Goserelin Buserelin	Oedema Headache Mood changes Acne Sweats Vaginitis Sweating
		Anti-androgens block androgen receptors Cyproterone	Hepatotoxicity Adrenal failure Thrombosis
Biological and immunomodulatory therapies	Recombinant human cytokines such as interleukin-2 and interferon-alpha as well as tumour vaccines and antitumour monoclonal antibody preparations are used to attempt to enhance the cytotoxic immune system's kill rate of malignant cells. In addition, monoclonal antibodies may be used to block the receptors downregulating cytotoxic T cells	IL-2 Interferon-alpha BCG Ipilimumab Dendritic cell vaccines	

tends to be given in single undivided doses. By directing the radiation beam through multiple planes which intersect within the tumour, it is possible to minimize irradiation of surrounding tissues whilst maximizing damage to the tumour.

- *Radioactive implants* may also be stereotactically placed into tumours (brachytherapy) in order to provide continuous irradiation for a predetermined period with a maximum dose to the tumour and a lower dose to surrounding previously healthy tissues. The implants may be left *in situ* if their radioactive half-life is sufficiently short or may be removed if the half-life is long. When radioactive sources are *in situ*, there may be limits placed on the duration of contact with the patient to minimize radiation exposure to others. Thus, it is important to consider the postoperative care required for a patient based on their history and comorbidities; if the patient warrants admission to the intensive care or high dependency unit, it is possible that the patient will not be suitable for the modality of brachytherapy planned. Good communication with the clinical oncology and surgery teams is recommended to avoid this becoming apparent only once the sources have been ordered and involved and unnecessary planning undertaken.

- *Total body irradiation (TBI)* may be undertaken to facilitate donor cell engraftment in haemopoietic stem cell transplant procedures. In high-dose therapy, marrow ablation and residual tumour cell death are facilitated whereas in lower-dose therapy, immunosuppression rather than marrow ablation is anticipated. Both high-dose and lower-dose therapy can have deleterious effects on the patient and both require medical supportive therapy to minimize subsequent morbidity and mortality.

Systemic side effects of chemotherapy and radiotherapy

Even with fractionation of doses and minimization of exposure of healthy tissues, certain tissue types have a poorer recovery following radiation exposure than others. Wherever possible, radiation doses to the kidney, brain, lung, small intestine, and spinal cord should be minimized for this reason. However, even with careful planning, long-term damage to healthy tissues can arise and side effects of radiotherapy which are pertinent to the anaesthetist or intensive care physician may develop. The side effects of chemotherapy are less predictable than those of radiotherapy and a higher proportion of the damage caused will reverse with time.

As a general principle, whenever two therapies or treatment modalities with similar side-effect profiles are used in combination, both the risk of realizing a side effect and the severity of the side effect will increase.

Cardiovascular

Cardiovascular side effects of chemotherapeutic agents are relatively common but generally minor such as flushing or relative hypotension around the time of administration. However, some important and potentially lethal side effects are seen such as:

- Venous and arterial thromboses
- Myocardial ischaemia

- Arrhythmias
- Pericarditis and pericardial fibrosis
- Tamponade
- Myocardial fibrosis
- Cardiomyopathy
- Heart failure
- Hypotension and hypertension.

These side effects are generally associated with specific therapeutic agents and may be dose limiting such as cardiac failure as with anthracyclines and imatinib or hypertension and ischaemia with cisplatin. The use of several cardiotoxic treatments in one patient increases the likelihood of each individual cardiotoxic effect and thus dose modification may be required when using combinations of drugs such as anthracyclines and taxanes or trastuzumab. Similarly, the use of chest radiotherapy increases the likelihood of developing cardiac toxicities associated with adjuvant chemotherapy.

As well as causing direct cardiotoxicity per se, many drugs increase the metabolic demands on the heart and make the unveiling of pre-existing underlying ischaemic heart disease more likely. Whilst most cardiotoxic side effects are seen around the time of treatment administration, late cardiotoxicity such as dilated cardiomyopathies can develop months or years later.

Radiotherapy to the chest which passes through the mediastinum can result in both acute and chronic cardiac problems. Acute pericarditis, arrhythmias, acute coronary artery thrombosis, and cardiac effusions even to the extent of tamponade can occur. In the longer term, constrictive pericarditis and coronary artery stenoses even in the absence of other risk factors can develop. This risk increases rather than diminishes with the passage of time and latent ischaemic heart disease should always be considered during the assessment even of apparently fit patients when they have a history of past chest radiotherapy, e.g. for breast cancer or lymphoma.

Risk factors for the development of cardiac damage following chest radiotherapy include left-sided therapy, concomitant smoking, concomitant cardiotoxic chemotherapy, and higher dose treatments.

Respiratory

Respiratory side effects during chemotherapy are relatively common (around 10% of patients). They can be directly related to the drugs administered or indirect, e.g. the development of infective complications secondary to drug-induced immunosuppression or pulmonary embolism secondary to drug-induced thromboses.

General drug-induced complications include:

- Bronchospasm
- Pleurisy
- Pneumonitis

- Fibrosing alveolitis
- Pleural effusions.

Frequently, at the time of acute presentation, there is no indication as to the underlying respiratory problem and tests are required to differentiate inflammation secondary to infection from inflammation secondary to adverse drug reactions. Chest computed tomography (CT), bronchoalveolar lavage and bacteriological and immunological tests for viruses, bacteria, and fungi are indicated. An open mind should be kept to several different factors coexisting such as there being a drug-induced pneumonitis with secondary bacterial infection. Rare infecting organisms such as *tuberculosis, Pneumocystis,* and *Aspergillus* are all relatively common pathogens in immunosuppressed patients and need to be excluded. Similarly, herpes, cytomegalovirus (CMV), respiratory syncytial virus, and influenza should be excluded as causes of inflammation as specific treatments are available for each.

When presented with a patient in respiratory failure whilst on chemotherapy, establishing the cause not only allows appropriate treatment but also reduces the risk of further harm such as a massive intraoperative thromboembolism which might have been prevented by preoperative inferior vena cava filter insertion or the development of worsening fibrosing alveolitis secondary to the use of unnecessary oxygen supplementation in a patient with previous bleomycin exposure (Figure 15.1). Except for emergency procedures, undertaking anaesthesia on such patients without first elucidating the cause of the problem and instituting appropriate treatment is unwarranted.

The likelihood of developing pulmonary toxicity secondary to chemotherapy is also increased whenever concomitant radiotherapy has also been administered to the chest.

The majority of patients with radiation to their chest will develop a degree of acute inflammation which may result in a dry cough and mild dyspnoea which resolves over a period of 2–3 months. Unfortunately, as many as 10% of patients following radical chest radiotherapy will develop symptomatic radiation pneumonitis. This is a progressive chronic pneumonitis which may onset several months to over a year post-irradiation.

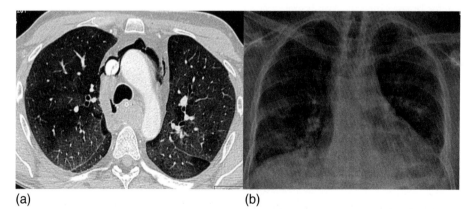

(a) (b)

Fig. 15.1 Heterogenous interstitial inflammatory changes seen in acute bleomycin lung toxicity in (a) a CT scan and (b) chest X-ray (CXR). Note the presence of air in the anterior mediastinum and the relative normality of the CXR if only a cursory assessment is undertaken.

This may result in progressive respiratory failure and needs to be differentiated from other treatable pulmonary pathologies such as radiation-induced lung tumours or bronchiectasis, infection, and recurrent chest malignancy. Asymptomatic deterioration in pulmonary function tests is common and should be considered when managing such patients perioperatively for unrelated conditions.

Acute and chronic X-ray changes are common and should be confined to the radiation fields. These may include ground-glass opacification, consolidation and effusions in the acute phase, and consolidation with volume loss and bronchiectasis in the late phase. Enlarging pleural effusions several weeks after radiotherapy has finished are indicative of a separate pathology and should not be attributed to radiotherapy.

In any patient with a history of breathlessness and past chest-radiotherapy, pulmonary function tests including gas transfer should be considered before embarking on anaesthesia. In addition, a thorough cardiac assessment is also warranted.

Renal

Renal tract damage may arise directly as a result of nephrotoxic, glomerulotoxic, or cystotoxic effects of chemotherapeutic drugs as they are filtered or excreted and concentrated in the urine or indirectly through metabolic disturbances secondary to dehydration as a result of reduced intake or diarrhoea and vomiting. Tubular damage may be permanent or temporary and may be exacerbated by the co-administration of other agents such as nephrotoxic antibiotics and non-steroidal anti-inflammatory analgesics. Renal tubular acidosis, Fanconi's syndrome, nephrogenic diabetes insipidus, and hypomagnesaemia are all recognized long-term complications. In addition, rarely, haemolytic-uraemic syndrome and thrombotic thrombocytopenic purpura may result from cisplatin, gemcitabine, and mitomycin administration. This significantly worsens a patient's prognosis during therapy.

Gastrointestinal

Gastrointestinal side effects of chemotherapy are common and varied including:

- Nausea and vomiting
- Diarrhoea
- Constipation
- Mucositis
- Xerostomia (dry mouth)
- Colitis
- Bowel perforation
- Hepatic dysfunction.

Nausea and vomiting are the commonest side effects after chemotherapy and can be acute, delayed, or anticipatory. Prevention and treatment using multiple classes of drugs including steroids, 5HT$_3$ receptor antagonists, and anticholinergics may increase the risk of adverse interactions and events. Examples of problems include the unmasking of relative adrenal insufficiency following protracted dexamethasone administration and acute serotonergic syndromes following high-dose $5HT_3$ receptor antagonist administration combined with fentanyl and tramadol administration during anaesthesia.

Diarrhoea secondary to gastrointestinal mucosal damage is common and if severe (>6 loose stools per day) may become life threatening requiring admission to intensive care for rehydration, electrolyte correction, and management of shock and renal insufficiency. After exclusion of infective causes, administration of high-dose loperamide and octreotide therapy may help to stabilize the patient. Despite intervention, death or long-term gastrointestinal dysfunction may result; post-chemotherapy lactose intolerance and irritable bowel syndrome are both recognized.

Constipation can arise as a (usually) temporary neuropathic effect of vinca alkaloids and thalidomide but more usually results from the administration of opioids and hypomotility agents such as $5HT_3$ receptor antagonist antiemetics and antispasmodics. Obstruction, pseudo-obstruction, and paralytic ileus need to be excluded before aperients and prokinetic agents are administered if an increased risk of bowel perforation is to be avoided.

Mucositis arises when chemotherapy results in damage to the mucous membranes of the oropharynx causing inflammation and ulceration. Secondary infection with *Candida* or herpes simplex virus (HSV) may further exacerbate the problem and prophylactic acyclovir and antifungals are often given. When severe, the risks of malnutrition, dehydration and aspiration are all increased and should be considered when planning anaesthesia or supportive care.

Colitis is an uncommon but potentially life-threatening complication of chemotherapy. *Clostridium difficile* colitis may develop following chemotherapy administration alone but is more common in combination with antibiotics. Other causes of infective colitis should also be considered from common food-poisoning with *Salmonella* and *Campylobacter* to more specific infections with CMV in neutropenic patients. Neutropenic colitis or typhlitis (Figure 15.2) may affect small or large bowel and usually involves the caecum too. It is believed to result from micro-organisms infecting the bowel wall having entered through areas of mucosa damaged by chemotherapy. Infarction, haemorrhage, and perforation may all result. Mortality is high and bowel resection commonly required.

Bowel perforation may result from rapid tumour necrosis after chemotherapy (a hole is left in the bowel wall where previously there was tumour) or, more commonly, an ischaemic perforation may occur secondary to administration of an antiangiogenesis chemotherapeutic agent such as bevacizumab.

Hepatic dysfunction may vary from mild elevations of biochemical markers of liver dysfunction to progressive hepatic venous occlusion with fulminant liver failure and death. In addition, reactivation of viral infections with agents such as EBV, CMV, HSV, and adenovirus as well as *de novo* infections may all occur in immunocompromised patients. Full investigations for infection, thrombotic processes, and cholestasis are required for all but the most minor disturbances of liver function and should include radiological imaging of the liver. Support of blood coagulation, glucose homeostasis, and renal function may all become necessary whilst the underlying problem is managed more specifically.

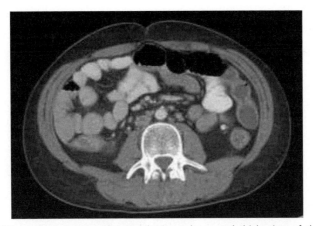

Fig. 15.2 Typhilitis or neutropenic colitis results in oedema and thickening of the caecum and either colon or ileum. Stranding is often seen in the mesentery and mucosal enhancement may be apparent.

Radiation damage to the gastrointestinal tract tends to be localized to the site of delivery. Radiation mucositis, colitis, proctitis, and xerostomia are all well described and can be highly debilitating. Following radiation therapy, the bowel heals with scarring. Attenuation of the mucosal blood supply and localized inflammation may result in perforation or fistula formation. Surgery on bowel that has been previously irradiated is more likely to be associated with bleeding and anastomotic failure.

Neurological

Neurological injury may result from:

♦ The malignant disease process

♦ A direct effect of a chemotherapeutic agent

♦ An infective process secondary to immunosuppression

♦ A consequence of prothrombotic or antithrombotic (usually thrombocytopenic) effects of the chemotherapy.

Peripheral neuropathies including autonomic neuropathies can cause a variety of effects from paraesthesia and pain to cardiac arrhythmias. Central injuries vary from permanent leucoencephalopathy through posterior reversible encephalopathy syndrome (PRES—Figure 15.3) to transient transverse myelitis. Manifestations are extremely diverse and include reduced consciousness, behavioural disturbances, blindness, seizures, and ataxia.

Whenever symptoms of neurological injury are present, full investigations should be conducted to elucidate the aetiology and to guide management and prognosis. Where doubt exists, even if disability is sudden and profound, full supportive intensive therapy should be offered until such time as reversibility has been excluded. As one example, the seizures, blindness, and reduced consciousness seen with PRES can resolve completely but may take several months to do so.

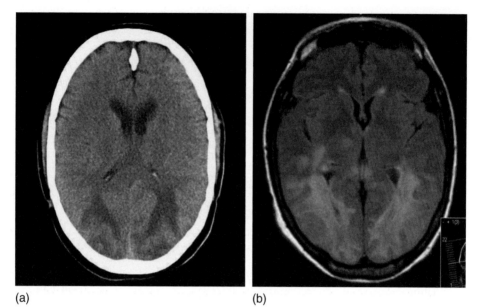

(a)   (b)

Fig. 15.3 Posterior reversible encephalopathy syndrome: (a) CT shows bilateral low attenuation in the posterior parietal and occipital lobes whereas MRI (b) demonstrates hyperintensity (T_2-weighted images). Cisplatin and cyclosporine are both recognized precipitants of PRES.

Haematopoietic

Bone marrow depression is a common sequelae of many different chemotherapeutic and occasionally of radiotherapeutic treatments and causes anaemia, leucopenia and thrombocytopenia. When protracted neutropenia is expected, GM-CSF (granulocyte macrophage colony stimulating factor) may be administered daily or PEG-GCSF administered weekly to reduce the period of neutropenia and thereby the risk of infection. Occasionally, in patients who have had an allogeneic stem cell transplant, donor leucocytes may be transfused to treat relapse of the primary host disease or to fight immunosuppression-related infections or tumours.

Erythropoietin may be used to stimulate red cell production and to counteract therapy-induced anaemia reducing the associated fatigue and dyspnoea. However, erythropoietin may also increase tumour cell growth and tumour angiogenesis thereby reducing long-term survival and successful disease cure. Thus, in the UK, anaemia is more commonly treated by blood transfusion.

Thrombocytopenia is also commonly seen and platelet counts as low as 20 may be tolerated provided no evidence of active bleeding is found. In general, the platelet count is raised above 75 if surgical procedures are to be undertaken and above 50 for line insertion or removal involving the femoral or internal jugular veins. Some patients require single donor platelets to avoid immune-mediated destruction of transfused platelets and very occasionally, human leukocyte antigen (HLA) matched platelets are required. Recombinant human thrombopoietin has been used in studies to increase the yield of platelets from donors and also in patients with bone marrow suppression. However, a number of patients developed an autoantibody to their endogenous thrombopoietin with subsequent thrombocytopenia. Thrombopoietin is therefore only available for use in clinical trials at the present time.

Myelosuppression may also follow radiotherapy although this tends to be less severe than with chemotherapy (excepting TBI pre-transplant). Leucopenia, thrombocytopenia, and anaemia can occur and should be excluded whenever a patient undergoing radiotherapy presents for surgery.

Immunological

Immunological disturbance during chemotherapy is not mediated by effects on the bone marrow alone. Cytotoxic drugs may cause immunosuppression by direct action against immunocytes per se:

♦ Steroids reduce the sequestration of white cells to sites of inflammation, increase white cell apoptosis, and reduce cytokine release from white cells.

♦ Monoclonal antibodies such as alemtuzumab and rituximab are directed against white cell epitopes and are used to treat lymphoid cancers by reducing white cell populations.

♦ Immunosuppressive therapies such as cyclosporine or mycophenolate may be deliberately administered to recipients of allogeneic stem cell transplants to modulate the severity of graft-versus-host disease.

In immunosuppressed patients with leucopenia, sepsis, shock, and proven or suspected hypogammaglobulinaemia, intravenous immunoglobulin therapy may aid recovery. However, in most instances, reduction of immunosuppressive treatment, administration of GM-GCSF where there is neutropenia and high-dose, broad-spectrum antimicrobial treatments are the mainstays of management.

Apart from TBI, radiotherapy tends to be less systemically immunosuppressive than chemotherapy but commonly damages mucosal barriers which provide innate immunity and may result in local infection at the damaged site or systemic infection secondary to translocation of pathogens.

Hypersensitivity reactions may also follow the administration of chemotherapeutic agents.

Metabolic disturbances

These may arise secondary to irradiation of the pituitary, thyroid, adrenals, gut, or kidney. Hypoadrenalism, hypothyroidism, and hypopituitarism should always be considered in any patient who has undergone radiation treatment in the vicinity of these glands. It may be that an endocrine insufficiency is relative and will only become unmasked at the time of exposure to a surgical stress. Equally, radiation-induced damage to the intestine or kidneys can result in lasting impairment to water and electrolyte absorption resulting in fluid balance and biochemical derangements which must be corrected preoperatively and monitored closely postoperatively. Mild cranial diabetes insipidus following radiotherapy to the brain may pass unnoticed if patients merely drink more to compensate for their water loss. Similarly, a patient with radiation damaged bowel and diarrhoea may supplement their fluid and nutritional intake to compensate. However, under anaesthesia or in ICU where a patient loses the ability to regulate their own fluid intake, metabolic disturbances may quickly become apparent.

Physical impairment

Whilst radiation burns are relatively infrequently seen with the use of fractionation and computer planning, long-term muscle fibrosis and tissue retraction still occur and can lead to physical distortion, pain, and limitation of movement. This is most commonly seen in head and neck radiotherapy where mouth opening can become very limited, the tongue relatively immobile, and the larynx fixed, making intubation extremely difficult or impossible with conventional laryngoscopy. A full airway assessment, ideally with review of recent CT scans of the mouth and larynx should be undertaken as a matter of routine. Similarly, positioning of the head during surgery should be undertaken with great care as, even with the use of neuromuscular blockade, it may have a relatively fixed deformity which will result in neck strain if appropriate supports are not used to spread the load evenly.

Bibliography

1. Andreyev HJ (2007). Gastrointestinal problems after pelvic radiotherapy: the past, the present and the future. *Clin Oncol (R Coll Radiol)* **19**(10):790–9.
2. Cappell MS (2004). Colonic toxicity of administered drugs and chemicals. *Am J Gastroenterol* **99**(6):1175–90.
3. Cavaliere R, Schiff D (2006). Neurologic toxicities of cancer therapies. *Curr Neurol Neurosci Rep* **6**(3):218–26.
4. Choi YW, Munden RF, Erasmus JJ, *et al.* (2004). Effects of radiation therapy on the lung: radiologic appearances and differential diagnosis. *RadioGraphics* **24**:985–97.
5. Daniel D, Crawford J (2006). Myelotoxicity from chemotherapy. *Semin Oncol* **33**(1):74–85.
6. Dimopoulou I, Bamias A, Lyberopoulos P, Dimopoulos MA (2006). Pulmonary toxicity from novel antineoplastic agents. *Ann Oncol* **17**(3):372–9.
7. Fernandez A, Brada M, Zabuliene L, Karavitaki N, Wass JAH (2009). Radiation-induced hypopituitarism. *Endocr Relat Cancer* **16**(3):733–72.
8. Healey Bird BRJ, Swain SS (2008). Cardiac toxicity in breast cancer survivors: Review of potential cardiac problems. *Clin Cancer Res* **14**:14.
9. Humphreys BD, Soiffer RJ, Magee CC (2005). Renal failure associated with cancer and its treatment: An update. *J Am Soc Nephrol* **16**:151–61.
10. Sul JK, Deangelis LM (2006). Neurologic complications of cancer chemotherapy. *Semin Oncol* **33**(3):324–32.
11. Yeh ET, Tong AT, Lenihan DJ, *et al.* (2004). Cardiovascular complications of cancer therapy: diagnosis, pathogenesis, and management. *Circulation* **109**(25):3122–31.
12. Zitvogel L, Apetoh L, Ghiringhelli F, *et al.* (2008). The anticancer immune response: indispensable for therapeutic success? *J Clin Invest* **118**(6):1991–2001.

Chapter 16

Interactions between critical illness management and cancer growth and spread

Paul Kelly

Introduction

Cancer patients may present to a critical care unit with obvious primary and clinically relevant metastatic lesions. In addition they may have an unknown number of circulating tumour cells and clinically undetectable micrometastases. While in critical care, subsequent proliferative, angiogenic, invasive and metastatic properties of these different cancer cell populations may be inadvertently influenced by the course of the critical illness and its management.

The impact of critical illness and its management on cancer growth has not been fully studied and only recently described. The purpose of this chapter is to explore this theoretical phenomenon in more detail.

When cancer and critical care collide . . .

During the course of critical illness there are numerous physiological alterations, supportive interventions, and pharmacological interventions that may theoretically modulate cancer cell growth.

Physiological alterations

Inflammation

The link between inflammation and carcinogenesis is well established and not surprising as the cellular pathways involved in inflammation, healing, and carcinogenesis are intricately entwined. Key transcription factors, including nuclear factor kappa B (NFκB) and hypoxia-induced transcription factor (HIF) are shared by these processes.

NFkB is a group of transcription factors responsible for regulating over 150 genes whose products are responsible for controlling inflammatory responses, cellular proliferation, and apoptosis. Its activation has been shown to be central to the development of:

- Acute respiratory distress syndrome (ARDS)
- Multiple organ dysfunction syndrome (MODS)
- Promotion of tumour cell survival, proliferation, vascularization, invasion, and metastasis.

Of the cytokines, tumour necrosis factor alpha (TNFα) and interleukin (IL)-1B, IL-6, IL-7, and IL-17 have all been shown to influence cancer growth and spread at multiple sites.

Inflammation may occur secondary to infection or trauma. There is some evidence that inflammation caused by physical trauma can modify cancer growth. In mice, experimental metastases have been shown to preferentially implant in healing wounds. In humans, there have been anecdotal reports and case reports of local trauma stimulating cancer growth at the site of trauma. There have been several theoretical articles written about surgical modification of cancer growth or 'oncotaxis'. Epidemiological studies have demonstrated an early peak in death post mastectomy compared to those treated conservatively yet the cause of this putative post-traumatic effect is not clear. One theory suggests that the primary tumours, metastases, and undetected, dormant micrometastases are stimulated by a post-traumatic inflammatory storm. Indeed, 5-year survival after lung surgery is reduced if the patient experienced a systemic inflammatory response syndrome (SIRS) response. Excessive inflammatory responses result in high levels of circulating cytokines and other inflammatory products (including chemokines, nitric oxide, and prostaglandins).

Another theoretical cause for surgically-induced modification of cancer growth is the potential spillage of tumour cells into the circulation as a result of tumour manipulation at the time of surgery. Circulating tumour cells have indeed been demonstrated to increase at the time of cancer surgery. These circulating cells may be attracted to distant capillary beds through chemokine receptor/ligand interactions.

In addition to excessive inflammatory responses, critically ill patients may also have inadequate responses. This may result in immunosuppression and an inability to maintain effective surveillance of defective cells. Immune cells, such as NK cells and cytotoxic T cells, capable of detecting and destroying cancer cells may be reduced in number and function in critically ill patients. This would apply to primary tumours, metastatic lesions, micrometastases, and circulating tumour cells.

Neuroendocrine

The neuroendocrine components of the stress response are initially activated by nociceptive and sympathetic nerve signals from the site of injury or infection. These, in turn, activate the neuroendocrine response via the hypothalamic–pituitary–adrenal (HPA) axis, the sympathetic nervous system and the renin angiotensin aldosterone axis with consequent hormone release from the hypothalamus, pituitary and extracranial glands. These hormones include corticotropin-releasing hormone, adrenocorticotropic hormone, cortisol, β endorphin, growth hormone, thyroid stimulating hormone, prolactin, luteinizing hormone, follicle-stimulating hormone, antidiuretic hormone, epinephrine, and norepinephrine. These hormones have widespread physiological consequences. In critical illness, as seen in inflammation, the neuroendocrine responses may be excessive or inadequate. An excessive response from the HPA axis may have direct and indirect effects on carcinogenesis.

- Direct effects may be mediated via endocrine receptors, such as adrenoreceptors and glucocorticoid receptors, present on tumour cells. Catecholamines and glucocorticoids, often abundant in critically ill patients, have been shown to directly influence tumour cell growth, angiogenesis, invasion, and metastasis.

- Indirect effects are likely to be immune mediated. Immune cells also possess adrenoreceptors and glucocorticoid receptors. Almost immediately following trauma such as surgery, cells involved in cell-mediated immunity (NK cells, cytotoxic CD8+ T cells, TH1 cells) are suppressed in both number and function. Catecholamines reduce NK cell and cytotoxic T lymphocyte (CTL) activity *in vitro*. In animal studies, blocking the sympathetic response with spinal anaesthesia or β-blockade reduced metastases following surgery. Retrospective human studies suggest that perioperative blockade of the sympathetic response by nerve blocks or epidurals may reduce cancer recurrence after primary excision. One can speculate that such blockade may facilitate detection and killing of circulating tumour cells and hence reduce subsequent metastases. In addition, nerve blockade reduces perioperative opioid requirements. Opioids may also contribute to perioperative immunosuppression.

Metabolic

Critically ill patients endure considerable metabolic derangement including hyperglycaemia, insulin resistance, hyperinsulinaemia, and high insulin-like growth factor (IGF-1) levels. These derangements are similar to those seen in diabetics, particularly type II diabetics. A series of recent studies and meta-analyses confirm that the risk for several solid and haematological malignancies (including liver, pancreas, colorectal, kidney, bladder, endometrial, and breast cancers and non-Hodgkin's lymphoma) is increased in diabetics. Potential mechanisms are multifactorial. Hyperglycaemia-induced cellular stress promotes free radical production and DNA damage. High glucose levels also lead to activation of NFκB which may influence cancer growth and spread directly or indirectly via its effects on the immune system. High insulin and insulin-like growth factor (IGF-1) levels may play significant roles as potent mitogenic growth factors. Insulin also has anti-inflammatory properties. Glucose control has been shown to be advantageous in diabetics and the critically ill. In terms of cancer, diabetics have a worse prognosis once diagnosed and improved control may increase the chance of remission. It is possible, therefore, that efforts to reduce insulin resistance and control hyperglycaemia in the critically ill cancer patient could reduce cancer growth and spread.

Hypoxia

Hypoxia is common feature of critical illness. Hypoxia induces an intracellular signalling cascade to promote survival. A key hypoxia-induced transcription factor is HIF that controls gene products involved in cell growth, survival, vascularization, and migration. It is recognized as a major promoter of tumour cell growth. Its expression is increased as tumour cells grow faster than the blood supply with resultant local hypoxia. Increased HIF expression is associated with accelerated vascularization. In critical illness profound hypoxia may enhance this process increasing vascularization of primary tumours and metastases. HIF also increases the expression of chemokines on cancer cells and may therefore improve their ability to target distant organs. To further consolidate this theory, mutations in von Hippel–Lindau (VHL) factor, a suppressor protein responsible for the degradation of HIF, have been identified in several tumour cell lines.

Hypoxia is also immunosuppressive. Reduced function of NK cells and cytotoxic T cells has been demonstrated in hypoxic conditions. Resultant defective immunosurveillance may tip the balance towards tumour cell growth.

Supportive interventions

Physiological interventions are an integral component of critical care management. These include ventilation, inotropic support, renal replacement therapy, and blood transfusion which may all modulate inflammatory and immune processes.

Ventilation

Ventilation is a recognized cause of lung injury. Long-term ventilation causes inflammation within the lung. Primary or metastatic tumours in the lung may be influenced by this response. In addition circulating cancer cells may be attracted and entrapped. However, the inflammatory response to ventilation is not restricted to the lung. Inflammatory products, such as cytokines, spill out into the peripheral circulation and are hypothesized to contribute to the pathogenesis of MODS. These inflammatory products may influence peripheral tumour cells and promote their growth and spread. The degree of this inflammatory response varies with the mode of ventilation. The choice of ventilation strategy may therefore influence local and distant growth and spread.

Inotropic support

Immune cells and cancer cells have adrenoreceptors and dopamine receptors. High levels of circulating endogenous or exogenous agonists may influence cancer growth through a number of mechanisms.

- β_2-adrenoreceptors are present on lymphocytes and NK cells. NK cell function is reduced *in vitro* by β_2 stimulation. In addition in animal models stress-induced metastases are increased by β_1 and β_2 stimulation and blocked by β-blockers. Noradrenaline infusions have also been shown to increase metastatic spread in the animal model. However, this effect is also blocked by β-blockers and may therefore be mediated via β-adrenoreceptors. Catecholamines may also directly influence cancer cells growth and spread. β_2-adrenoreceptors have been identified on several cancer cell lines including breast, colon, and prostate.

- Dopamine has widespread anti-inflammatory effects, reducing proinflammatory cytokine production, T-cell proliferation, and antibody responses. In addition to acting directly on immune cell dopamine receptors, dopamine may act indirectly by reducing pituitary prolactin production. Dopamine has no direct effects on the growth and survival of tumour cells yet it does have potent antiangiogenic effects mediated by inhibiting proliferation and migration of tumour endothelial cells through suppression of the vascular endothelial growth factor (VEGF) receptor.

Phosphodiesterase inhibitors, such as milrinone, may also have benefits in the cancer cell population by promoting cancer cell death and inhibiting proliferation.

Renal replacement therapy

Cancer is known to be more common in those suffering from end-stage renal failure. This may be secondary to impaired DNA repair or suppressed immune function. In acute renal failure increases in both pro-inflammatory and anti-inflammatory products are also seen. This may be due to decreased clearance of enhanced inflammation secondary to uncleared organic and inorganic compounds. Renal replacement therapy could theoretically influence cancer growth through adsorption of circulating cancer cells and inflammatory products, removal of tumour-secreted growth and immunosuppressive products, and inappropriate immune activation in the extracorporeal circuit. This theory has been tested in an animal model of tumour growth, where animal survival and NK cell activity was demonstrated to increase following adsorption-based filtration.

Blood transfusion

Several meta-analyses and studies now exist which suggest that blood transfusion is an independent risk factor for increasing cancer recurrence particularly after surgery. However, the mechanism remains elusive. Blood transfusions are known to have immunosuppressive effects including reduction in NK-cell and cytotoxic T-cell activity. It has been suggested that high levels of VEGF in stored blood may contribute towards increased tumour angiogenesis. A recent animal study showed the erythrocytes rather than soluble factors were responsible for the cancer-promoting effects. In addition the duration of storage appeared to be critical. The authors hypothesized that the host's innate immune system is occupied by the deteriorating erythrocytes leaving the residual tumour cells unchecked.

Pharmacological interventions

Given the vast array of drugs used in the course of critical illness it would not be surprising to find that some may have a significant effect on cancer growth.

Sedation

Most commonly used sedatives have immunomodulatory properties that may influence cancer growth. Propofol has significant anti-inflammatory properties yet may possess anticancer properties. The mechanism is unknown but may involve NFκB and cycloxygenase inhibition. Clinically relevant concentrations have been shown to decrease the metastatic potential of human cancer cells, inhibit pulmonary metastasis of murine osteosarcoma, inhibit growth and induce apoptosis in human leukaemic cells, significantly suppress tumour growth and enhance cytotoxic T-cell activity in mice.

Analgesia

Despite their use for the treatment of cancer-related pain, opioids may have direct tumour-promoting properties. A few recent trials and observations illustrate this potential. In 2002 a palliative care trial demonstrated an increased survival with spinal rather than systemic analgesia. Similarly, cancer patients taking the selective opioid antagonist methylnaltrexone for constipation lived longer than expected. In addition, two recent retrospective studies suggested a survival advantage for patients undergoing breast and prostate surgery with regional rather than systemic analgesia. Whether this is an opioid-sparing phenomenon or due to a reduction in stress response is unknown. μ receptor agonism has been shown to increase tumour proliferation, vascularization, migration, and decrease barrier function allowing increased penetration. These effects are reversed by opioid antagonists.

Antibiotics

In 2004 an epidemiological study was published that suggested an increased risk of breast cancer was associated with increased antibiotic use. Although there appears to be an association, it is not clear if it is due to a direct effect or related to indirect effects on inflammatory responses or the illnesses necessitating antibiotic usage. There is some evidence that antibiotics are able to directly influence cancer growth. Macrolides appear to have antiangiogenic properties. Lung cancer patients treated with clarithromycin have been shown to have a survival advantage. In addition, tetracyclines are associated with an increased expression of cyclooxygenase-2 (COX-2) and prostaglandin E2. Overexpression of COX-2, as seen in several cancers including breast, prostate, and colorectal, is associated with increased motility and invasiveness.

Conclusion

The pathogenesis of cancer and critical illness is far from being understood. What is apparent is that their pathways merge at vital junctions. The course of critical illness is likely to affect cancer cell proliferation, angiogenesis, invasion, and metastasis. In addition, critical care management has the inadvertent potential to both negatively and positively influence this effect. Further research and understanding will hopefully unravel this mystery and aid the selection of critical care interventions aimed at improving cancer prognosis.

Bibliography

1. Armaiz-Pena G, Lutgendorf S, Cole S, Sood A (2009). Neuroendocrine modulation of cancer progression. *Brain, Behav, Immun* **23**(1):10–15.
2. Atzil S, Arad M, Glasner A, *et al.* (2008). Blood transfusion promotes cancer progression: A critical role for aged erythrocytes. *Anesthesiology* **109**(6):989–97.
3. Beutler B (2003). Science review: key inflammatory and stress pathways in critical illness – the central role of the Toll-like receptors. *Crit Care* **7**(1):39–46.

4. Biki B, Mascha E, Moriarty DC, Fitzpatrick JM, Sessler DI, Buggy DJ (2008). Anesthetic technique for radical prostatectomy surgery affects cancer recurrence: a retrospective analysis. *Anesthesiology* **109**(2):180–7.

5. Cavaillon J, Annane D (2006). Compartmentalization of the inflammatory response in sepsis and SIRS. *J Endotoxin Res* **12**(3):151–70.

6. Chakroborty D, Sarkar C, Basu B, Dasgupta PS, Basu S (2009). Catecholamines regulate tumor angiogenesis. *Cancer Research* **69**(9):3727–30.

7. Clark JA, Coopersmith CM (2007). Just the right amount of JNK: How nuclear factor-kappaB and downstream mediators prevent burn-induced intestinal injury. *Crit Care Med* **35**(5):1433–4.

8. Coffey J, Smith M, Wang J, Bouchier-Hayes D, Cotter T, Redmond H (2006). Cancer surgery: risks and opportunities. *Bioessays* **28**(4):433–7.

9. El Saghir N, Elhajj I, Geara F, Hourani M (2005). Trauma-associated growth of suspected dormant micrometastasis. *BMC Cancer* **5**(1):94.

10. Exadaktylos AK, Buggy DJ, Moriarty DC, Mascha E, Sessler DI (2006). Can anesthetic technique for primary breast cancer surgery affect recurrence or metastasis? *Anesthesiology* **105**(4):660–4.

11. Giovannucci E, Michaud D (2007). The role of obesity and related metabolic disturbances in cancers of the colon, prostate, and pancreas. *Gastroenterology* **132**(6):2208–25.

12. Gottschalk A, Sharma S, Ford J, Durieux ME, Tiouririne M (2010). Review article: the role of the perioperative period in recurrence after cancer surgery. *Anesth Analg* **110**(6):1636–43.

13. Gupta K, Kshirsagar S, Chang L, *et al.* (2002). Morphine stimulates angiogenesis by activating proangiogenic and survival-promoting signaling and promotes breast tumor growth. *Cancer Res* **62**(15):4491–98.

14. Krone CA, Ely JTA (2005). Controlling hyperglycemia as an adjunct to cancer therapy. *Integr Cancer Ther* **4**(1):25–31.

15. Kushida A, Inada T, Shingu K (2007). Enhancement of antitumor immunity after propofol treatment in mice. *Immunopharmacol Immunotoxicol* **29**(3–4):477–86.

16. Moss J, Israel RJ (2009). Effects of anesthetics on cancer recurrence. *J Clin Oncol* **27**(25):e89.

17. Porta C, Larghi P, Rimoldi M, *et al.* (2009). Cellular and molecular pathways linking inflammation and cancer. *Immunobiology* **214**(9–10):761–77.

18. Pouyssegur J, Dayan F, Mazure NM (2006). Hypoxia signalling in cancer and approaches to enforce tumour regression. *Nature* **441**(7092):437–43.

19. Rakoff-Nahoum S (2006). Why cancer and inflammation? *Yale J Biol Med* **79**(3–4):123–30.

20. Sarkar C, Chakroborty D, Chowdhury UR, Dasgupta PS, Basu S (2008). Dopamine increases the efficacy of anticancer drugs in breast and colon cancer preclinical models. *Clin Cancer Res* **14**(8):2502–10.

21. Velicer CM, Heckbert SR, Lampe JW, Potter JD, Robertson CA, Taplin SH (2004). Antibiotic use in relation to the risk of breast cancer. *JAMA* **291**(7):827–35.

22. Weckermann D, Polzer B, Ragg T, *et al.* (2009). Perioperative activation of disseminated tumor cells in bone marrow of patients with prostate cancer. *J Clin Oncol* **27**(10):1549–56.

23. Yoshimura A (2006). Signal transduction of inflammatory cytokines and tumor development. *Cancer Sci* **97**(6):439–47.

Chapter 17

Ethics and law in critical care of the cancer patient

Andrew Lawson and Paul Farquhar-Smith

Introduction

In the past decade it was commonly held that haematological or metastatic malignancy was considered a relative contraindication to admission to critical care units (CCUs), with restriction of level of treatment or even refusal of admission being commonplace. In one prospective French study half of those with a diagnosis of cancer who were considered for intensive care were refused because of chronic illness and lack of options for the treatment of their malignancy. Previously the situation was worse, one prospective study concluded that 'The majority of patients with solid tumours and haematological cancers admitted to the intensive care unit die before discharge, or, if they survive the hospital admission, they spend a minimal amount of time at home before dying. This limited survival is achieved at considerable cost'. However, as de Jonge and Bos pointed out recently 'the times they are a changing'. Advances in the treatment of solid tumours and in haematological malignancies have led to significant improvements in life expectancy and it is now recognized that patients with malignant disease may do better than expected on CCUs (see Chapter 14). Where once intensive care was considered futile it is now recognized that prognostic models commonly used in CCUs cannot reliably predict adverse outcomes in cancer patients. Cancer patients collectively account for approximately 10% of patients in general CCUs. Mortality is related to organ failure not the nature or stage of malignancy. This chapter reviews the major ethical issues relevant to the management of patients with cancer in the critical care setting.

Ethics and law

Ethics, or moral philosophy, is a branch of philosophy concerned with what ought or what not ought to be done under given sets of circumstances. It would be convenient if the law was the source for our ethical needs. The law is important and the practice of healthcare takes place within a framework of laws and regulations relevant to the particular jurisdiction. However, the fact that something is legal does not necessarily imply that it is morally permissible, nor is the converse true. The American jurist Earl Warren put the relationship succinctly: 'In civilized life, law floats in a sea of ethics. Each is indispensable to civilization. Without law, we should be at the mercy of the least scrupulous; without ethics, law could not exist.'

Thus ethics is the bedrock of our professional and legal relationship with patients, no more or less so on the CCU than on the general ward.

Law in the CCU

The law holds for patients with cancer on CCU as it does with any other patient and there are no specific caveats. Healthcare professionals have a duty of care for their patients and they are obliged to provide treatment where medically indicated. This duty is a statutory but not an absolute duty. It is accepted in law that resources are finite and thus doctors are not obligated to provide services that are beyond reasonable grounds.

A principal legal concern for those working in critical care is that of the position of the law on the withdrawal of treatment. It is clear in law that a doctor is not required to provide treatment that is not in the patient's best interests and that under exceptional cases it may not be in the patient's best interests to receive life-saving treatments. In the 1990s (Airedale NHS Trust v Bland) Lord Wilkinson commented that continuing life-support systems where not in the best interest of the patient would 'constitute the crime of battery and the tort of trespass to the person'.

Why do we need ethics? How do we decide what is right?

Right and compassionate decisions can be made in the absence of formal ethical teaching and knowledge, but an understanding of ethical principles (now a mandatory part of undergraduate training) can assist in decision-making, especially in situations where there is potential for a conflict of interests as may be the case in CCUs.

Recourse to religious principles might seem an attractive solution to what is right. In popular conceptions of morality there is often an assumed link with religion, equating moral principles with divine revelation. However philosophically, there is a problem with 'religion'. Is the good 'good' because a deity commands it, or does a deity command it because it is good? If the former is true then morality is mere obedience to an arbitrary will. If the latter is true then morality is independent of the will of God, limiting the use of religion in ethics.

Another frequent criticism of ethics is that it is subjective and that commonsense will find the answer. Indeed in day-to-day practice doctors and nurses have for generations worked in an ethical manner. With a few notorious exceptions, the training and self-selection of people in the caring professions ensures a high level of 'ethical conduct'. However we are more often now presented with problems which common sense cannot solve. In the event of a pandemic flu how will we decide whom to ventilate? Would it be morally correct (if illegal) to assist the death of a suffering patient at their request? A key question is what is the difference (if any) between withholding and withdrawing treatment? These problems are not commonsensical and require an ethical approach to resolve them.

The goals of medicine and capacity for benefit

To guide our ethical management, we need to consider what the goals are for a patient with malignant disease on CCU. The progress of medicine has increased life expectancy, but does living longer risk taking longer to die? Longevity has brought with it a plethora of end of life decisions around so-called 'life-saving technology'. Putting patients on life support machines may support life, but for how long and at what cost? Hardwig discusses the idea of dying at the right time. He accepts the tragedy of a premature end of life but asserts that death can come too late because of what continuing on living on entails. What is the purpose of medicine when applied to people who may near the end of their lives? Quality of life needs to be taken into account rather than just prolonging life whatever the cost.

What are the needs of patients with cancer on CCU? For a vitalist, survival is the key but it is highly unlikely people would wish to survive at any cost. A more realistic need might be to survive to leave hospital and have a reasonable quality of life. This goal of medicine can be described as a capacity to benefit. If a patient can gain no benefit, would that justify not offering intensive care? Not intervening could infringe a patient's rights to healthcare but does a need for healthcare translate into a right to healthcare? Is this right tenable? Accepting a need for healthcare does not necessarily mean patients must be treated. A need may exist, but may be contingent on capacity to benefit. If the patients have no capacity to benefit then their need is unmeetable and an unmeetable need cannot be a right. It is unfortunate, not unfair, that the need cannot be met. The assessment of the capacity to benefit is therefore key in the decision-making for intensive treatment for cancer patients.

Cassel and Neugarten have characterized the goals of medicine around two distinct models, the heroic and humanistic. The goal of the heroic model are saving life and curing diseases. The humanistic model is concerned primarily with improving the quality of life. Intensive care is perhaps the most 'heroic' of medical endeavours. The two goals are not necessarily mutually exclusive though, as measures that have a principal aim of improving quality of life will more often than not prolong life. The difficulty with applying a humanistic goal of medicine is that of making quality of life judgements. Whereas it is possible in conscious autonomous patients to engage them in discussions of quality of life, how do we come to the right conclusions for a ventilated or heavily sedated patient? It is clear that doctors may have a statistical sense of what the quality of life is likely to be for a patient, but that is difficult to use as a reason not to treat a specific patient.

On a practical level, six proper goals of medicine have been described:

◆ Restoration of health
◆ Relief of symptoms
◆ Restoration and maintenance of function
◆ Saving or prolonging of life
◆ Avoiding harm
◆ Education and counselling of patients.

Most of these goals ascribe to the humanistic model and reinforce the tenet that improvement of quality of life (imbued in capacity to benefit) is paramount rather than prolongation of life. These six goals seem to be a good working model of what doctors do on a day-to-day basis and fit within the four principles approach to medical ethics being subsets of beneficence (doing good) and non-maleficence (not doing harm). In the four principles approach, considerations of respect for autonomy and considerations of justice temper these goals of medicine.

Balance of meeting needs and benefits

The balance of beneficence and non-maleficence is perhaps the most relevant aspect for a non-autonomous patient on CCU. Doctors have a special obligation to benefit their patients but also to avoid harm. Even in patients with advanced malignant disease short-term survival may in fact be the objective for the patient and their family. As such, CCU care may be considered appropriate on the grounds of beneficence. Active treatment may also have a great symbolic and emotional significance for relatives and staff and may be an expression of society's desire to help those in greatest need.

Considerations of justice form the fourth of the four principles; this will be in terms of the fairness of resource allocation (distributive justice) as well as the fairness of the treatment for their particular disease. A principal aim of medicine has been described as 'the well working of the whole', the same author commenting that if preventing death was the primary reason for medicine then the ideal would be 'bodily immortality' which it clearly is not. Attempting to restore the well working of the whole is consistent with these patients and this model of medicine. Medicine is also about responding to suffering which seems to be an immediate response of those who care for the ill. This has been considered to be a perfect duty. Ignoring suffering according to Emmanuel Levinas 'jeopardizes the agent's moral being'.

The British Medical Association (BMA) has declared 'The primary goal of medical treatment is to benefit the patient by restoring or maintaining the patient's health as far as possible, maximizing benefit and minimizing harm'. The benefits to the patient may include prolonging life but not under all circumstances and quality of life is also a relevant issue. The fact that the expected quality of life that might be obtained can be considered when making treatment decisions has been accepted into UK law. The position of the BMA seems to have a consequentialist thread to it, implicitly involving benefit/harm analysis and rejecting vitalist claims of the sanctity of life. Where the primary goal of medicine cannot be achieved and no net benefit can be achieved then the BMA consensus is that the justification for treatment no longer stands.

Roman Catholic teaching has parallels with a beneficence/non-maleficence model which includes a capacity to benefit. It distinguishes between proportionate and disproportionate means of preserving one's life or health. The former are morally required, the latter are optional. Disproportionate means are those which 'do not offer a reasonable hope of benefit or entail an excessive burden'. This stance takes into account a wide array of benefits and burdens. In respect of the benefit to a patient the whole condition of the patient is considered and not just the targeted ailment. For example, one is not morally obliged to undergo open heart surgery if one has terminal cancer. Disproportionate means also recognizes that the range of burdens includes those on the community. Such burdens might be said to include economic burdens, which include the cost of treating such patients. The Catholic position also does not view mortal life as an absolute good, due to the belief in an eternal destiny. Omitting extraordinary means of treatment in this context means a patient understands the value of life is not absolute.

Balancing goals and needs with costs

As resources are limited it might be acceptable to restrict access to intensive care to those who would benefit most or those whose needs were meetable. If a need cannot be met then there may not be an obligation to meet it. This has contemporary resonance in the establishment of organizations such as the National Institute for Health and Clinical Excellence. If there is no reliable evidence that a treatment works, then that treatment cannot be said to be able to meet a healthcare need and as such its provision is not obligatory. Using needs to determine goals of medicine also produces another problem, how do we balance out competing needs, especially in an individual patient? There may be a hierarchy of needs, to live but not to live with disability, for example.

In any medical endeavour there is a degree of benefit/harm analysis. For example, the side effects of new drugs are weighed against the beneficial effects. This consequentialist (utilitarian, maximizing benefit) approach is mirrored in a view of the goals of medicine, that of maximizing the quality of life of a population overall. This is exemplified by the QALY (quality-adjusted life year) approach. In essence, the QALY approach looks at cost-effectiveness aggregated over time to produce an integer (a QALY) with which to compare different healthcare interventions.

Doctors on the whole seem averse to financial quantification, feeling that it lacks humanity, but we cannot ignore fiscal limitation anymore than we can ignore symptoms and signs. Morreim has argued that physicians must work within a resource nexus and has introduced the concept of a 'standard of resource use' which encompasses the fiscal resources that physicians are expected to utilize for their patients. Working within this system physicians would have an implicit obligation to keep one eye on cost. There would be a minimum level of resource that each citizen would be entitled to, and it would seem that above that level the fiduciary responsibilities of the physician are diluted by other considerations. Physicians cannot 'commandeer resources', nor are they obliged to, but rather they are obliged firstly to act as advocates for their patients. Morreim though adds another duty, that of acting as an advocate for all patients to improve resource policies. This second duty implies a shift from the dyadic doctor–patient relationship to a more general duty of a doctor to think beyond the individual patient. Williams has said that 'we need to inculcate a sense of statistical compassion' commenting that 'behind the mere statistics there are a lot of real people who do have names and addresses and worried loved ones'.

When a doctor decides to admit a patient to CCU he or she must make a sort of calculus of outcome probability and cost-effectiveness. This would seem impossible on a day-to-day basis, yet in practice doctors often make inferences under conditions of uncertainty to guide decision-making. It might then be possible to come to a common sense, best guess calculation. It should not be true that a physician need take no note of cost when deciding on treatment. There is thus a tension between their role as fiduciary agent of the patient and gatekeeper of healthcare resources. Can a physician involved in making what have been termed 'tragic choices' be expected to consider cost? When dealing with limited supplies of highly expensive drugs, doctors do exactly that, this has been acknowledged for some years. The American Thoracic Society (ATS) stated in 1997 'Marginally beneficial intensive care may be justifiably limited on the basis of societal consensus that its cost is too high in relation to the value of its outcome'. Hospitals, doctors, and health budgets are societal resources and the ATS has stated 'extraordinary expenditures of resources for marginal gains unfairly compromise the availability of a basic minimum level of health care services for all'. Issues of cost in this setting are principally concerned with distributive justice and may be balanced using a utilitarian tool like the QALY. However, autonomy and issues of beneficence, justice, and non-maleficence do not lend themselves to a solution based on integers. Decisions about healthcare are not made on cost alone. Again, the key assessment is that of capacity to benefit which leads the ethical decision-making.

End of life care for the cancer patient

The intensivist whilst balancing all the above principles may have additional issues to deal with when dealing with the cancer patient. The principal goal of the intensivist is curative. In the patient with cancer the issues may become more complex. On the CCU the cancer patient may be being 'cured' of complications relating to treatment, having supportive care during chemotherapy, treatment of problems unrelated to diagnosis, and treatment of the underlying disorder or a form of intensive palliation. At some point for many patients there is a shift from curative to end of life care. At this point critical care and palliative care start to merge. Whilst it may be appropriate to move patients from the CCU to the general ward or hospice there will be patients in whom such a transfer would be inappropriate where they are not expected to live for long following removal of supportive therapy.

Five domains of good end of life care have been identified:

◆ Adequate pain and symptom control
◆ Avoidance of inappropriate prolongation of dying
◆ Achieving a sense of control
◆ Relieving of burdens, and
◆ Strengthening relationships with loved ones.

Of prime importance to the dying patient is symptom control, particularly pain. Beyond that the intensivist should tailor the degree of sedation to the patient's wishes, both physical and spiritual, in concert with attending relatives and or friends. Whilst the autonomy of the patient should remain paramount consideration should be given to the needs of those relatives or friends who are in attendance as part of a family-centred approach to the care of the dying.

As well as addressing the needs of the patient and the family the needs of the clinical team looking after the cancer patient dying on the CCU should be addressed. It may be challenging for staff used to the heroic and curative ethic to switch to the palliative care ethic.

Communication between different members of the CCU team should be clear. Some studies have documented a dissonance between the physician members of the CCU team and the nurses caring for the patients with regard to this shift from curing to caring and this should be avoided. Regular team meetings and regular meetings between the various specialties involved and the CCU team are essential.

Conclusion

The management of a patient with malignant disease on the CCU entails thinking ethically about the process of treatment but sadly also at times thinking ethically about the process of dying. As with patients with non-malignant disease a conception of the goals of medicine helps clarify decisions.

Bibliography

1. ATS Bioethics Task Force (1997) Fair allocation of intensive care unit resources. *Am J Respir Crit Care Med* **156**(4):1282–301.
2. Brenner H (2002). Long-term survival rates of cancer patients achieved by the end of the 20th century: a period analysis. *Lancet* **360**(9340):1131–5.
3. British Medical Association (2007). *Withholding and withdrawing life-prolonging medical treatment: guidance for decision making.* Oxford: Blackwell.
4. Calabresi G, Bobbitt P (1978). *Tragic Choices: The Conflicts Society Confronts in the Allocation of Tragically Scarce Resources.* New York: W. Norton.
5. Darmon M, Thiery G, Ciroldi M, *et al.* (2005). Intensive care in patients with newly diagnosed malignancies and a need for cancer chemotherapy. *Crit Care Med* **33**(11):2488–93.
6. de Jonge E, Bos M (2009). Patients with cancer on the ICU: the times they are changing. *Crit Care* **13** (2):122–3.
7. Gillon R (1995). Medical ethics: four principles plus attention to scope. *BMJ* **310**(6974):261–2.
8. Hardwig J (2000) Dying at the right time. In Hardwig J (ed) *Is there a duty to die?*, p.81. New York: Routledge.
9. McGrath S, Chatterjee F, Whiteley C, Ostermann M (2010). ICU and six-month outcome of oncology patients in the intensive care unit. *Q J Med* **103**:397–403.
10. Metnitz PG, Moreno RP, Almeida E, *et al.* (2005). SAPS 3 investigators: SAPS 3–from evaluation of the patient to evaluation of the intensive care unit. Part 1: Objectives, methods and cohort description. *Intensive Care Med* **31**:1336–44.
11. Morreim E (1989). Stratified Scarcity: Redefining the standard of care. *Law, Med Health Care* **17**:356–67.
12. Namendys-Silva SA, Texcocano-Becerra J, Herrera-Gómez A (2010). Prognostic factors in critically ill patients with solid tumours admitted to an oncological intensive care unit. *Anaesth Intensive Care* **38**(2):317–24.
13. Schapira D, Studnicki J, Bradham D, Wolff P, Jarrett A (1993). Intensive care, survival, and expense of treating critically ill cancer patients. *JAMA* **269**(6):783–6.
14. Thiéry G, Azoulay E, Darmon M, *et al.* (2005). Outcome of cancer patients considered for intensive care unit admission: A hospital-wide prospective study. *J Clin Oncol* **23**(19):4406–13.
15. Williams A (2001). How economics can extend the scope of ethical discourse. *J Med Ethics* **27**:251–5.

Part 4

Cancer and pain

Chapter 18

Acute pain management in cancer patients taking regular opioid medication

John E. Williams

Introduction

Patients who present for cancer surgery on high doses of opioids need to be recognized prior to surgery because they may be tolerant to the effects of opioids given postoperatively and require larger than normal doses. Failure to recognize these patients may lead to poor pain control and precipitation of withdrawal phenomena. The mainstay of management is:

◆ Systematic patient recognition

◆ Formulation of a perioperative analgesic plan

◆ Maintenance of baseline opioid requirements

◆ Treatment of breakthrough pain with short-acting opioids

◆ Concomitant use of non-opioid drugs and techniques.

Population at risk

There are two groups of patients who present for cancer surgery on high-dose opioids:

◆ Cancer/chronic pain patients

◆ Recreational opioid abusers.

Both groups of patients need to be recognized prior to surgery as they may be relatively tolerant to opioids given around the time of a surgical procedure.

Cancer/chronic pain patients

Many patients with cancer receive opioids for the management of associated cancer-related pain. This pain could be as the result of tumour pressure, tumour infiltration of nerve roots or viscera, or related to chemotherapy, radiotherapy, or surgery. Some patients take opioids for a short period of time (e.g. following painful oral mucositis), others may be taking opioids for longer periods of time (e.g. patients with bone metastases).

In addition, as the cancer survivor population is increasing as a result of improvements in cancer treatments, many of these patients have pain problems requiring the use of opioids, e.g. for the treatment of chronic back and neck pain.

Most cancer/chronic pain patients use opioid medication appropriately and adhere to an opioid prescribing treatment plan which includes instructions about dosages and side effects and outlines the benefits of treatment expressed in terms of improved physical functioning.

Recreational opioid abusers

A small number of patients who present for cancer surgery may be taking opioids for 'recreational' purposes. It is important to recognize this group as they too may have different opioid requirements around the time of their operation. According to a recent Home Office Report, recreational opioid abusers account for about 1.1% of the UK population and it is therefore possible that some of these patients may present for cancer surgery. It is often difficult to assess the extent of drug use in individual patients, as these drugs will have been obtained via illicit means. Emotionally and behaviourally this group may be difficult to manage perioperatively, as such patients are often sophisticated users of the healthcare system and may be suspicious and distrustful of the service provided.

The term 'pseudoaddiction' refers to patients who in many ways behave in a similar drug-seeking way to opioid abusers, but who in fact have real pain problems that have been undertreated. Once this group is given appropriate analgesics their drug-seeking behaviour diminishes.

Opioid drugs

Patients who present for cancer surgery may be on many different types of opioid for varying periods of time (e.g. morphine, oxycodone, methadone, hydromorphone, pethidine, etc.) which may be modified release (e.g. Zomorph, fentanyl patch) or immediate release preparations (e.g. Sevredol, Oramorph, OxyNorm). The route of delivery may be oral, subcutaneous via a syringe pump, transdermal, or neuraxial. The dosage of opioids in cancer patients can show a wide variation.

Pharmacological changes

Tolerance

Tolerance is a phenomenon in which exposure to a drug results in the diminution of an effect or the need for a higher dose to maintain an effect. It may develop 1–2 weeks or more after initiation of opioid therapy. A larger dosage of perioperative opioid will be required to achieve the desired effect and there is a risk of underdosing which may result in uncontrolled pain and opioid withdrawal symptoms.

Physiological dependence and withdrawal

Patients on high-dose opioids may have developed a physiological dependence requiring the continued administration of opioids. If opioid therapy is abruptly stopped or given in inadequate doses, such as at the time of a surgical operation, then the body reacts with a combination of sympathetic and parasympathetic responses characterized by symptoms such as fatigue, malaise, abdominal cramps, fever, and shaking, also known as a 'withdrawal reaction' or 'abstinence syndrome'. The time course of opioid withdrawal symptoms onset and peak intensity is variable depending on the opioid used. Short-acting opioids such as fentanyl or pethidine have a more rapid onset of withdrawal symptoms and an earlier peak intensity than longer acting drugs such as diamorphine and methadone.

The issues of tolerance, physical dependence, and withdrawal only relate to patients who have been on World Health Organization (WHO) Step 3 strong opioids such as morphine or oxycodone for more than 1–2 weeks preoperatively. These issues are not likely to be a problem in patients taking WHO Step 2 analgesics such as codeine or tramadol unless the patient is taking larger than normal doses. In general, the higher the daily opioid dose requirement, the greater is the degree of tolerance development.

Acute pain management

Assessment

Patients should be identified preoperatively and a distinction should be made between opioid abusing patients and patients who are taking opioids for legitimate medical reasons. Some patients may deny or under-report the level of opioid intake. This group is at risk of poor postoperative pain control and may result in such patients having a longer than expected hospital stay following surgery.

Patients will present for surgery taking many opioid formulations (e.g. oral transmucosal fentanyl, transdermal buprenorphine) at different dosages and it is important that these drugs are recognized prior to surgery.

A 'perioperative analgesic plan' should be devised after discussions with the patient's opioid prescriber and with the acute pain team. This plan will include a calculation of anticipated perioperative opioid dosage requirements and use of non-opioid analgesic drugs and techniques.

It is not appropriate to attempt a deliberate reduction in opioid drug dosages or rehabilitation in the perioperative period. This should only be done when the patient has fully recovered from the effects of surgery and is in a stable condition.

Preoperative management

There have not been any randomized controlled trials evaluating different management options of the opioid-dependent patient prior to surgery. Therefore management is derived from case reports and clinical experience.

- ◆ Opioids should be continued prior to surgery and in this way the patient's 'baseline opioid requirement' is satisfied. This means that patients on sustained release opioid preparations such as Zomorph or morphine sulphate continus or transdermal fentanyl should continue on these drugs prior to surgery. Similarly patients on neuraxial opioids should continue with the usual pump settings. Patients who have stopped taking or who are unable to take their regular opioid drugs (e.g. after trauma, or patients with an acute abdomen) may need to be prescribed short-acting oral opioids prior to surgery, or parenteral opioids on induction of anaesthesia.

◆ Additional short-acting opioids given intravenously should be used intra- and post-operatively to manage surgical pain.

Intraoperative management

◆ During the operation preoperative transdermal opioid patches can be continued. Additional doses of short-acting opioids can be given intraoperatively at a higher dosage to compensate for the effects of tolerance.

◆ Patients on methadone maintenance for opioid addiction have been managed by continuing their baseline methadone dosage and adding in other short-acting strong opioids to treat the postsurgical pain.

◆ Non-opioid analgesic drugs and techniques should be used whenever possible. Typically doses of intraoperative, intravenous opioids will need to be 25–100% higher than doses used in opioid naïve patients. Patients on high doses of preoperative opioids (e.g. >100mg of oral morphine per day) may need more opioid intraoperatively compared with patients on lower doses.

◆ Neuraxial (epidural and intrathecal) opioid and local anaesthetic mixtures have been used successfully to treat postoperative pain in this group of patients. However, there may also be some tolerance to the effect of neuraxial opioids in opioid-dependent patients and larger than normal doses may be required. Use of neuraxial local anaesthetic and clonidine will have a beneficial opioid-sparing effect. Indeed a plain local anaesthetic epidural infusion is favoured by some anaesthetists, with baseline and breakthrough opioid doses given parenterally.

◆ Regional anaesthetic techniques should be used wherever possible. The potential benefit being improved pain control via a non-opioid technique and improved peripheral blood flow from any sympathetic blockade.

◆ Non-steroidal anti-inflammatory drugs, cyclo-oxygenase-2 (COX-2) antagonists, and paracetamol have demonstrable analgesic and opioid-sparing effects, without any concomitant sedative effects, and can be used, assuming no contraindications, in combination with regular opioid medication.

Postoperative management

Effect of surgery on opioid requirements

Surgery itself will have a variable effect on opioid requirements. The effect of surgery may be to increase pain as a result of local tissue trauma with increases of 20% or more above the baseline opioid requirement reported, depending on the surgical procedure. Conversely pain may be reduced after surgery, e.g. reduction in pain due to removal of direct tumour pressure effects on local structures such as the lumbosacral plexus. In such cases baseline doses of opioid may need to be reduced by as much as 50–75%.

Minor surgery

For minor surgery it may be appropriate to manage initial postoperative pain with small doses of intravenous short-acting opioid such as fentanyl in the recovery room. Once the patient is stabilized then the patient should resume taking oral opioids to satisfy baseline opioid requirements with supplementary doses added depending on the magnitude of the surgery performed. Patients unable to take oral opioids postoperatively will require an equivalent parenteral dose calculated to cover baseline requirements, with additional intravenous or subcutaneous opioids given for breakthrough pain. Opioid dosage converters calculate dosage equivalents with adjustments for drug type, route of delivery, and incomplete cross tolerance.

Major surgery

Following major surgery an intravenous patient-controlled analgesia (PCA) machine could be used, with a background infusion delivered according to the patient's baseline opioid requirement calculated from their preoperative opioid dose.

Patient-controlled analgesia

PCA has been used successfully in opioid-dependent patients. The advantage is that dosages and lock-out intervals can be adjusted according to need. To compensate for opioid tolerance, higher than normal bolus doses of morphine, and a background infusion rate equivalent to the patient's baseline opioid requirement should be considered.

It may be appropriate to use intravenous or oral benzodiazepines to treat fear and anxiety in the postoperative period.

Conclusion

Acute pain management of the cancer patient who is taking regular opioids is complex and currently lacks an evidence-based evaluation. Patients need to be identified prior to surgery and an appropriate management plan needs to be devised with the anaesthetist and acute pain team. It is important that the patient's baseline opioid requirements are maintained perioperatively to prevent a withdrawal reaction. Supplemental opioids may be required at larger than normal doses which take into account the effects of tolerance. Such patients are best managed in a recovery or high dependency area. Non-opioid analgesic drugs and techniques such as neuraxial or regional blocks should be utilized whenever possible.

Bibliography

1. Aust R, Sharp C, Goulden C (2002). *Prevalence of drug use: key findings from the 2001/2002 British Crime Survey Home Office Research Findings.* London: Home Office.
2. de Leon-Casasola OA, Lema MJ (1992). Epidural sufentanyl for acute pain control in a patient with extreme opioid dependency. *Anesthesiology* **76**:853–6.
3. Kouyanou K, Pither CE, Wessely S (1997). Medication misuse, abuse and dependence in chronic pain patients. *J Psychosom Res* **43**:497–504.
4. Laulin JP, Celerier E, Larcher A, Le Moal M, Simmonet G (1999). Opiate tolerance to daily heroin administration : an apparent phenomenon associated with enhanced pain sensitivity. *Neuroscience* **89**:632–6.

5. Lewis N, Williams JE (2005). Acute pain management in patients receiving opioids for chronic and cancer pain *Contin Educ Anaesth Crit Care Pain* **5**:127–9.
6. Macintyre PE (2001). Safety and efficacy of patient controlled analgesia. *Br J Anaesthesia* **87**:36–46.
7. May JA, White HC, Leonard-White A, Warltier DC, Pagel PS (2001). The patient recovering from alcohol or drug addiction: special issues for the anesthesiologist. *Anesth Analg* **92**:160–1.
8. Mehta V, Langford RM (2006). Acute pain management for opioid dependent patients. *Anaesthesia* **61**:269–76.
9. Mitra S, Sinatra RS (2004). Perioperative management of acute pain in the opioid-dependent patient. *Anesthesiology* **101**:212–27.
10. Narcotic opioid converter: http://www.globalrph.com/narcoticonv.htm.
11. O'Brien CP (2001). Drug addiction and drug abuse. In Hardman JG, Limbird LE (eds) *Goodman and Gilman's The Pharmacological basis of Therapeutics*, 10th edn, pp.621–42. New York: McGraw-Hill.
12. Portenoy R (1990). Chronic opioid therapy in non-malignant pain. *J Pain Symptom Manage* **5**:S46–62.
13. Weissman DE, HaddoxJD (1989). Opioid pseudoaddiction: an iatrogenic syndrome. *Pain* **36**:363–6.
14. Zenz M, Strumph M, Tryba M (1992). Long-term oral opioid therapy in patients with chronic non-malignant pain. *J Pain Symptom Manage* **7**:69–77.

Chapter 19

Cancer-induced bone pain

Catherine Urch

Introduction

Cancer-induced bone pain (CIBP) is a common clinical problem with more than 60% of cancer inpatients reporting acute flares of pain. CIBP is correlated with an increased morbidity, reduced performance status, increased anxiety and depression, and a reduced quality of life. The pain is comprised of a triad of:

- Tonic (background) ache/pain
- Spontaneous pain
- Movement-induced pain (often, though confusingly, referred to as breakthrough pain).

Although treatment has been revolutionized in the past 20 years with the introduction of bisphosphonates, and a greater variety of fast-acting opioids, there have been no novel therapeutic approaches to the persistent problem of movement-induced or spontaneous bone pain. In part this was due to a lack in understanding of the basic pathophysiology of CIBP and identification of therapeutic targets. Over the last two decades, animal models of CIBP have been developed which have allowed a greater insight into the unique pathophysiology, and a wider understanding of cancer pain. Peripheral neural and bone research has demonstrated the complex pathological interaction between cancer cells, osteoblasts, and osteoclasts, leading to bone destruction, abnormal remodelling, inflammation, and deafferentation. In addition extensive unique changes in dorsal horn of the spinal cord in both neuronal and glial pathways lead to a dynamic excited state, with abnormal and attenuated inhibition. CIBP appears to be a unique pain state, both inflammatory and neuropathic, with an array of potential novel therapeutic targets to be exploited.

CIBP arises from primary bone sarcomas or secondary cancer metastases (most commonly breast, prostate, lung, and myeloma with metastases invading bone in 60–84% of cases). CIBP has a huge impact on patients' lives, and more so now patients are living longer as cancer survivors as well as living longer with cancer and sequelae. It is difficult to estimate the prevalence of CIBP, as it will vary between cancer types, but also because it is poorly defined and often mixed in with 'breakthrough' pain (which may be neuropathic or end-of-dose failure). Studies vary with one reporting 180/200 advanced cancer patients had movement-related pain, another found 93% of consecutive hospice admissions (243 patients) had episodic pain, whilst in ambulatory cancer outpatient populations it was reported that over 60% had 'breakthrough' pain.

Animal models of CIBP

Previous animal models of CIBP have relied on the systemic injection of cancer cells, which resulted in unwell animals and random and multiple sited bone deposits. In the late 1990s, a method of local infusion of cancer into a single bone, with no systemic spread was reported. Osteosarcoma cells were infused into a mouse femur and whilst the animals remained systemically well, they displayed progressively severe nocifensive (pain) behaviour. Over 21 days movement-induced pain behaviours, lack of weight bearing of the limb, and eventually pathological fracture correlated with the degree of bone destruction. The model was rapidly refined, with plugging of bone after cell infusion, and further models were developed using breast carcinoma cells within the rat tibia, fibrosarcoma, melanoma, or adenocarcinoma cells within the mouse humerus or femur. The animal model parallels the clinical course of bone metastases, with progressive bone destruction leading to a pathological fracture (Figure 19.1) accompanying progressive limping, guarding, spontaneous flinching and vocalization on palpation, reduced movement, secondary hyperalgesia, and allodynia (Figure 19.1).

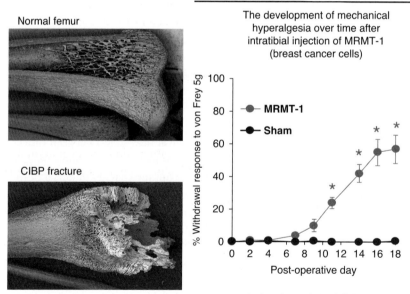

Animal model of CIBP

Fig. 19.1 Results of intratibial injection of MRMT-1 breast cancer cells in rat model of CIBP. Left-hand panel shows two scanning electron microscope pictures of a normal rat tibia (top) and the pathological fracture (bottom) after d20, note abnormal bone resorption (osteoclast action), and abnormal bone formation (osteoblast action). The right-hand panel demonstrates the withdrawal response to von Frey 5g filament over d0–18 post MRMT1 injection (grey) and sham injection (black). Note the significant withdrawal from d11, indicating hyperalgesia in cancer model (CIBP).

Why is tumour-induced bone destruction painful?

Primary afferents

In the past it was suggested that tumour-induced bone pain may be due to vascular occlusion, compression of the bone or peripheral nerve, or due to mechanical instability. The input of primary afferents within the bone itself was considered of little importance as the periosteum was thought to be the only innervated structure. Changes in the preparation of bones allowed the extent of intermedullary penetration of primary afferents and sympathetic fibres to be demonstrated. These neural networks transmit non-noxious (Aβ fibres) and noxious stimuli (Aδ and C fibres) to the dorsal horn of the spinal cord. There the signals undergo extensive excitatory and inhibitory modulation, before being relayed to higher centres in the brain.

The primary afferents to bone are comprised of:

- Neuropeptidergic C fibres expressing calcitonin gene related peptide (CGRP), neuropeptide Y (NPY), vasoactive intestinal peptide (VIP), vallinoid receptor (VR1), and Trk A receptors
- Aδ fibres (similar expression pattern to C fibres)
- Sympathetic neurons (SNS).

Neuropeptides are important in regulating bone metabolism and osteoclast function, such that neonatal ablation of C fibres and SNS resulted in a 21% and 45% reduction in osteoclasts.

Pro-excitatory factors released within the bone

Tumours invade and grow within the bone medulla, directly affecting primary afferents and bone osteoclast/osteoblast balance. Tumour cells release numerous growth factors (such as nerve growth factor (NGF), which binds to Trk A receptor on C fibres), cytokines (such as tumour necrosis factor (TNF), which binds to the ubiquitous p75 and TNF receptors on C fibres), prostinoids (bind to prostinoid receptors), interleukins, and others. These factors have direct excitatory effects on the peptidergic C fibres, as well as immune-recruiting functions. In addition tumour cells are rapidly growing and dying, releasing ATP amongst other intracellular stimulators of primary afferents. The complex interactions between tumour cells, recruited immune cells, osteoclasts, and primary afferents are vital to understanding the peripheral contribution to CIBP.

Cytokines are small soluble proteins that activate receptors in autocrine and paracrine actions to produce numerous reactions via superfamilies of receptors and cytokines. In CIBP cytokines are responsible for 'pre-setting' an excitatory neuronal background, peripherally and centrally. TNF is upregulated and anti-TNF therapy has been reported to markedly reduce resistant CIBP. Growth factors, such as NGF, have come under intense scrutiny given their role in C-fibre activation in inflammatory pain. NGF is released by tumour cells and recruited activated macrophages within bone medulla, and

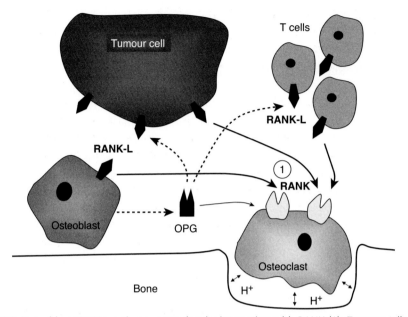

Fig. 19.2 Osteoblast RANK-L activates osteoclast by interaction with RANK (1). Tumour cells, and inflammatory T cells add to this activation increasing bone destruction (1). Activated osteoblasts release OPG which normally inhibits osteoclasts by interaction with RANK. Sequestration of OPG by tumour cells (dotted line) reduces this inhibition and further increases bone destruction.

binds to Trk A receptors expressed on 90% of bone C fibres. This property has been exploited by the use in animal models of a Trk A-sequestering antibody, which significantly attenuated pain behaviours in a CIBP-osteosarcoma model. Clinical trials are needed to further explore this effect.

The expression of endothelins (ETs) by tumour cells is required in order to metastasize through vascular endothelium, regulate tumour cell signal transduction, mitogenesis, endothelial cell growth, and angiogenesis. In addition, ETs are implicated in inflammatory pain via C fibres expression of ET receptors. A mouse model of osteolytic carcinoma demonstrated a correlation between peak pain behaviours and elevation of ET-1 secretion, furthermore blockade of ET_A receptors attenuated this response. In clinical prostate cancer ET levels correlate with bone pain, and the use of ET_A receptor antagonists have demonstrated a reduction in bone metastases and reduction in bone pain.

Osteoclast activation: acidosis and RANK

Osteoclasts act to resorb bone from the bone surface. Osteoclast formation and activation requires macrophage colony stimulating factor (M-CSF) and the binding of the receptor activator for nuclear factor κB (RANK), expressed on osteoclast precursors, with RANK ligand (RANK-L), which is expressed on several cell types including osteoblasts, and an acid environment (pH <6).

The RANK–RANK-L interaction is crucial for normal balanced activation of osteo-clasts and osteoblasts. To limit the forward feeding cycle, osteoblasts secrete a cytokine, osteoprotegerin (OPG), which binds and sequesters RANK-L preventing RANK binding and therefore reduces osteoclast activation (Figure 19.2). OPG is part of the TNF super-family and binds to a variety of receptors inducing apoptosis. Invading cancer cells and recruited T cells also express RANK-L, so an imbalance in osteoclast–osteoblast activation is induced, as well as sequestering OPG. In humans RANK-L cancer expression (high in myeloma and low in prostate cancer) is correlated with osteolytic damage, and low circulat-ing OPG levels. In one study, 225 patients with myeloma were shown to have serum OPG levels 18% lower than normal controls, correlating with extensive painful metastases.

Activated osteoclasts absorb mineralized bone at an abnormal rate in CIBP. The destruction can be extensive, with on occasion loss of the bone cortex and fracture. Even new bone formation is disordered. This extensive resorption leads to secondary destruc-tion of primary afferent terminals, producing a classic deafferentation pattern.

OPG is a potential therapeutic target for CIBP analgesia. In mouse models, infusion of OPG significantly attenuated pain behaviours, and virtually eliminated bone destruction by reducing osteoclast activation. In addition OPG-Fc fusion protein has been adminis-tered to patients with myeloma, with minimal side effects and a significant reduction in markers of bone turnover equivalent to intravenous pamidronate.

Acid pH is another potent peripheral C-fibre trigger (resulting in pain). Activated osteoclasts reduce the pH to less than 5, to facilitate bone resorption. In addition, rapidly growing cancers generate a hostile acid environment with an accumulation of acid metab-olites, ischaemia, apoptosis, and phagocytosis. This in turn can directly activate acid sens-ing ion channels (ASIC) such as transient receptor potential vanilloid type 1 (TRPVR1) and the ASIC 3, which have been demonstrated on bone C fibres. Rodent models have demonstrated a significant attenuation of pain behaviours with TRPV-1 receptor antago-nist, but an increase in thermal hyperalgesia. Clinical studies are underway.

Dorsal horn changes

The dorsal horn is a vital centre for primary afferent input modulation. In all types of pain the dorsal horn is responsible for extensive up- or downregulation of the input. Modulation is intrinsic to the dorsal horn, such as tonic inhibition (via cannabinoid and endorphin systems), to 'wind-up' and central sensitization, and extrinsic such as descend-ing inhibition and facilitation from supraspinal levels. Neuropathic and inflammatory noxious stimuli induce specific changes within the dorsal horn, whilst both excitatory the pattern of neuroreceptor expression alters. In CIBP the dorsal horn has a unique signa-ture, neither inflammatory nor neuropathic. Primary afferent stimuli are mixed (inflam-matory via immune cells, cytokines, prostinoids, and neuropathic via deafferentation). The dorsal horn undergoes significant alteration in neuronal receptor expression, intrinsic excitation, loss of inhibition, and glial activation.

Rodent models have demonstrated an upregulation in dynorphin expression (not VIP or CGRP and others), and an extensive glial hypertrophy and activation. The extent may be tumour type dependent; however it is extensive and persistent. This results in a pro-excitatory state demonstrated by increased neuronal response at lower threshold. Uniquely to CIBP, dorsal horn neurons lamina I change from being predominately nociceptive specific (NS), (responding only to noxious stimuli) to wide-dynamic range (WDR) (responding to noxious and non-noxious stimuli) (Figure 19.3). This is of particular importance as lamina I is the main termination point for nociceptive Aδ fibres on the classical pain pathway. In addition lamina V, also demonstrates hyperexcitability, more in keeping with inflammatory stimuli and important for the ultimate modulation of C-fibre input.

In terms of pain behaviours, the rodent model closely parallels the clinical state. A period of no pain is followed by a sudden and prolonged increase with reduction in weight-bearing limb and movement (movement-induced pain), tonic and spontaneous pain, and ultimately pathological fracture. The alteration in lamina I excitation is correlated with the sudden expression of pain behaviours, and attenuation of lamina I response directly leads to a reduction of pain behaviours in rodent models. Systemic gabapentin has been shown to normalize lamina I response, and normalize the ratio of NS:WDR neurons and attenuate pain behaviours (Figure 19.4). This demonstrated the importance of a dynamic response in the dorsal horn in facilitating pain, which bodes well for clinical analgesia.

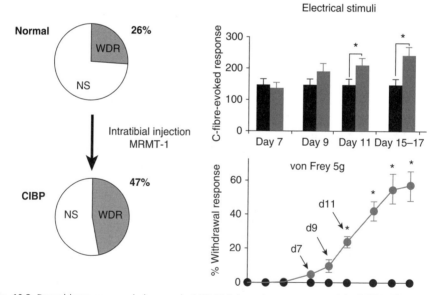

Fig. 19.3 Dorsal horn neuronal changes in MRMT-1 breast cancer rat model of CIBP. The left-hand panel demonstrates the ratio of nociceptive specific (NS) to wide-dynamic range (WDR) in normal (or sham) and in CIBP (from d15 onwards). It can be seen that the percentage of WDR neurons increases from 25% to almost 50%. The right-hand panel demonstrates the neuronal response in lamina 1 neurons to electrical (top panel) and von Frey 5g filament. For both stimuli there is a significant response in the MRMT-1 group as compared to control.

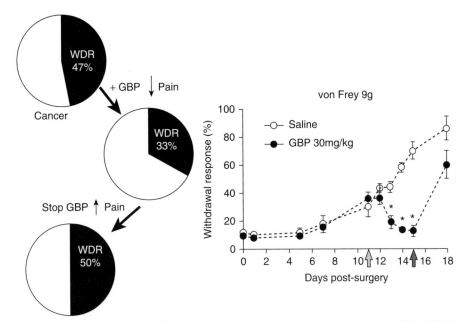

Fig. 19.4 Dorsal horn neuronal changes and behavioural response to noxious stimuli in MRMT-1 breast cancer rat model CIBP treated with systemic gabapentin (GBP) 30mg/kg between d11–15. The left panel shows the changes in lamina I NS and WDR neurons, with an increase in WDR to 50% in CIBP, falling back to 25% (equivalent to normal dorsal horn) during gabapentin treatment, but reverting to 50% once gabapentin has stopped. This is mirrored in the right panel showing behavioural response, with a significant normalization of response (reduced percentage withdrawal to von Frey 9g filament compared to saline treated), which then reverts to no treatment response once gabapentin is withdrawn.

What is unknown is whether the increased excitation seen in lamina I is due to direct increased excitation or a loss of inhibition. Work from a pancreatic rodent model, suggests that it is the loss of tonic opioid inhibition which is the switch from 'no-pain to pain'. Other work suggests that the intrinsic cannabinoid system is important in maintaining tonic inhibition, and loss is also related to increased pain behaviours. Descending facilitatory pathways, and/or reduction of descending inhibitory pathways also influence dorsal horn excitation. The lamina I excitatory response can be attenuated by the addition of 5-hydroxy-tryptophan-3 receptor antagonist (ondansetron) intrathecally in a rat model of CIBP. This receptor is part of the descending facilitatory pathway and demonstrates the excitatory impact of this pathway in CIBP.

More recently the role of glial cells in the generation and maintenance of pain pathways has been demonstrated. Far from being merely bystander cells, whose role was only to support neurons, it has now been acknowledged that astrocytes and the immune-derived microglia play as an intrinsic role in pain pathways as neurons. In neuropathy and inflammatory models glia activation has been demonstrated, and attenuation of hyperalgesic response via glia inhibitors. In addition in CIBP the significant astrocyte and microglia activation implies a central role. CIBP has been shown to increase spinal pro-inflammatory mediators including interleukin 1 (IL-1), that activate microglia. IL-1 antagonists can attenuate CIBP. In addition early administration of systemic minocycline (a potent inhibitor of microglia) significantly delayed the development of CIBP behaviours, but not when administered at a later time point. This indicates a role for microglia in the induction and generation of neuronal excitation and pain pathway, but less of role in maintenance.

Supraspinal processing

Neuroimaging studies using fMRI (functional magnetic resonance imaging) techniques have made a huge impact on the understanding of supraspinal pain pathways in humans. The complex neural networks (pain matrix) span prefrontal cortex, subcortical, thalamic, hippocampal, and brainstem areas that produce the sensory-discriminative integration of pain. In addition data supports the importance of the descending modulatory system and the regulation of tonic inhibition/excitation, with respect to background and spontaneous pain. As yet no studies have been reported in CIBP patients, so the long-term remodelling, or contributions of descending modulation, or cortical areas have not yet been revealed.

Current treatment

Satisfactory analgesia is difficult to achieve given the speed of onset of movement or spontaneous pain, intensity, and short duration. Animal models and clinical CIBP have demonstrated sensitivity to opioids, which can deliver satisfactory analgesia for both background and flares of pain, however the delivery and half-life of most opioids preclude them from being clinically effective. Thus the dose that successfully treats background pain is not sufficient to control flares of pain, but continuous doses of opioids sufficient to control the flares of pain, render the patient toxic and sedated between flares. This dilemma is often addressed by a low background dose of opioids and as-required fast-acting (often transmucosal) opioid. Non-steroidal anti-inflammatory drugs (NSAIDs) are often prescribed for CIBP with little or no evaluation of efficacy and increased exposure of the patient to serious side effects. There is no published trial of NSAID efficacy in CIBP although spinal COX II enzyme has been shown to expressed constitutively on neurons and glia in the rat lumbar spinal cord and animal models of CIBP acute treatment with a highly selective COX II inhibitor MF tricyclic attenuated pain behaviours (and reduced tumour burden).

Other current analgesics include local radiotherapy or systemic isotopes for hemibody metastases. The former has been demonstrated to achieve at least 50% pain relief in 50% of patients by 8 weeks, although there is no difference between dosing schedules (single or multiple fractions). Systemic bisphosphonate treatment has risen in popularity, as they have been shown to reduce the development of bone metastases, delay the time to first fracture, and reduce pain. A Cochrane review demonstrated some evidence for their use as analgesics with a delayed effect with a NNT (number needed to treat) of seven by 12 weeks.

Conclusion

After decades of being ignored, CIBP is coming to the forefront of research and clinical awareness. The development of reliable animal models where animals remained well, with localized, reproducible pain development which closely parallels the human situation, has allowed elucidation of some of the basic mechanisms that may underlie this pain state. It is apparent that CIBP is a unique pain state, arising from complex interactions between tumour cells, osteoclasts, recruited immune cells, and destruction of primary afferents. A range of novel targets have been demonstrated in animal models to be of potential therapeutic benefit, with some promising preliminary clinical data. Central pathophysiology is unique, the dorsal horn excitation resulting from glial activation, reduction of inhibition, descending facilitation, and intrinsic pro-excitatory neuroreceptor upregulation. Together these factors lead to a complex clinical pain state, with a triad of pains—background, spontaneous, and movement related, the last two remaining resistant to current therapies. The explosion of knowledge and acknowledgement of the complexity of cancer-induced bone pain may yet yield new more effective analgesics.

Bibliography

1. Bjurholm A, Kreicbergs A, Terenius L, Goldstein M, Schultzberg M (1988). Neuropeptide Y-, tyrosine hydroxylase- and vasoactive intestinal polypeptide-immunoreactive nerves in bone and surrounding tissues. *J Auton Nerv Syst* **25**(2–3):119–25.
2. Caraceni A, Portenoy RK (1999). An international survey of cancer pain characteristics and syndromes. IASP Task Force on Cancer Pain. International Association for the Study of Pain. *Pain* **82**(3):263–74.
3. Carducci MA, Padley RJ, Breul J, *et al.* (2003). Effect of endothelin-A receptor blockade with atrasentan on tumor progression in men with hormone-refractory prostate cancer: a randomized, phase II, placebo-controlled trial. *J Clin Oncol* **21**(4):679–89.
4. Coyle N, Adelhardt J, Foley KM, Portenoy RK (1990). Character of terminal illness in the advanced cancer patient: pain and other symptoms during the last four weeks of life. *J Pain Symptom Manage* **5**(2):83–93.
5. Davar G, Hans G, Fareed MU, Sinnott C, Strichartz G (1998). Behavioral signs of acute pain produced by application of endothelin-1 to rat sciatic nerve. *Neuroreport* **9**(10):2279–83.
6. Donovan-Rodriguez T, Dickenson AH, Urch CE (2005). Gabapentin normalizes spinal neuronal responses that correlate with behavior in a rat model of cancer-induced bone pain. *Anesthesiology* **102**(1):132–40.
7. Fairhurst M, Wiech K, Dunckley P, Tracey I (2007). Anticipatory brainstem activity predicts neural processing of pain in humans. *Pain* **128**(1–2):101–10.
8. Honore P, Luger NM, Sabino MA, *et al.* (2000). Osteoprotegerin blocks bone cancer-induced skeletal destruction, skeletal pain and pain-related neurochemical reorganization of the spinal cord. *Nat Med* **6**(5):521–8.
9. Kong YY, Yoshida H, Sarosi I, *et al.* (1999). OPGL is a key regulator of osteoclastogenesis, lymphocyte development and lymph-node organogenesis. *Nature* **397**(6717):315–23.
10. Laughlin TM, Bethea JR, Yezierski RP, Wilcox GL (2000). Cytokine involvement in dynorphin-induced allodynia. *Pain* **84**(2–3):159–67.
11. Luger NM, Sabino MA, Schwei MJ, *et al.* (2002). Efficacy of systemic morphine suggests a fundamental difference in the mechanisms that generate bone cancer vs. inflammatory pain. *Pain* **99**(3):397–406.

12. Luger NM, Mach DB, Sevcik MA, Mantyh PW (2005). Bone cancer pain: from model to mechanism to therapy. *J Pain Symptom Manage* **29**(5 Suppl):S32–46.

13. McNicol E, Strassels SA, Goudas L, Lau J, Carr DB (2005). NSAIDS or paracetamol, alone or combined with opioids, for cancer pain. *Cochrane Database Syst Rev* **1**:CD005180.

14. McQuay HJ, Collins SL, Carroll D, Moore RA (2000). Radiotherapy for the palliation of painful bone metastases. *Cochrane Database Syst Rev* **2**:CD001793.

15. Mercadante S, Fulfaro F, Casuccio A (2002). A randomised controlled study on the use of anti-inflammatory drugs in patients with cancer pain on morphine therapy: effects on dose-escalation and a pharmacoeconomic analysis. *Eur J Cancer* **38**(10):1358–63.

16. Schwei MJ, Honore P, Rogers SD, *et al.* (1999). Neurochemical and cellular reorganization of the spinal cord in a murine model of bone cancer pain. *J Neurosci* **19**(24):10886–97.

17. Sezer O, Heider U, Zavrski I, Kuehne CA, Hofbauer LC (2002). RANK ligand and osteoprotegerin in myeloma bone disease. *Blood* **7**:7.

18. Suzuki K, Yamada S (1994). Ascites sarcoma 180, a tumor associated with hypercalcemia, secretes potent bone resorbing factors including transforming growth factor alpha, interleukin 1 alpha and interleukin 6. *Bone Miner* **27**(3):219–33.

19. Swanwick M, Haworth M, Lennard RF (2001). The prevalence of episodic pain in cancer: a survey of hospice patients on admission. *Palliat Med* **15**(1):9–18.

20. Watkins LR, Maier SF (2002). Beyond neurons: evidence that immune and glial cells contribute to pathological pain states. *Physiol Rev* **82**(4):981–1011.

21. Watkins LR, Wiertelak EP, Furness LE, Maier SF (1994). Illness-induced hyperalgesia is mediated by spinal neuropeptides and excitatory amino acids. *Brain Res* **664**(1–2):17–24.

22. Watkins LR, Hutchinson MR, Rice KC, Maier SF (2009). The 'toll' of opioid-induced glial activation: improving the clinical efficacy of opioids by targeting glia. *Trends Pharmacol Sci* **30**(11):581–91.

23. Wong R, Wiffen PJ (2002). Bisphosphonates for the relief of pain secondary to bone metastases. *Cochrane Database Syst Rev* **2**:CD002068.

Chapter 20

Breakthrough cancer pain

Andrew N. Davies

Introduction

It is 20 years since the phenomenon of breakthrough pain was first characterized by Portenoy and Hagen. In the intervening period, there has been an increasing recognition of the morbidity caused by breakthrough pain, and also of the health economic impact of breakthrough pain. Furthermore, we are now seeing the emergence of therapeutic interventions, which have been specifically developed to treat breakthrough cancer pain (BTCP), e.g. oral transmucosal opioid formulations, intranasal opioid formulations.

Definition

Currently, there is no universally accepted definition for breakthrough pain. Recently, an expert group from the UK suggested the following definition of breakthrough pain: 'a transient exacerbation of pain that occurs either spontaneously, or in relation to a specific predictable or unpredictable trigger, despite relatively stable and adequately controlled background pain'.

On the basis of the above, the term breakthrough pain should not be used to describe episodes of pain that occur during the initiation or titration of opioid analgesics, since the patient clearly does not have controlled background pain in this situation. Such episodes of pain should be termed either a 'background pain flare', or simply an 'exacerbation of background pain'.

Similarly, the term breakthrough pain should not be used to describe episodes of pain that occur before the administration of opioid analgesics ('end-of-dose failure'), since the patient again does not have controlled background pain in this situation. However, end-of-dose failure is regarded as a subtype of breakthrough pain by some experts in the field.

Figure 20.1 shows the diagnostic algorithm developed by the aforementioned expert group from the UK.

Epidemiology

Breakthrough pain is a common problem in patients with cancer. The prevalence of breakthrough pain has been reported to be 19–95% amongst various groups of patients.

DOES THE PATIENT HAVE BACKGROUND PAIN?

[Background pain = pain present for ≥ 12 hr/day during previous week (or would be present if not taking analgesia)]

↓

YES (If no, patient does not have breakthrough pain)

↓

IS THE BACKGROUND PAIN ADEQUATELY CONTROLLED?

[Adequately controlled = pain rated as "none" or "mild", but not "moderate" or "severe" for ≥ 12 hr/day during previous week]

↓

YES (If no, patient does not have breakthrough pain)

↓

DOES THE PATIENT HAVE TRANSIENT EXACERBATIONS OF PAIN?

↓

YES (If no, patient does not have breakthrough pain)

↓

PATIENT HAS BREAKTHROUGH PAIN

Fig. 20.1 Algorithm for diagnosing patients with breakthrough cancer pain.

This disparity reflects a number of factors, including differences in the definition and methodology utilized, and in the populations studied.

Interestingly, an International Association for the Study of Pain (IASP) survey of cancer pain characteristics and syndromes found that pain specialists from English-speaking (North America, Australasia) and Northern/Western European countries reported more breakthrough pain than pain specialists from South American, Asian, and Southern/Eastern European countries.

Breakthrough pain appears to be more common in patients with:

- Advanced disease
- Poor performance status
- Pain originating from the vertebral column (and to a lesser extent other weight-bearing bones/joints)
- Pain originating from the nerve plexuses (and to a lesser extent nerve roots).

Aetiology

The aetiology of the breakthrough pain is usually the same as that of the background pain. Thus, breakthrough pain may be due to:

1 Direct effect of the cancer (i.e. anatomical effect of the cancer)
2 Indirect effect of the cancer (i.e. physiological effect of the cancer)

3 Effect of the anticancer treatment

4 Effect of a concomitant illness.

The pathophysiology of the breakthrough pain is also usually the same as that of the background pain. Thus, breakthrough pain may be nociceptive, neuropathic, or mixed (i.e. nociceptive and neuropathic).

Classification

Breakthrough pain is usually classified according to its relationship/lack of relationship to specific events:

◆ Spontaneous pain (also known as 'idiopathic pain')—this type of pain occurs unexpectedly.

◆ Incident pain (also known as 'precipitated pain' or 'movement-related pain')—this type of pain is related to specific events, and can be subclassified into three categories:

1 Volitional incident pain—precipitated by a voluntary act (e.g. walking)

2 Non-volitional incident pain—precipitated by an involuntary act (e.g. coughing)

3 Procedural pain—related to a therapeutic intervention (e.g. wound dressing).

End-of-dose failure describes an exacerbation of pain that occurs prior to the next dose of the background analgesic, and reflects declining levels of the background analgesic. However, many experts now believe that end-of-dose failure is not a subtype of breakthrough pain, since they perceive that end-of-dose failure represents inadequately controlled breakthrough pain (see 'Definition' section).

Clinical features

Breakthrough pain is not a single condition, but a spectrum of very different conditions. The clinical features vary from individual to individual, and may vary within an individual. Nevertheless, breakthrough pain is usually reported to be frequent in occurrence, acute in onset, short in duration, and moderate-to-severe in intensity. For example, Zeppetella et al. reported a mean number of four episodes per day (range 1–14), whilst Gomez-Batiste et al. reported a mean duration of 34min (range 1–180min). The clinical features of the breakthrough pain are often related to the clinical features of the background pain.

Breakthrough pain may result in a number of physical problems (related to reduced activity and movement), psychological problems (including increased levels of anxiety and depression), and social complications, such as decreased levels of working and social interaction. Hence, the presence of breakthrough pain can have a significant negative impact on the quality of life of the patient and the quality of life of the patient's family and carers.

Assessment

The successful management of breakthrough pain depends on adequate assessment of the patient. Patients with pain should be assessed for the presence of breakthrough pain, and patients with breakthrough pain should have this pain specifically assessed.

The objectives of assessment are to determine the aetiology of the pain, the pathophysiology of the pain, and any factors that would indicate or contraindicate specific interventions. Inadequate assessment may lead to ineffective, or even inappropriate, treatment (and so continuance of the breakthrough pain).

The assessment of breakthrough pain is similar in nature to that of the background pain, and depends primarily on basic clinical skills, i.e. taking a detailed history and performing a thorough examination. Currently there is no validated clinical breakthrough pain assessment tool.

Management

The management of breakthrough pain should be individualized. The optimal management of breakthrough pain depends on a variety of pain-related factors including:

◆ The aetiology of the pain: cancer-related, treatment-related, concomitant illness

◆ The pathophysiology of the pain: nociceptive, neuropathic, mixed

◆ The clinical features of the pain.

Furthermore, the management of breakthrough pain depends on a variety of patient-related factors, including the stage of the disease, the performance status of the patient, and the personal preferences of the patient.

The management of breakthrough pain includes treatment of the underlying cause of the pain, avoidance/treatment of the precipitating factors of the pain, modification of the background analgesic regimen ('around the clock medication'), use of rescue medication ('breakthrough medication'), use of non-pharmacological methods, and use of interventional/anaesthetic techniques. However, the evidence for most of these strategies is from small non-analytical studies, or so-called 'expert opinion'.

Modification of the background analgesic regimen ('around-the-clock medication')

Modification of the background analgesic regimen has been shown to be a useful approach in managing breakthrough pain, and may involve one or more of the following treatment strategies:

◆ Titration of opioid analgesics: titrating the opioid has been shown to be effective in reducing the intensity and/or frequency of movement-related volitional incident pain. However, this strategy is often limited by the dose-dependent adverse effects (e.g. sedation).

◆ Switching of opioid analgesics: switching the opioid or the route of administration of the opioid has also been shown to be effective in reducing the severity of movement-related volitional incident pain.

◆ Addition of 'adjuvant analgesics': adjuvant analgesics are agents which provide pain relief in certain circumstances. This strategy can be effective in reducing the impact of specific breakthrough pain syndromes (e.g. anticonvulsants for neuropathic pain, antispasmodics for visceral pain).

◆ Addition of other 'adjuvant drugs': adjuvant drugs are agents whose function is not analgesia, but which provide relief from the adverse effects of analgesic drugs or the complications of the pain. This strategy can be effective in allowing titration of the analgesic drugs, which in turn can be effective in reducing the impact of breakthrough pain, such as psychostimulants for opioid-related sedation.

◆ Other strategies: in theory, alteration and/or addition of non-opioid analgesic drugs could also lead to improvements in breakthrough pain (e.g. paracetamol, non-steroidal anti-inflammatory drugs).

Use of rescue medication ('breakthrough medication')

The mainstay of the management of breakthrough pain episodes is the use of so-called 'rescue medication' or 'breakthrough medication'. Rescue medication is taken as required, rather than on a regular basis: rescue medication should be taken at the onset of the pain, although may be taken in advance of pain in cases of volitional incident pain or procedural pain.

The characteristics of an 'ideal' rescue medication include:

◆ Good efficacy

◆ Rapid onset of action

◆ Short duration of effect

◆ Good tolerability

◆ Easy to use

◆ Acceptable to the patient

◆ Available and affordable.

In most cases the most appropriate rescue medication will be an opioid analgesic, rather than a non-opioid or an adjuvant analgesic. However, it is important to use an appropriate opioid formulation, and an appropriate (titrated) dosage of the opioid formulation.

Oral rescue medication

Traditionally, the most common form of rescue medication has been a fixed dose of an oral 'immediate-release' formulation of morphine. However, the pharmacodynamic profile of oral morphine does not tend to mirror the temporal characteristics of most breakthrough pain episodes. Thus, the slow onset of action (onset of analgesia: 20–30min; peak analgesia: 60–90min) results in delayed or ineffective analgesia, whilst the prolonged duration of effect (3–6h) results in ongoing adverse effects (see Figure 20.2). Therefore, oral morphine is not the optimal rescue medication for most breakthrough pain episodes. These factors apply equally to the oral immediate-release formulations of similar opioid analgesics (e.g. hydromorphone, oxycodone).

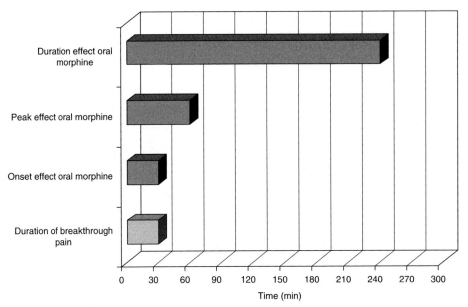

Fig. 20.2 Temporal relationship between breakthrough pain episode and oral morphine treatment.

Nevertheless, oral morphine may have a role in the management of breakthrough pain. It may be useful in the management of breakthrough pain episodes lasting for more than 60min, and may be considered in the pre-emptive management of volitional incident pain or procedural pain if taken at least 30min, and probably 60min, before the relevant precipitant of the pain. A novel effervescent oral formulation of morphine has been developed and has been reported to have a quicker onset of analgesia than conventional oral formulations.

Parenteral rescue medication

Parenteral opioids are frequently used in the management of breakthrough pain in the secondary care setting (i.e. hospital, hospice), and sometimes in the primary care setting (i.e. home, nursing home). Parenteral opioids are associated with a rapid onset of analgesia (5–10min), but can be associated with a prolonged duration of effect (see above). However, their use is limited by practical issues, and, to a lesser extent, by the reluctance of patients to use parenteral routes of administration.

Oral transmucosal rescue medication (i.e. buccal, sublingual)

The oral transmucosal routes of administration are well established in the management of breakthrough pain episodes. A number of commercial formulations have been developed utilizing these routes of administration, including a fentanyl lozenge on stick (buccal administration), a fentanyl buccal tablet, a fentanyl sublingual tablet, and a fentanyl buccal soluble film. Data from clinical studies suggest that these products have a quicker onset of action than oral opioids (resulting in a greater efficacy than oral opioids), and cause typical opioid-related adverse effects with little local toxicity. However, some patients have difficulty in using these products due to coexisting oral problems such as salivary gland dysfunction.

Intranasal rescue medication

The intranasal route of administration is also well established in the management of breakthrough pain episodes. A couple of commercial formulations have been developed utilizing this route of administration, including a fentanyl spray, and a fentanyl-pectin spray. These products may have a quicker onset of action than oral opioids and than oral transmucosal opioids. They also cause typical opioid-related adverse effects but with little local toxicity. Coexisting nasal problems may preclude their use, and some patients are reluctant to use this route of administration.

Intrapulmonary rescue medication

The intrapulmonary route of administration has also been used in the management of breakthrough pain episodes. A number of commercial formulations are being developed utilizing this route of administration. Currently, there is limited data on the efficacy or tolerability of these formulations.

Conclusion

The successful management of breakthrough pain depends on adequate reassessment of the patient. Patients with breakthrough pain should have this pain specifically reassessed. The objectives of reassessment are to determine the efficacy of the treatment, the tolerability of the treatment, and any change in the nature of the breakthrough pain. Inadequate reassessment may lead to continuance of ineffective or inappropriate treatment and continuing breakthrough pain. The reassessment of breakthrough pain is similar in nature to that of the background pain.

- ◆ BTCP is a common problem in patients with cancer pain.
- ◆ BTCP is associated with significant morbidity, and a variety of physical, psychological, and social complications.
- ◆ The management of BTCP involves adequate assessment, appropriate treatment, and adequate re-assessment.
- ◆ The treatment of BTCP involves a number of different strategies, although the mainstay of treatment is the use of rescue medication (generally an opioid analgesic).
- ◆ Oral opioids are often ineffective in the treatment of BTCP, as the pharmacodynamic profile of these drugs does not match the temporal characteristics of these pains.

Bibliography

1. Bailey F, Farley A (2006). Oral opioid drugs. In Davies A (ed) *Cancer-related breakthrough pain*, pp.43–55. Oxford: Oxford University Press.
2. Breakthroughcancerpain.org http://www.breakthroughcancerpain.org.

3. Bruera E, Fainsinger R, MacEachern T, Hanson J (1992). The use of methylphenidate in patients with incident cancer pain receiving regular opiates. A preliminary report. *Pain* **50**(1):75–7.

4. Caraceni A, Portenoy RK (1999). An international survey of cancer pain characteristics and syndromes. *Pain* **82**(3):263–74.

5. Caraceni A, Martini C, Zecca E, *et al.* (2004). Breakthrough pain characteristics and syndromes in patients with cancer pain. An international survey. *Palliat Med* **18**(3):177–83.

6. Colleau SM (1999). The significance of breakthrough pain in cancer. *Cancer Pain Release* **12**(4), 1–4.

7. Dale O (2006). Opioid drugs via other routes. In Davies A (ed) *Cancer-related breakthrough pain*, pp.73–82. Oxford: Oxford University Press.

8. Davies A (2006a). Introduction. In Davies A (ed) *Cancer-related breakthrough pain*, pp.1–11. Oxford: Oxford University Press.

9. Davies A (2006b). General principles of management. In Davies A (ed) *Cancer-related breakthrough pain*, pp.31–42. Oxford: Oxford University Press.

10. Davies AN, Vriens J (2005). Oral transmucosal fentanyl citrate and xerostomia (dry mouth). *J Pain Symptom Manage* **30**(6):496–7.

11. Davies AN, Vriens J, Kennett A, McTaggart M (2008). An observational study of oncology patients' utilisation of breakthrough pain medication. *J Pain Symptom Manage* **35**(4):406–11.

12. Davies AN, Dickman A, Reid C, Stevens AM, Zeppetella G (2009). The management of cancer-related breakthrough pain: recommendations of a task group of the Science Committee of the Association for Palliative Medicine of Great Britain and Ireland. *Eur J Pain* **13**(4):331–8.

13. Enting RH, Oldenmenger WH, *et al.* (2002). A prospective study evaluating the response of patients with unrelieved cancer pain to parenteral opioids. *Cancer* **94**(11):3049–56.

14. Fortner BV, Okon TA, Portenoy RK (2002). A survey of pain-related hospitalizations, emergency department visits, and physician office visits reported by cancer patients with and without history of breakthrough pain. *J Pain* **3**(1):38–44.

15. Fortner BV, Demarco G, Irving G, Ashley J, Keppler G, Chavez J, *et al.* (2003). Description and predictors of direct and indirect costs of pain reported by cancer patients. *J Pain Symptom Manage* **25**(1):9–18.

16. Freye E, Levy JV, Braun D (2007). Effervescent morphine results in faster relief of breakthrough pain in patients compared to immediate release morphine sulfate tablet. *Pain Pract* **7**(4):324–31.

17. Gannon C, Davies A (2006). Non-opioid drugs. In Davies A (ed) *Cancer-related breakthrough pain*, pp.83–96. Oxford: Oxford University Press.

18. Gómez-Batiste X, Madrid F, Moreno F, *et al.* (2002). Breakthrough cancer pain: prevalence and characteristics in patients in Catalonia, Spain. *J Pain Symptom Manage* **24**(1):45–52.

19. Hwang SS, Chang VT, Kasimis B (2003). Cancer breakthrough pain characteristics and responses to treatment at a VA medical center. *Pain* **101**(1–2):55–64.

20. Kalso E, Heiskanen T, Rantio M, Rosenberg PH, Vainio A (1996). Epidural and subcutaneous morphine in the management of cancer pain: a double-blind cross-over study. *Pain* **67**(2–3):443–9.

21. Laverty D, Davies A (2006). Assessment. In Davies A (ed) *Cancer-related breakthrough pain*, pp.23–30. Oxford: Oxford University Press.

22. Mercadante S, Radbruch L, Caraceni A, *et al.* (2002). Episodic (breakthrough) pain. Consensus conference of an Expert Working Group of the European Association for Palliative Care. *Cancer* **94**(3):832–9.

23. Mercadante S, Villari P, Ferrera P, Casuccio A (2004). Optimization of opioid therapy for preventing incident pain associated with bone metastases. *J Pain Symptom Manage* **28**(5):505–10.

24. Portenoy RK (1997). Treatment of temporal variations in chronic cancer pain. *Sem Oncol* **5** (Suppl 16):S16–7–12.

25. Portenoy RK, Hagen NA (1990). Breakthrough pain: definition, prevalence and characteristics. *Pain* **41**(3):273–81.

26. Portenoy RK, Payne D, Jacobsen P (1999). Breakthrough pain: characteristics and impact in patients with cancer pain. *Pain* **81**(1–2):129–34.

27. Skinner C, Thompson E, Davies A (2006). Clinical features. In Davies A (ed) *Cancer-related breakthrough pain*, pp.13–22. Oxford: Oxford University Press.

28. Walker G, Wilcock A, Manderson C, Weller R, Crosby V (2003). The acceptability of different routes of administration of analgesia for breakthrough pain. *Palliat Med* **17**(2):219–21.

29. Zeppetella G (2006). Oral transmucosal opioid drugs. In Davies A (ed) *Cancer-related breakthrough pain*, pp.57–71. Oxford: Oxford University Press.

30. Zeppetella G, Ribeiro MD (2003). Pharmacotherapy of cancer-related episodic pain. *Expert Opin Pharmacother* **4**(4):493–502.

31. Zeppetella G, O'Doherty CA, Collins S (2000). Prevalence and characteristics of breakthrough pain in cancer patients admitted to a hospice. *J Pain Symptom Manage* **20**(2):87–92.

Chapter 21

Opioid switching and the genetics of opioid sensitivity

Joanne Droney and Julia Riley

Introduction

Morphine is recommended by the World Health Organization as the first-line strong opioid of choice for cancer pain. Since introducing the Cancer Pain Relief Programme, the global use and availability of morphine has increased dramatically. Most patients who are treated with morphine for cancer pain respond well: they achieve adequate pain relief without troublesome side effects. A significant proportion of patients, however (up to 30%), do not respond well to morphine. These patients present in a number of ways:

- Inadequate analgesia despite escalating morphine doses
- Adequate analgesia but intolerable side effects
- Inadequate analgesia because of dose-limiting side effects
- A further small group of patients appear to experience neither analgesia nor side effects on morphine.

There is also considerable variability in the dose of morphine required to achieve adequate analgesia. Variability in response to opioids other than morphine also occurs, although it is less well documented. Recognition of this substantial interindividual variation in response to morphine for cancer pain has resulted in the emergence of two clinical phenomena. Firstly 'opioid switching' as a clinical manoeuvre to redress the balance between analgesia and side effects has become widely accepted. Secondly there has been a surge of interest in the mechanisms underlying interindividual variation in morphine response with a number of clinical studies being carried out in this area.

The following chapter refers to interindividual variation in response to morphine for cancer pain, although variability has also been demonstrated in the non-cancer, postoperative, and healthy volunteer setting.

Opioid switching

Opioid switching and opioid rotation

Opioid switching and opioid rotation are terms which are used interchangeably in the literature. Opioid switching refers to the clinical practice of changing a patient from one opioid to another with the aim of improving the analgesia and side-effect profile. Patients who require opioid switching are those patients who have not responded well to the original opioid. Opioid rotation refers to the substitution of one opioid for another or the rotation from one route of opioid administration to another because of patient or physician preference, opioid/route availability or cost. Patients who undergo opioid rotation are not necessarily non-responsive to the original opioid.

Opioid switching: clinical evidence

A Cochrane review on opioid switching (in which the term 'switching' was used interchangeably with 'rotation') reviewed 23 case reports, 15 retrospective studies or audits, and 14 prospective uncontrolled studies and found there was no substantial evidence to support the practice of opioid switching. To date there are no reported randomized controlled trials of opioid switching in cancer patients. However, the currently available evidence indicates that when applied judiciously, opioid switching is a powerful tool in cancer pain management. One systematic review suggested that opioid switching results in an improvement in symptoms in at least 50% of patients. Two more recent prospective studies suggest that in fact the success rate may be in the order of 80–90%. In both a small proportion of patients required more than one switch.

Opioid switching: patient characteristics

There is wide variation in the dose of the initial opioid which the patient is taking when the decision is made to switch to an alternative opioid. In one study in which patients were switched from morphine to methadone, the median daily morphine dose was 200mg (range 30–1000mg). There is also variation in the duration of the initial opioid therapy. In one study the median duration of the initial opioid was 44 days with a range of 20–240 days. In another study patients were on the initial opioid for a mean of 25.8 weeks (180.6 days) (range 1–104 weeks).

There appears to be two broad groups of patients which require opioid switching:

- ◆ Patients that require switching shortly after initiation of the initial opioid, when the opioid dose is relatively low, reflecting that not all drugs are efficacious in all patients. 'Heterogeneity of treatment effects' is seen with most pharmaceutical medications and may be explained in part by individual pharmacokinetic or pharmacodynamic factors.

- ◆ Patients who appear to become non-responsive to the initial opioid at either higher doses or after chronic opioid therapy. This may be due to development of physical tolerance to the initial opioid.

Incomplete cross-tolerance

At a population level there is no evidence that there are any major differences between the opioids in terms of analgesia or side effects. Furthermore, most opioids commonly used in clinical practice have a similar mode of action via the μ-opioid receptor. Therefore the scientific rationale underlying the beneficial effects of opioid switching is not yet fully understood. One factor likely to contribute to the success of opioid switching (to redress the balance between pain and side effects in patients who are poorly responsive to the initial opioid) is incomplete cross-tolerance. The degree to which an individual is tolerant to the effects of one opioid will not necessarily be the same for the alternative opioid probably due to differences in the opioid pharmacokinetics and pharmacodynamics. Incomplete cross-tolerance may affect both opioid-induced analgesia and side effects. Thus opioid switching in the setting of incomplete cross-tolerance may facilitate improved analgesia and dose titration with a reduction in opioid side effects.

Opioid switching: dosing regimens

Incomplete cross-tolerance also contributes to one of the main challenges in switching from one opioid to another: deciding on the starting dose of the alternative opioid. Equianalgesic opioid dose tables exist but when switching from one opioid to another, these are merely rough guides. These tables were generally derived from single-dose administrations. Over-reliance on these tables does not take into account the complexities associated with cancer pain management or incomplete cross-tolerance between opioids, and the actual dose ratio between two opioids varies widely. There appears to be no direct relationship between the dose of the initial opioid which the patient is taking at the point of switching and the final dose of the alternative opioid. For example, the generally accepted equianalgesic dose ratio between oral morphine and oral oxycodone is usually in the region of 1.5:1 or 2:1. In a prospective cohort study in which morphine non-responders were switched to oral oxycodone, the actual ratio of oral morphine:oxycodone ranged from 0.25–12. Therefore for some patients the final opioid

---

Box 21.1 Guidelines for safe, effective switching between opioids in patients with cancer pain

1   Conservative use of equianalgesic dose ratios. In order to take into account incomplete cross tolerance, an initial dose reduction of 25–50% is recommended. Recent recommendations from an interdisciplinary expert panel suggest that the larger reduction (up to 50%) should be applied if the patient is on higher doses of opioids, is elderly or medically frail.

2   Careful assessment of the reasons for opioid switching. The choice of initial dose of the alternative opioid may vary depending on whether or not the patient is experiencing severe pain or serious opioid-related side effects.

3   Individual dose titration up or down according to the patient's level of pain relief/side effects.

4   After switching between one opioid and another it may take a number of days to achieve a good outcome in terms of analgesia and side effects. The time to stabilization on the second opioid may be slightly longer if the patient was switched because of both pain and side effects.

> ### Box 21.2 Some of the main factors to consider in order to optimize the likelihood of achieving a good outcome after opioid switching
>
> Is the pain opioid responsive?
>
> Some pains e.g. neuropathic pain may be better treated using an antidepressant or antiepileptic medication. However in these cases opioid switching may be worth trying, especially as cancer pain is usually of mixed origin.
>
> Have other factors which may be contributing to the intolerable side effects been considered?
>
> Cancer patients are often prescribed a many concomitant medications and many of these have side effects similar to those of opioids, especially drowsiness. Furthermore factors relating to the disease itself may be responsible for the apparent opioid side effects including hypercalcaemia and brain metastases.

dose is higher than that of the original, while in others the final dose is much lower. Dose ratios between opioids may also change according to the initial opioid dose (especially when switching between morphine and methadone) and even according to the direction of the opioid switch. For example, in a recent study of 54 cancer patients who were switched from morphine to methadone, the morphine:methadone dose ratio varied from 3:1 in patients who were switched for pain and were on a daily morphine dose of less than 300mg to 9.1:1 in patients who were switched because of side effects and who were taking more than 300mg morphine per day.

Clinical factors associated with interindividual variation in response to opioids

A number of studies have examined the role of different clinical factors on interindividual variation in morphine response. Gender may be influential, perhaps due to neurohormonal differences. The evidence, however, is inconsistent and often conflicting. There is some evidence that older patients require lower doses of opioids and experience less pain than younger patients but again this finding is not replicated in all studies. One prospective cohort study compared 186 morphine responders and 47 morphine non-responders and identified seven factors which were independently associated with morphine non-response:

- Weight
- Total white cell count
- Taking a β-blocker
- Taking a proton-pump inhibitor
- Taking a 5-HT$_3$ antagonist antiemetic

- Having received chemotherapy within the previous 14 days
- Having a tumour of the lower gastrointestinal tract.

As the authors stated, such modelling is not applicable to clinical practice without prospective testing and further validation. Little or no data exist on the impact of diet, psychological, or social factors on morphine response. To date the only clinical factor which has been consistently associated with variability in morphine response is renal impairment. Morphine and its metabolites morphine-3-glucuronide and morphine-6-glucuronide are eliminated via the kidneys. Patients with renal impairment are more susceptible to the effects of morphine. However, even patients with normal renal function exhibit variation in opioid response.

Pharmacogenetics and personalized prescribing

The search for factors to explain and account for interindividual variation in morphine response is driven by the quest for personalized prescribing. Prospective prediction of the correct opioid at the correct dose for each individual patient holds promise of more rapid pain control, reduced morbidity due to side effects, and overall improvement in patient care. In recent years much attention has been focused on pharmacogenetics: the impact of an individual's genetic make-up on their response to a drug (Table 21.1). One of the most well-known examples of pharmacogenetics in clinical practice is that of response to codeine. The clinical effects of codeine are mediated through its metabolism to morphine by the CYP2D6 enzyme. A proportion of patients have genetically-mediated variations in the levels of activity of this enzyme and thus exhibit marked variation in response to codeine for pain. Up to 10% of Caucasians are known as 'poor metabolizers' in that they lack CYP2D6 activity and thus do not experience any analgesia from codeine. At the other end of the spectrum are 'extensive metabolizers' who, through genetic variation in the gene coding for CYP2D6, are more susceptible to both the beneficial and adverse effects of codeine.

Single nucleotide polymorphisms (SNPs)

All published genetic association studies of variation in response to opioids for cancer pain involve analysis of SNPs. SNPs are the most common type of genetic variant at a

Table 21.1 The main genes studied in terms of variability in response to morphine

Gene symbol	Gene name	Gene product/function
OPRM	μ opioid receptor	The main site of action of morphine and other opioids
COMT	Catechol-O-methyltransferase	An enzyme involved in catecholamine metabolism
MDR1	Multidrug resistance gene	This gene codes for p-glycoprotein which is involved in the transport of morphine and other drugs across the blood–brain barrier
ARRB2	β-arrestin2	A protein involved in opioid receptor signalling
UGT2B7	Uridine diphosphate-Glu-curonosyltransferase 2B7	The main enzyme involved in the hepatic catabolism of morphine to its metabolites

There has also been some study of genes coding for cytokines including TNF-α, IL-6, and IL-8.

DNA level. A SNP is a point change in the nucleotide sequence along the strand of DNA. The different variants that a polymorphism may take are called alleles. In most cases there are two (but sometimes more) possible alternative alleles; the common allele, which is carried by most people in the population, and the variant allele. Each SNP has a unique identifier, often known as an 'rs number' (reference SNP number). SNPs are also often given names which are derived from their location in the gene and the amino acid change they are associated with. SNPs may be associated with a change in the structure or function of the protein coded for by that gene, either directly through interference with the processes of transcription and translation or indirectly through non-random association (linkage disequilibrium) with another true-susceptibility SNP. Genetic association studies search for a link between the clinical outcome measured (phenotype) and these genetic variants.

OPRM and response to opioids

The most frequently studied gene in terms of interindividual variation in response to morphine is *OPRM*. Of the hundreds of known SNPs spanning this gene, the most commonly studied is rs1799971. Depending on the ethnicity of the population studied, up to 46% of the population carry this variant allele. This SNP occurs in the region of the gene which codes for the extracellular portion of the μ-opioid receptor. The polymorphism involves substitution of a G (guanine) in place of the A (adenine) nucleotide at this position along the DNA, therefore this SNP is also known as A118G. This in turn is associated with an amino acid change from asparagine to aspartic acid in the protein structure coded for by the gene. There is a resultant loss of a potential N-glycosylation site at this point on the μ-opioid receptor which may have implications for ligand binding. Experimental data on the functional consequences of this SNP however are inconsistent.

In cancer patients A118G has been associated with higher morphine dose requirements and a reduced analgesic response. The numbers of patients homozygous (with two copies) of the variant G allele in these studies, however, tended to be low. Another study in cancer patients, however, did not find any association between this SNP and overall morphine response. To complicate matters even more, one study suggested that carriers of the variant G allele required lower, not higher opioid doses. A recent meta-analysis of the influence of *OPRM* A118G on pain treatment concluded there is only a weak association between this SNP and opioid dose requirements and that data do not support personalized prescribing of opioids based on genotyping of this polymorphism.

Opioids for cancer pain: results of pharmacogenetic studies to date

The results from studies involving other genes in terms of response to morphine for cancer pain are also inconsistent. The most commonly studied SNP in *COMT* is called Val158Met. This SNP is associated with an amino acid change (valine to methionine) and reduced activity of the catechol-O-methyltransferase enzyme. Early studies in non-cancer patients suggested an association between this SNP and variability in pain sensitivity but these findings were not replicated in other studies. One study has demonstrated that cancer patients carrying the variant allele at this position require lower morphine doses than those with the common allele.

Overall the results of genetic association studies in cancer patients on opioids have, as yet, not yielded any marker which can be conclusively used to explain interindividual variation in response to opioids or indeed to prospectively predict opioid response. There may be a number of reasons for this:

- Firstly there have been relatively few studies in this area. Publication bias may lead to the publication of small positive studies at the expense of relevant negative studies.

- Over 12 million SNPs have been identified, yet the number of SNPs and indeed the number of genes studied in this field has been miniscule. To date, all published genetic association studies involving response to opioids for cancer pain have used the candidate gene approach. Genes included in the analyses were chosen because their end product (the protein they code for) is known to play a role in opioid response. Although hypothesis-driven and resource-friendly, candidate gene studies provide limited information because 1) a limited number of SNPs along a single gene are studied, 2) a limited number of genes are examined, and 3) the amount of data, and especially the amount of new information generated, is limited by the breadth of current biological and genetic knowledge. The first genome-wide association study (GWAS) in pain was published in 2009 in 221 patients undergoing oral surgery. 255,785 SNPs spanning the entire genome were simultaneously analysed in this study. The study outcomes included maximum postoperative pain, postoperative pain onset, and time to analgesia post ketorolac administration. No such GWAS has been yet published in patients taking opioids for cancer pain.

- Most studies of the genetics of response to opioids have focused on variation at a DNA level. However, genetic variability is not confined to DNA alone. It may also occur via post-transcriptional modification at an RNA level through processes such as alternative splicing. In this way a single stretch of DNA can result in a number of different protein products. Alternative splicing of OPRM has been associated with the production of a number of μ-opioid receptor subtypes, with different structures and functions. The implication of these so-called 'splice variants' has not been tested directly in cancer patients on opioids because of the practical challenges of obtaining fresh brain RNA from patients. There has been one study, however, in which a DNA SNP in OPRM was found to be associated with alternative splicing. This SNP was also associated with variability in pain perception. It was not however found to be associated with variation in response to morphine but the numbers of patients in this analysis was small.

- Most of the genetic association studies in cancer patients taking opioids have involved single genes (even single SNPs). Response to opioids, however, is likely to be a complex trait, resulting from multiple gene–gene and gene–environment interactions. Some studies have examined the influence of SNP–SNP interactions on morphine response including combinations of OPRM/MDR1, OPRM/COMT, and COMT/MDR. In each of these studies, combinations of two SNPs at a time have been examined.

There is huge potential to further explore the interaction between multiple SNPs across multiple genes, with increasing complexities in terms of sample size, analytical approaches, and corrections for multiple testing.

♦ Interpretation of results of is made difficult by the different and incomparable outcome measures (clinical phenotypes) used. One group has examined the role of genetic variants on the daily dose of morphine, another on whether or not patients require switching from morphine to an alternative opioid. Another group has examined the change in pain scores between baseline and 1 week after initiation of morphine therapy. Differences in phenotype definition is a common reason for failure to replicate in genetic association studies.

♦ A further challenge is recruitment of adequate numbers of patients for genetic association studies. Two of the factors determining the necessary sample size are the frequency of the genetic variant and the strength of the association between the genetic variant and the outcome of interest. The largest genetic association study in cancer patients taking opioids has included 228 patients but some have published with as few as 99 subjects, too small to identify rare genetic associations with smaller effect size.

Conclusion

Interindividual variation in response to opioids is common and presents a number of challenges in the management of cancer pain. Opioid switching as a technique to improve the analgesic and side-effect profile of opioids is widely used in clinical practice yet the current evidence regarding efficacy and methodology of opioid switching is sparse. Furthermore the scientific rational underpinning variability in opioid response has yet to be elucidated. The potential for further research in this area is enormous. This includes increasing the number of carefully designed, adequately powered studies, examination of a larger number and breadth of genetic variants, and exploration of response to opioids other than morphine. The potential benefits of pharmacogenomics are immense, as can be seen by the successes for predicting response to drugs such as warfarin, irinotecan, and abacavir. For the reasons above, however, it is too early to be able to use the results of genetic association studies in clinical management of cancer pain with opioids.

Bibliography

1. Anderson R, Saiers JH, Abram S, Schlicht C (2001). Accuracy in equianalgesic dosing. conversion dilemmas. *J Pain Symptom Manage* **21**(5):397–406.
2. Benitez-Rosario MA, Salinas-Martin A, Guirre-Jaime A, Perez-Mendez L, Feria M (2009). Morphine-methadone opioid rotation in cancer patients: analysis of dose ratio predicting factors. *J Pain Symptom Manage* **37**(6):1061–8.
3. Campa D, Gioia A, Tomei A, Poli P, Barale R (2008). Association of ABCB1/MDR1 and OPRM1 gene polymorphisms with morphine pain relief. *Clin Pharmacol Ther* **83**(4):559–66.
4. Cherny N, Ripamonti C, Pereira J, *et al.* (2001). Strategies to manage the adverse effects of oral morphine: an evidence-based report. *J Clin Oncol* **19**(9):2542–54.

5. Diatchenko L, Nackley AG, Slade GD, *et al.* (2006). Catechol-O-methyltransferase gene polymorphisms are associated with multiple pain-evoking stimuli. *Pain* **125**(3):216–24.

6. Fine PG, Portenoy RK (2009). Establishing 'best practices' for opioid rotation: conclusions of an expert panel. *J Pain Symptom Manage* **38**(3):418–25.

7. Hirschhorn JN, Daly MJ (2005). Genome-wide association studies for common diseases and complex traits. *Nat Rev Genet* **6**(2):95–108.

8. Innocenti F, Undevia SD, Iyer L, *et al.* (2004). Genetic variants in the UDP-glucuronosyltransferase 1A1 gene predict the risk of severe neutropenia of irinotecan. *J Clin Oncol* **22**(8):1382–8.

9. Kim H, Ramsay E, Lee H, Wahl S, Dionne RA (2009). Genome-wide association study of acute post-surgical pain in humans. *Pharmacogenomics* **10**(2):171–9.

10. Klepstad P, Rakvag TT, Kaasa S, *et al.* (2004). The 118 A > G polymorphism in the human mu-opioid receptor gene may increase morphine requirements in patients with pain caused by malignant disease. *Acta Anaesthesiol Scand* **48**(10):1232–9.

11. Knotkova H, Fine PG, Portenoy RK (2009). Opioid rotation: the science and the limitations of the equianalgesic dose table. *J Pain Symptom Manage* **38**(3):426–39.

12. Mercadante S, Bruera E (2006). Opioid switching: a systematic and critical review. *Cancer Treat Rev* **32**(4):304–15.

13. Mercadante S, Ferrera P, Villari P, Casuccio A, Intravaia G, Mangione S (2009). Frequency, indications, outcomes, and predictive factors of opioid switching in an acute palliative care unit. *J Pain Symptom Manage* **37**(4):632–41.

14. Quigley C (2004). Opioid switching to improve pain relief and drug tolerability. *Cochrane Database Syst Rev* **3**:CD004847.

15. Rakvag TT, Klepstad P, Baar C, *et al.* (2005). The Val158Met polymorphism of the human catechol-O-methyltransferase (COMT) gene may influence morphine requirements in cancer pain patients. *Pain* **116**(1–2):73–8.

16. Reyes-Gibby CC, Shete S, Rakvag T, *et al.* (2007). Exploring joint effects of genes and the clinical efficacy of morphine for cancer pain: OPRM1 and COMT gene. *Pain* **130**(1–2):25–30.

17. Riley J, Ross JR, Rutter D, *et al.* (2006). No pain relief from morphine? Individual variation in sensitivity to morphine and the need to switch to an alternative opioid in cancer patients. *Support Care Cancer* **14**(1):56–64.

18. Ross JR, Riley J, Taegetmeyer AB, *et al.* (2008). Genetic variation and response to morphine in cancer patients: catechol-o-methyltransferase and multidrug resistance-1 gene polymorphisms are associated with central side effects. *Cancer* **112**:1390–403.

19. Ross JR, Rutter D, Welsh K, *et al.* (2005). Clinical response to morphine in cancer patients and genetic variation in candidate genes. *Pharmacogenomics J* **5**(5):324–36.

20. Shabalina SA, Zaykin DV, Gris P, *et al.* (2008). Expansion of the human μ-opioid receptor gene architecture: novel functional variants. *Hum Mol Genet* **18**(6):1037–51.

21. Sindrup SH, Brosen K, Bjerring P, *et al.* (1990). Codeine increases pain thresholds to copper vapor laser stimuli in extensive but not poor metabolizers of sparteine. *Clin Pharmacol Ther* **48**(6):686–93.

22. Slatkin NE (2009). Opioid switching and rotation in primary care: implementation and clinical utility. *Curr Med Res Opin* **25**(9):2133–50.

23. Walter C, Lötsch J (2009). Meta-analysis of the relevance of the OPRM1 118A>G genetic variant for pain treatment. *Pain* **146**(3):270–5.

24. Wang WY, Barratt BJ, Clayton DG, Todd JA (2005). Genome-wide association studies: theoretical and practical concerns. *Nat Rev Genet* **6**(2):109–18.

25. Wirz S, Wartenberg HC, Elsen C, Wittmann M, Diederichs M, Nadstawek J (2006). Managing cancer pain and symptoms of outpatients by rotation to sustained-release hydromorphone: a prospective clinical trial. *Clin J Pain* **22**(9):770–5.

26. World Health Organization (1996). *Cancer pain relief*, 2nd edn. Geneva: World Health Organization.

Chapter 22

Cancer pain management in children

Stefan J. Friedrichsdorf

Introduction

The majority of children with cancer experience medium to severe pain, which may be disease or treatment- (including procedure/intervention) related somatic, visceral, neuropathic, and/or spiritual pain. Data reveals a significant undertreatment of pain in children with cancer in the developed world.

However, children and parents expect pain to be relieved and parents' greatest distress is failing to protect their child from pain. The younger children are, the less likely it is that they receive appropriate analgesia. State-of-the-art pain management requires that pharmacological management must be combined with integrative, non-pharmacological therapies to manage a child's cancer pain effectively.

Broad-spectrum analgesia

In the management of intractable cancer pain in children it may be necessary to combine non-opioids, opioids, integrative therapies, adjuvant analgesia and anaesthetic, or neurosurgical interventions in order to achieve excellent analgesia without oversedation (Figure 22.1).

Pain assessment

Regular pain assessment followed by appropriate analgesia is necessary to adequately relieve the children's suffering. One-dimensional self-report measures (e.g. visual analogue scales with the anchor points 0 = no pain, 10 = worst possible pain, or faces scale, Figure 22.2) provide easy pain assessment of alert and responsive children communicating with the caregiver. For infants and children younger than 4 years of age several pain assessment tools have been validated. Independent observers record the physical behaviours, as well as the frequency of their occurrence. Behavioural observation measures to assess pain in cognitively impaired children are increasingly used, including the Non-communicating Children's Pain Checklist – Revised.

As children may suffer from different pains, a single pain rating may not be sufficient to assess the whole dimension of pain and may require a more detailed focus to evaluate the different pain aspects. Examples could include: 'How would you rate your constant achy pain, and how would you rate the occasional shooting pain'.

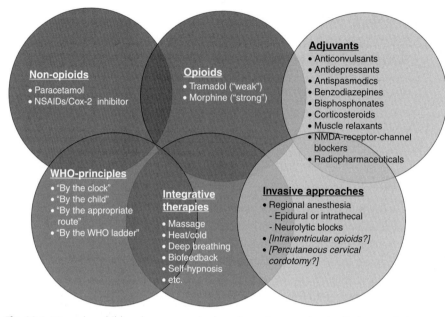

Non-opioids
• Paracetamol
• NSAIDs/Cox-2 inhibitor

Opioids
• Tramadol ("weak")
• Morphine ("strong")

Adjuvants
• Anticonvulsants
• Antidepressants
• Antispasmodics
• Benzodiazepines
• Bisphosphonates
• Corticosteroids
• Muscle relaxants
• NMDA-receptor-channel blockers
• Radiopharmaceuticals

WHO-principles
• "By the clock"
• "By the child"
• "By the appropriate route"
• "By the WHO ladder"

Integrative therapies
• Massage
• Heat/cold
• Deep breathing
• Biofeedback
• Self-hypnosis
• etc.

Invasive approaches
• Regional anesthesia
  - Epidural or intrathecal
  - Neurolytic blocks
• [Intraventricular opioids?]
• [Percutaneous cervical cordotomy?]

Fig. 22.1 Managing children in cancer pain: broad-spectrum analgesia. Dark grey circles: standard approach; light grey circles: advanced management in selected cases.

Integrative pain management

Pharmacological management is no longer the sole approach to the management of a child's pain and suffering. Integrative therapies, used alone or with pharmacology, include cognitive behavioural techniques (such as guided imagery, hypnosis, abdominal breathing, distraction) and physical methods (such as cuddle/hug, massage, transcutaneous electrical nerve stimulation (TENS), comfort positioning, heat, cold, aromatherapy) as well as acupuncture. Children cope better with pain when they understand what is happening and when they are encouraged fully in the process to attain pain relief. Comprehensive pain control requires tailoring to the needs of the individual child and integrating methods of pain management.

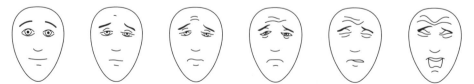

Fig. 22.2 Faces Pain Scale Revised (FPS-R). Please check the website http://www.painsourcebook.ca for correct administration and translations into many languages of these instructions.

Pharmacological pain management

World Health Organization principles

Applying the World Health Organization (WHO) principles of pain management results in good pain relief for the large majority of children with cancer pain:

- 'By the analgesic ladder'
- 'By the clock'
- 'By the appropriate route'
- 'With the child'.

'By the analgesic ladder'

The choice of analgesic drugs should be based on the WHO analgesic ladder (Figures 22.3 and 22.4).

An assessment of pain severity dictates the choice of analgesic. Severe acute cancer pain requires opioids and should be commenced immediately. The usefulness of a step 2 is debatable, especially as codeine often proves to be a rather unfavourable choice (see below). Some authorities argue to discontinue step 2, using lower doses of 'strong' opioids of step 3 instead.

'By the clock'

Regular scheduling ensures a steady blood level, reducing the peaks and troughs of PRN dosing. Commonly used opioid drug regimens include immediate release oral morphine

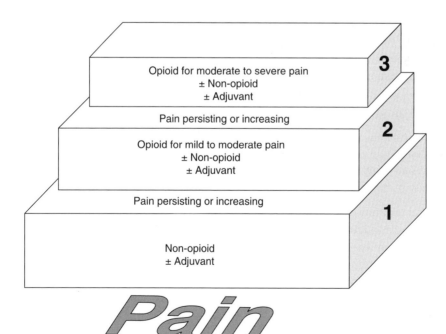

Fig. 22.3 The WHO three-step analgesic ladder.

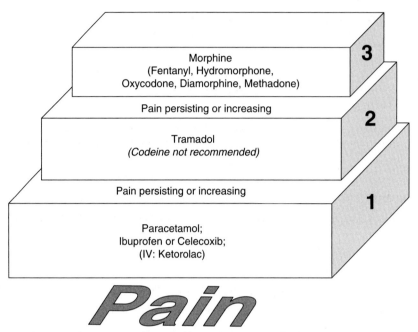

Fig. 22.4 The WHO three-step analgesic ladder with paediatric first-line drug suggestions.

every 4 hours (or controlled-release morphine twice daily) plus (for both strategies) at least 10% (up to 16%) of the 24-hour morphine requirement as an hourly fast-release breakthrough pain medication as needed (Table 22.1).

'By the appropriate route'

The least invasive route of administration, often chosen by the child, should be used, making intramuscular administration obsolete.

- The oral route (or via nasogastric/percutaneous endoscopic gastrostomy tube) is convenient, non-invasive, and usually preferred by the children and their care providers.

- The sublingual application of opioids (morphine, fentanyl, oxycodone, hydromorphone, and methadone) appears safe and well liked by children and caregivers. Bioavailability varies widely for the different opioids from 20% for oxycodone to 65% for sublingual fentanyl.

- Oral transmucosal fentanyl—the fentanyl lozenge is a solid drug matrix with berry flavour providing oral transmucosal fentanyl citrate (OTFC) and absorption across the oral mucosa directly into the systemic blood is rapid. OTFC has been used for children 3 years of age and above. Recent studies in opioid-naïve children showed typical opioid side effects of OTFC including respiratory depression. Earlier paediatric trials, which reported higher rates of respiratory depression, either used high doses of OTFC (>20mcg/kg) and/or treated cardiosurgical patients, including children with cyanotic heart defects. Some paediatric trials reported nausea and vomiting commonly, others rarely or not at all. Due to these adverse effects, OTFC is indicated exclusively for the treatment of breakthrough pain in cancer patients and is no longer used for sedation or pre-medication.

♦ Transdermal fentanyl patches are contraindicated for acute pain management due to a long onset time (it may take more than 60 hours to reach peak concentrations in children), inability to rapidly titrate drug delivery and long elimination half-life (up to 24 hours). Patches can be applied on intact, healthy skin every (48–)72 hours. Children should be on the equivalent of 30–60mg oral morphine/24 hours to safely rotate to a fentanyl patch and immediate release breakthrough (rescue) opioid is required. Transdermal fentanyl has its role in chronic, stable pain.

♦ Intranasal application of opioids is pain free and safe. Fentanyl can be diluted in normal saline solution (0.9%) and may be applied as a nasal spray or in drops. The pharmacokinetic profile of intranasal fentanyl seems to be similar to intravenous fentanyl. Reported intranasal fentanyl doses in children (1–1.5mcg/kg) are similar to suggested intravenous doses (see Table 22.1).

♦ Rectal application is often unpopular and may deliver a wide variability in blood levels through variable absorption. However good analgesia can be achieved in children when suppositories or liquid opioids via a small catheter are administered rectally.

♦ The intravenous administration of opioid may be feasible, especially when there is central access. Patient-controlled analgesia/nurse controlled-analgesia (PCA/NCA) with a continuous background often provides excellent pain management (Table 22.2). Alternatively the opioid analgesics can be applied subcutaneously in the same dose as intravenously. With the necessary support, children can be made comfortable in terminal care with a subcutaneous or intravenous PCA/NCA in the home setting.

'With the child'

The analgesic treatment should be individualized according to the child's pain, response to treatment, frequently reassessed, and modified as required. Some children may require extremely high doses of opioids to control severe pain. Adjuvant drugs may be appropriate in the pain management of the individual child.

Non-opioids

The most frequently used non-opioids are paracetamol and the non-steroidal anti-inflammatory drugs (NSAIDs):

♦ Paracetamol (10–15mg/kg PO/PR Q4–6h; dose limit: <2 years: 60mg/kg/day, >2 years: 90mg/kg/day)

♦ Ibuprofen (10mg/kg PO TDS–QID; dose limit 2400mg/day)

♦ IV ketorolac should be rotated to oral ibuprofen as soon as tolerated (<2 years= 0.25mg/kg TID; >2 years: 0.5mg/kg q6h; max. 30mg/dose; recommended dosing no longer than 5 days).

Table 22.1 Opioid analgesics: usual starting doses (doses for children >6 months of age and are capped at 50 kg body weight)

Drug (route of administration)	Equianalgesic dose (parenteral)	Starting dose IV	IV:PO ratio	Starting dose PO (transdermal)	Starting dose controlled release
Morphine (PO, SL, IV, SC, PR)	10mg	Bolus dose: 50–100mcg/kg every 2–4h. Continuous infusion: 10–30mcg/kg/h	1:3	0.15–0.3mg/kg every 4h	0.45–0.9mg every 12h
Fentanyl (IV, SC, SL, transdermal, buccal)	100–250mcg	Bolus dose: 1–3mcg/kg (slowly over 3–5min—fast bolus may cause thorax rigidity) Continuous infusion: 1–2mcg/kg/h	1:1 (IV to trans-dermal)	12mcg/h patch (must be on the equivalent of at least 30mg oral morphine/24 hours, before switched to patch)	n/a
Hydromorphone (PO, SL, IV, SC, PR)	1.5mg	Bolus dose: 15–20mcg/kg every 4h Continuous infusion: 5mcg/kg/h	1:5	60mcg/kg every 3–4 h	180mcg/kg every 12h– currently not available in USA
Oxycodone (PO, SL, PR)	5–10mg	n/a	n/a	0.1–0.2mg/kg every 4–6h	0.3–0.9mg/kg every 12h
Codeine (not recommended)	120mg	n/a	n/a	0.5–1mg/kg every 3–4h	n/a
Tramadol (PO, PR)	100mg	IV not available in USA (Bolus dose: 1mg/kg every 3–4h Continuous Infusion: 0.25mg/kg/h)	1:1	1–2mg/kg every 3–4h, max. of 8mg/kg/day (>50kg: max. of 400mg/day)	2–4mg/kg every 12h

Calculated rescue (breakthrough) dose: 10–16% of 24-h opioid dose to be given every 1–2h as needed.

IV = intravenous; PO = by mouth; PR = rectal; SL = sublingual; SC = subcutaneous; n/a = not applicable.

Table 22.2 Usual starting doses for patient (or nurse)-controlled analgesia (PCA) pumps—dose escalation usually in 50% increments both for continuous and PCA bolus dose (Pain Medicine & Palliative Care, Children's Hospitals and Clinics of Minnesota, USA). Doses for children >6 months of age and are capped at 50kg body weight

	Continuous infusion (mcg/kg/h)	PCA bolus (mcg)	Lock-out time (minutes)	Maximum number of boluses/hour
Morphine	20 (max. 1000)	20 (max. 1000)	5–10	4–6
Hydromorphone	3–5 (max. 250)	3–5 (max. 250)	5–10	4–6
Fentanyl	1 (max. 50)	1 (max. 50)	5	4–6

Although widely used in paediatric oncology, the cyclo-oxygenase-2 (COX-2) inhibitor celecoxib (4mg/kg/day in one or two doses, max. 200mg/day) is not approved in paediatrics and as yet there are no published paediatric randomized controlled trials (RCTs) regarding safety and efficacy.

'Weak' opioids

Codeine and tramadol are frequently used for mild–moderate pain and are commonly called 'weak opioids' due to their ceiling effect (increasing above recommended dosing does increase adverse effects, but does not increase analgesia).

Codeine, cannot be recommended in paediatric analgesia anymore:

◆ Codeine has less efficacy than ibuprofen.

◆ Codeine has a very high incidence of nausea and vomiting.

◆ Codeine produces its analgesic effect only through its metabolite morphine produced by activity of the enzyme cytochrome CYP 2D6. Slow metabolizers and intermediate metabolizers (up to a third of children) do not achieve analgesia. Conversely, around 5% of white Caucasians (29% Ethiopians) have multiple copies of CYP 2D6 and are ultra-rapid metabolizers, and therefore metabolize unusually high doses of morphine which can result in significant respiratory depression and deaths have been recorded.

Tramadol has been trialled in neonates and children (mainly postoperative) and shown to be safe and effective. Tramadol (a weak mu-receptor agonist) analgesia is augmented by inhibiting monoamine neurotransmitter (noradrenaline/serotonin) reuptake. Although tramadol is metabolized by CYP 2D6 into the more potent O-desmethyltramadol, tramadol itself is a potent analgesic. For slow CYP 2D6 metabolizers the parent compound remains active, resulting in only a slightly diminished analgesia. Common adverse effects include nausea, vomiting, dizziness, constipation, and sedation. A rare, but severe side effect is the serotonergic syndrome. Tramadol appears not to increase the risk of idiopathic seizures, but patients with seizure tendency or on medication that lowers seizure threshold may be at increased risk. Tramadol appears fairly safe regarding respiratory depression with overdose: no symptoms noted in children younger than 6 years who ingested 10mg/kg or less.

'Weak' and 'strong' opioids should not be combined due to an unfavourable side effect profile.

'Strong' opioids

The most frequently used opioid in paediatrics for moderate to severe cancer pain remains morphine. Opioid-associated side effects have to be expected and treated accordingly, including a scheduled bowel regimen such as a stool softener such as lactulose plus/minus stimulant such as senna. Morphine undergoes first-pass metabolism and is metabolized into morphine-6 glucuronide (M6G) and morphine-3 glucuronide (M3G). M6G is a more potent analgesic with associated side effects. M3G is not analgesic with different adverse effects, especially hyperexcitability/neurotoxicity. The ratio of M6G/M3G thereby defines the analgesia to adverse effect profile in individuals. Children in renal failure have a higher risk of side effects. Neither fentanyl nor methadone are excreted renally, and are a better choice in this scenario.

If dose-limiting opioid toxicity occurs, an opioid rotation may be necessary. This may be necessary in up to 15% of children. A switch from one opioid to another often changes the balance between analgesia and side effects. A favourable change in opioid analgesia occurs if there is less cross-tolerance at the opioid receptors mediating analgesia than at those mediating adverse effects.

If a child becomes unconscious during the last days of life due to the underlying disease process (and not as an opioid toxicity), ceasing regular opioid analgesic drugs should not occur, as it will likely provoke unpleasant withdrawal.

Oxycodone is a selective mu-opioid receptor agonist. The potency of oral oxycodone to oral morphine is between 1:1 to 2:1. One advantage of oxycodone over morphine is the slightly longer half-life, frequently allowing every-6-hours dosing. Renal and hepatic impairment increases the oxycodone serum level.

Fentanyl is a popular choice for analgesia prior to painful procedures due to its rapid onset and its brief duration of action. It is also used for intra- and postoperative analgesia, in paediatric palliative care, and in sedation analgesia for ventilated children on the intensive care. Fentanyl provides a good alternative to morphine when dose-limiting side effects mandate a rotation of opioid drug.

Diamorphine has not been approved outside the UK by regulating authorities as an analgesic medication. This strong opioid is an excellent alternative to morphine and wildly used in the UK in paediatric cancer pain management.

Hydromorphone is another selective mu-opioid receptor agonist commonly used in paediatrics. Opioid hyperexcitability has been reported in patients with renal failure taking hydromorphone.

Methadone remains underutilized. It is a mu-opioid receptor agonist, a NMDA (N-methyl-D-aspartic acid) -receptor antagonist, and blocker of serotonin and noradrenaline re-uptake.

Table 22.3 Equianalgesic methadone chart

Total daily oral morphine dose	Estimated daily oral methadone requirement		
	Gazelle G (2002) www.eperc.mcw.edu	Roxane Laboratories, Inc. Columbus, OH 43216	Toombs JD (2005) Americ Family Physician 71(7):1353–8
<100mg	3:1	20–30%	33%
101–300mg	5:1	10–20%	20%
301–600mg	10:1	8–12%	10%
601–800mg	12:1	5–10%	8%
801–1000mg	15:1	5–10%	7%
>1000mg	20:1	<5%	5%

Advantages include:

◆ Long half-life (dosing twice or three times per day)

◆ Efficacy for chronic and neuropathic pain

◆ NMDA receptor antagonist mechanism (reduces tolerance)

◆ Lower incidence of constipation

◆ No active metabolites, safe in renal failure and stable liver disease

◆ Inexpensiveness.

Disadvantages include wide dosing variation, long half-life (accumulation; quick titration difficult), and more complex equianalgesic conversion, requiring longer and closer patient observation.

An equianalgesic conversion chart when switching to methadone is recommended (Table 22.3).

Methadone should not be prescribed by those unfamiliar with its use. Its effects should be closely monitored particularly when it is first started and after dose changes.

Fixed combination analgesia (paracetamol plus opioid) cannot be recommended in paediatric analgesia. Separate titration of paracetamol and an opioid is recommended.

Neuropathic pain and adjuvant analgesia

Although paediatric data is limited, evidence from treatment of adult neuropathic pain supports the use of strong opioids, tricyclic antidepressants, and anticonvulsants. Opioids are first-line analgesia in paediatric neuropathic cancer pain, but often require the combination with adjuvant drugs (Table 22.4).

Tricyclic antidepressants (TCAs)

Mechanism of action is by serotonin/noradrenaline re-uptake inhibition, stimulating descending inhibiting pathways. Adverse effects of all TCAs include arrhythmia and anticholinergic/antihistamine effects, such as dry mouth, constipation, urinary retention,

Table 22.4 Adjuvant analgesia in neuropathic paediatric pain management (Pain Medicine & Palliative Care, Children's Hospitals and Clinics of Minnesota)

Class	Medication	Dose	Route of administration
Tricyclic antidepressants (TCA)	Amitriptyline	Starting dose 0.1mg/kg OD(QHS), usually slowly titrated up to 0.5mg/kg (max 1–2mg/kg)	PO
	Nortriptyline	Starting dose 0.1mg/kg OD(QHS), usually titrated up to 0.5mg/kg (max 1mg/kg)	PO
Gabapentenoids	Gabapentin	Starting dose 2mg/kg OD(QHS), usually slowly titrated up to initial target dose of 6mg/kg/dose TID (max 300mg/dose TID). Max. dose escalation to 24mg/kg/dose TID (max. 1200mg/dose TID)	PO
	Pregabaline	Starting dose 0.3mg/kg OD(QHS), usually slowly titrated up to initial target dose of 1.5mg/kg/dose BID (max. 75mg/dose BID). Max. dose escalation to 6mg/kg/dose BID (max. 300mg/dose BID)	PO
Sodium channel blocker/local anaesthetic	Lidocaine 5%	Max. of 4 patches (in patients >50kg) 12h on/12h off	Transdermal patch
Glucocorticoid	Dexamethasone	0.1–1.5mg/kg (max. 10mg) starting dose, then 0.1–0.25mg/kg ×2/day (for < 14 days) (Malignant spinal cord compression (adult dose): Dexamethasone 16–96mg/day or equivalent)	PO, IV
NMDA-receptor anatgonist	Ketamine (racemic mixture of S(+)/R(−) enantiomers)	IV: 0.06–0.3mg/kg/h PO: 0.2–0.5mg/kg TID–QID and PRN	IV, PO, (SC, SL, intranasal, PR, spinally)

blurred vision, and sedation. Nortriptyline may be better tolerated than amitriptyline. Cases of the use of amitriptyline in paediatric cancer neuropathic pain have been reported but there are no RCT data.

Doses above 25mg/dose for teenagers (amitriptyline or nortriptyline) are rarely necessary. The TCA should be reduced gradually over 1–2 weeks to avoid withdrawal. Sedative effects (to improve sleep) may commence immediately, but analgesia may take days to weeks.

There is anecdotal evidence of sudden death in children using desipramine.

Gabapentinoids

Gabapentin is widely used in paediatric neuropathic and chronic pain management, usually second-line in combination with a first-line TCA. Adverse effects occur if dose is started too high or escalated too fast, but even with slow dose escalation side effects may occur. These include ataxia, nystagmus, myalgia, hallucination, dizziness, somnolence, aggressive behaviours, hyperactivity, thought disorder, peripheral oedema. When gabapentin is weaned, it should be decreased over 1–2 weeks. Analgesia may take days to weeks to occur.

If gabapentin is ineffective at maximum dose, or because of dose-limiting side effects, one may switch to pregabalin at a conversion rate of about 6:1. Patients who fail to benefit from gabapentin may benefit from pregabalin or vice versa. No data exist to suggest that either drug is better than the other one.

Sodium-channel blocker

The lidocaine 5% patch/plaster is effective for peripheral neuropathic pain conditions and allodynia. The patch is a matrix and can be cut to fit. The drug maker recommends 12 hours on/12 hours off to avoid tolerance; however a raised systemic lidocaine level is very unlikely even with extended usage.

NMDA-receptor antagonists

Ketamine is a dissociative anaesthetic, which is analgesic in subanaesthetic doses. Low-dose analgesic dose is 0.06–0.3mg/kg/h IV. The common adverse effects seen in anaesthetic usage (intracranial hypertension, tachycardia, and psychotomimetic phenomena such as euphoria, dsyphoria, vivid hallucinations) usually do not occur at low dose, but can be managed with a benzodiazepine. A short-term 'burst' treatment with ketamine may have long-term benefit. Steady-state oral/parenteral ratio is unclear, but estimated at about 3:1. The intravenous formulation of ketamine has a bitter taste, and when administered orally should be mixed with a flavour. There is anecdotal evidence, that the concurrent administration of low-dose ketamine and methadone has improved effectiveness.

Other adjuvants to analgesia

- ◆ Anti-inflammatory corticosteroids. Due to potentially serious side effects, administration should be short term
- ◆ Muscle relaxants (e.g. baclofen)
- ◆ Low-dose benzodiazepines

- Bisphosphonates for bone pain due to metastatic cancer (e.g. pamidronate)
- Antispasmodics (e.g. hyoscine, glycopyrrolate).

Conclusion

Many myths still remain and may be responsible for the inadequate pain management of many children in cancer care. In particular, infants and very young children as well as severely impaired children and teens often do not receive sufficient analgesia, because their discomfort is different from that of adults. It is fallacious to believe that children's nervous systems are immature and therefore unable to perceive experience pain.

- Providing a good pain management usually requires a holistic, interdisciplinary approach and the knowledge to apply appropriate analgesic drugs in combination with integrative non-drug therapies.
- The large majority of children with cancer would enjoy good to excellent pain management, if the four WHO principles would always be implemented.
- Children in moderate–severe acute pain usually need strong pain medication, i.e. morphine or other strong opioids.
- A dose-limiting side effect occurs in more than 10% of children and likely will require an opioid rotation of equianalgesic dose.
- The use of codeine is not recommended.
- Methadone is probably underutilized in paediatric cancer pain management, however it should not be prescribed by those unfamiliar with its use.
- Evidence supports other routes of opioid application: transmucosal, transdermal, and intranasal opioid applications are well tolerated, effective, and safe.
- A subgroup of children will benefit from the addition of adjuvant analgesia or invasive approaches.

Bibliography

1. Bamigbade TA, Langford RM (1998). The clinical use of tramadol hydrochloride. *Pain Rev* **5**:155–82.
2. Borland ML, Jacobs I, Geelhoed G (2002). Intranasal fentanyl reduces acute pain in children in the emergency department: a safety and efficacy study. *Emerg Med (Fremantle)* **14**(3):275–80.
3. Collins JJ, Dunkel IJ, Gupta SK, *et al.* (1999). Transdermal fentanyl in children with cancer pain: feasibility, tolerability, and pharmacokinetic correlates. *J Pediatr* **134**(3):319–23.
4. Desmeules JA (2000). The tramadol option. *Eur J Pain* **4**(Suppl A):15–21.
5. Drake R, Longworth J, Collins JJ (2004). Opioid rotation in children with cancer. *J Pall Med* **7**(3):419–22.
6. Elliott C, Jay SM, Woody P (1987). An observational scale for measuring children's distress during medical procedures. *J Ped Psych* **12**:543–51.
7. Friedrichsdorf S (2004). Fentanyl in pediatric pain management - novel routes of administration. *Suffering Child* **8**(2):24–9.
8. Friedrichsdorf SJ, Kang TI (2007). The management of pain in children with life-limiting illnesses. *Pediatr Clin North Am* **54**(5):645–72.

9. Hain RDW, Miser A, Devins M, Wallace HB (2005). Strong opioids in pediatric palliative medicine. *Paediatric Drugs* **7**:1–9.

10. Heubi JE, Barbacci MB, Zimmerman HJ (1998). Therapeutic misadventure with paracetamol: hepatotoxicity after multiple doses in children. *J Pediatr* **132**:22–7.

11. Hicks CL, von Baeyer CL, Spafford P, van Korlaar I, Goodenough B (2001). Faces Pain Scale-Revised: toward a common metric in pediatric pain measurement. *Pain* **93**:173–83.

12. Jay SM, Elliott C, Siegal S (1987). Cognitive, behavioral, and pharmacologic interventions for children's distress during painful medical procedures. *J Consult Clin Psych* **55**:860–5.

13. Koren K (2009). Codeine, ultrarapid-metabolism genotype, and postoperative death. *NEJM* **361**:827–8.

14. Kuttner L (2005). Integrative methods to relieve pain and suffering. In Goldman A, Hain RDW, Liben S (eds) *Textbook of Paediatric Palliative Care*, pp.332–41. Oxford: Oxford University Press.

15. Kuttner L, Bowman M, Teasdale M (1988). Psychological treatment of distress, pain and anxiety for children with cancer. *Develop Behav Ped* **9**:374–81.

16. Manjushree R, Lahiri A, Ghosh BR, Arpita L, Handa K (2002). Intranasal fentanyl provides adequate postoperative analgesia in pediatric patients. *Can J Anesth* **49**(2):190–3.

17. Rose JB, Finkel JC, Arquedas-Mohs A, *et al.* (2003). Oral tramadol for the treatment of pain of 7–30 days' duration in children. *Anesth Analg* **96**:78–81.

18. Schechter NL, Berde CB, Yaster M (2003). Pain in infants, children, and adolescents – An overview. In Schechter NL, Berde CB, Yaster M (eds) *Pain in infants, children, and adolescents*, 2nd edn, pp.3–18. Philadelphia, PA: Lippincott Williams & Wilkins.

19. Solodiuk J, Curley MA (2003). Pain assessment in nonverbal children with severe cognitive impairments: the Individualized Numeric Rating Scale (INRS). *J Ped Nursing* **18**:295–9.

20. Twycross R (2003). Analgesics. In Twycross R, Wilcock A, Charlesworth S, Dickman A (eds) *Palliative Care Formulary*, 2nd edn, pp.129–202. Oxford: Radcliff Medical Press.

21. Weinberg DS, Inturrisi CE, Reidenberg B, *et al.* (1988). Sublingual absorption of selected opioid analgesics. *Clin Pharmacol Ther* **44**(3):335–42.

22. World Health Organization (1999). *Cancer Pain Relief and Palliative Care in Children*. Geneva: WHO.

23. Yaster M, Kost-Byerly S, Maxwell LG (2003). Opioid agonists and antagonists. In Schechter NL, Berde CB, Yaster M (eds) *Pain in infants, children, and adolescents*, 2nd edn, pp.181–224. Philadelphia, PA: Lippincott Williams & Wilkins.

Chapter 23

Complementary therapies for cancer pain control

David O'Regan, Jonathan T.C. Yen, and
Jacqueline Filshie

Introduction

Orthodox treatment modalities for cancer such as surgery, chemotherapy, and radiation therapy have resulted in considerable success in reducing mortality rates, as well as providing increasing symptom relief in the palliative care setting. These treatments are evidence-based but are associated with numerous unpleasant symptoms and side effects, including pain, that are not always resolved by medical intervention. Increasing numbers of cancer patients are turning to complementary and alternative medicine (CAM) in an effort to lessen symptoms of cancer and their treatments. CAM therapies are perceived as being more 'natural', less aggressive, and potentially safer than their conventional counterparts. Unfortunately, these traits have been hijacked by some unscrupulous 'practitioners' to sell unproven treatments and exaggerate promises of success to vulnerable patients. Furthermore, many herbal/botanical preparations are far from being inert, and have the potential to interact in a non-beneficial way with conventional treatments. As more cancer patients choose CAM therapies, it is important for professional health care practitioners to be aware of the growing evidence base and be able to provide reliable information concerning efficacy and safety. CAM treatments therefore need to pass the same scientific scrutiny of evidence-based medicine as their conventional counterparts.

A summary of 26 surveys from 13 countries in 1998 found that the prevalence of CAM in oncology patients ranged from 7% to 64% (average of 30%). This tallies with a survey in 2007 of just over 23,000 adult cancer patients conducted in the USA, where 38% of patients were using some form of CAM. In European countries CAM has a prevalence of 15–73% (average 36%). Adults who used CAM tended to be female, younger in age, and of higher social class. Among children, rates up to 84% have been reported. Factors associated with CAM use in children with cancer included poor prognosis, higher parental education, previous CAM use, and religious faith.

The terms 'complementary', 'alternative', 'integrated', and 'holistic' medicine are often used interchangeably which can lead to confusion over terminology.

◆ Cochrane defines complementary medicine as 'diagnosis, treatment and/or prevention which complements mainstream medicine by contributing to a common whole, by satisfying a demand not met by orthodoxy or by diversifying a conceptual frame-work of medicine'.

- Alternative therapies, on the other hand, are a substitute for mainstream medical treatment, but have little or no evidence base for their efficacy.

- Integrated therapy is when conventional medical treatment is combined with CAM therapies of proven efficacy, with an emphasis on prevention and lifestyle changes. For example, most chronic pain clinics in the UK offer acupuncture, which has numerous positive systematic reviews and meta-analyses for pain and symptom control.

- Holistic medicine looks at the individual as a whole rather than the functional parts. However, good medical practice should do this anyway. Palliative care physicians, for example, do not focus on physical symptoms alone, but also offer psychological, social, and spiritual support.

In this chapter, complementary therapies with the widest clinical applications are discussed.

Acupuncture

Acupuncture has its origins in Traditional Chinese Medicine. It is based on the theory of regulation of the flow of 'Qi', or vital energy, by stimulation of certain points on the body with needles, or pressure in the case of acupressure. In the last 30 years there has been great interest in acupuncture and research that seeks to reconcile the practice of traditional acupuncture with modern medical thinking. The strength of current scientific evidence has made acupuncture more acceptable to Western-trained doctors and given birth to Western Medical Acupuncture. Medical acupuncturists first establish an orthodox diag-nosis, and then choose acupuncture points based on neurophysical and neuropharmaco-logical evidence. In pain, segmental points are used relating to the affected area or structure and trigger points are treated for myofascial pain. Certain traditional acupuncture points are also used, particularly those with an evidence base.

Scientific evidence points to the nervous system as the mediator of acupuncture's effects. Release of a myriad of neurotransmitters and changes in brain functional MRI (magnetic resonance imaging) signals are observed during treatment. Moreover, acupuncture can alter gene expression, upregulating opioid production. Acupuncture causes release of endogenous substances, such as β endorphin, enkephalins, and dynorphins, which act on μ, δ, and κ opioid receptors. Cholecystokinin, an endogenous opioid antagonist, is also released, which might explain why patients become tolerant after multiple treatments. Serotonin, oxytocin, and adrenocorticotropic hormone are also released. As the effects depend upon transmission in Aδ nerves, prior administration of local anaesthesia can block the effects of acupuncture.

A typical course of treatment for non-malignant chronic pain would be once a week for 6 weeks, with further top-up treatments as required. Six treatments have been shown to be the minimum number necessary for the relief of chronic pain of mixed origin.

Cancer patients need a more gentle approach, and treatment should be tailored to response. In a patient with a short life expectancy, treatment should be stopped if there is no pain relief after 3 weeks.

There have been numerous systematic reviews and meta-analyses that support the use of acupuncture for various non-malignant pain conditions compared with sham acupuncture or usual care. A systematic review by Sun et al. of acupuncture for postoperative pain showed it was an effective technique and resulted in a significant reduction in postoperative pain and opioid consumption. A 29% reduction in opioids peaked at 72 hours and led to a significant reduction in opioid adverse effects. In a double-blinded randomized controlled trial (RCT), using semipermanent intradermal needles preoperatively on patients undergoing major gastrointestinal surgery, there was a reduction of opioid consumption by 50% and of the incidence of postoperative nausea and vomiting by 30%. Another RCT of 250 cancer patients undergoing major abdominal surgery needed less conventional analgesia when they received electroacupuncture before and during surgery. An RCT of patients undergoing breast surgery with axillary lymph node removal showed reduced postoperative pain and increased mobility in the acupuncture group.

Clearly more RCT evidence for acupuncture in cancer pain is required. However, there are a number of non-RCT studies that show acupuncture can provide clinical relief for patients with cancer pain even in terminal cancer patients whose pain was opioid resistant or who had toxicity. Combined results from two extensive audits on the use of acupuncture on 339 cancer patients demonstrated that 52–56% of patients had long-lasting relief after three weekly sessions. There was a longer lasting effect for pain from anticancer treatment such as postsurgery breast pain or radiotherapy than pain of metastatic disease.

Recent RCTs in acupuncture suggest clinical benefit for oncology patients in control of other symptoms including nausea and vomiting, hot flushes, shortness of breath, fatigue, anxiety, depression, and insomnia. Whilst some of the trials have methodological flaws, the evidence currently available suggests that acupuncture is a safe, low-cost, and effective therapy.

Apart from occasional pain and bruising and mild sedation following acupuncture, serious complications are extremely rare in the hands of well-trained practitioners but include infection, trauma (e.g. pneumothorax in a cachetic patient), needle fracture, syncope, and drowsiness. Though those adverse events are rare, special consideration are suggested for cancer patients. Needles should be not be used in a limb that is prone to or has lymphoedema, such as after axillary lymph node dissection. Acupuncture should be avoided around any area of spinal instability, since this could theoretically reduce protective muscle spasm and result in cord compression.

Herbal/botanical medicine

Herbal and animal products have been used to treat a variety of diseases, including cancer. Over 50% of modern drugs come from natural sources. In one study of adult cancer patients in the UK, 51.6% of patients took herbal remedies and only 46.3% had discussed this with a healthcare professional. There is emerging evidence to support herbal medicine for cancer pain.

Cannabinoids are being intensively studied for a variety of beneficial effects including pain relief and reduction in nausea. One systematic review concluded that the analgesic effect of cannabinoids was equivalent to codeine, and reported that psychoactive central side effects limit its use. However, ongoing RCTs looking at the analgesic efficacy of cannabinoids may provide further information.

In an RCT, topical capsaicin cream (derived from chilli pepper) was reported to reduce scar pain in patients with post-breast cancer surgery pain.

Though they are labelled as natural remedies, herbal medicines are not necessarily safe or harmless. Many herbs (e.g. garlic and St John's Wort) have interactions with prescription medication, such as anticoagulants and sedatives as well as chemotherapy agents. Plant extracts contain numerous chemicals, so it is unsurprising that they could cause adverse effects and interact with orthodox medication. Commonly used herbal preparations have the potential to cause problems in the perioperative period. Echinacea has been shown to have immunostimulatory effects, and though there are no studies showing any interactions with immunosuppressive drugs, expert opinion warns against its concomitant use with these drugs. There has been a reported case of anaphylaxis from the use of echinacea. Garlic can inhibit platelet aggregation. One case report describes an elderly heavy user of garlic developing a spontaneous epidural haematoma. Ginseng also can inhibit platelet aggregation, and can affect clotting times. Some ginseng preparations have oestrogenic activity and are contraindicated in patients with oestrogen positive tumours.

Clinicians need to routinely enquire whether their patients are using herbal remedies or nutritional supplements. Guidelines from the American Society of Anaesthesiologists suggested that the patient should discontinue all herbal medication 2–3 weeks prior to surgery. However, there are concerns that withdrawal of herbal remedies may increase morbidity and mortality after surgery, just as for conventional medications.

Homoeopathy

Homoeopathy is based on the principle of 'similia similibus curantur' or 'likes are cured by likes'; diseases can be treated by the substance that produces the same symptoms and signs in an individual. These substances, derived from plant, animal, and mineral sources, are serially diluted until almost no active molecules of the original substance remain. Between dilutions, the solution is vigorously shaken, in a process termed potentization.

Such principles fuel scientific scepticism, and render homoeopathy a controversial alternative therapy. Nonetheless, it remains a popular treatment amongst patients who cite a high level of satisfaction when homoeopathy is included in their package of care. Homoeopathy consultations are long and non-specific effects are likely to contribute to the beneficial effects. Furthermore, each preparation needs to be tailored to the individual, as practitioners believe that each individual responds differently. Whilst this may increase the patient's feeling of being 'a unique case', it complicates the assessment of clinical trials within the field.

Patients with cancer generally use homoeopathic remedies for supportive care and symptomatic relief. There is limited evidence supporting the use of homoeopathy in the treatment of cancer pain. It might have a role in difficult cases, and has been used in the UK for pain including that of mucositis. A Cochrane review evaluated the effectiveness and safety of homeopathic medicines used to prevent or treat the adverse effects of cancer, and the authors concluded that their review 'found preliminary data to support' the use of homoeopathy, but also that it was 'difficult to draw firm conclusions because of the paucity of evidence, clinical heterogenicity and lack of repetition of the included trials'. Additionally, two remedies, which were supported by good evidence, were not highly diluted. If dilutions are prepared according to homeopathic rules, they are technically homeopathic remedies even if they are not highly diluted. Such concentrated remedies will retain pharmacological activity, and hence it is no surprise that they are effective. Concluding that homeopathic remedies are effective on this evidence could therefore be misleading. Overall the bulk of evidence shows that homoeopathy is not necessarily more beneficial than placebo.

Hypnosis and imagery

Despite their different names, hypnosis and imagery are quite similar in terms of practice. They both focus on the creation of mental representations through the recall of memories or creative imagination that change the desired outcome (e.g. symptom experience).

When subjects are hypnotized, they experience a distortion of time awareness, memories, and the perception of activities around them as well as a sense of dissociation from the environment, emotions, and sensation. In this state, suggestions can be implanted which can continue after the therapy: post-hypnotic suggestion. Hypnotisability is a measurable state. Up to two-thirds of the normal adult population are hypnotizable, and up to 10% are highly responsive. Inducing a hypnotic state relies more on the susceptibility of the subject rather than the skill of the practitioner.

Hypnosis can be used in cancer patients for reducing anxiety and with the displacement of pain or nausea. Hypnosis can also be used to change or even remove unpleasant memories. Self-hypnosis can be taught to both enhance self-control and to give the patients some control over their pain and other symptoms. Pleasant images are created to distract attention from a painful symptom, and conversely, images of an unpleasant symptom can be modified to change the symptom experience. Studies suggest that the body mimics neurohormonal responses to the mental images as if they were actually occurring.

Evidence suggests that hypnotic analgesia involves activation of endogenous descending inhibitory pain pathways. Naloxone does not inhibit hypnotic analgesia, suggesting that these descending pathways do not involve endogenous opioids.

One study found that healthy subjects had reduced pain sensation and unpleasantness of 30% and 40% respectively. Hypnotic analgesia involved descending pain inhibitory pathways at a spinal level which are not under voluntary control.

A recent review of hypnosis/imagery included RCTs with conventional treatments as controls. The majority of studies demonstrated support in relieving cancer-related pain. A separate study showed significant reductions in pain in patients with metastatic breast cancer. Here, the hypnosis treatment group lived for an average of 36 months as compared with 18 months in the control group. Superior pain control for mucositis of bone marrow transplantation has also been demonstrated with imagery/hypnosis. Hypnosis is widely used to reduce pain associated with procedures such as bone marrow aspiration in both adults and children.

An expert panel of the National Institutes of Health in the USA assessed the efficacy of different behavioural and relaxation techniques in the treatment of chronic pain. They concluded that there was strong evidence for the use of hypnosis in alleviating cancer pain and for the use of relaxation in reducing chronic pain.

Side effects can occur with hypnosis. A skilled hypnotherapist should be able to manage an involuntary purging of memories, known as catharsis, which can be distressing to the patient if it occurs during therapy. A retrospective survey of the use of hypnosis in palliative care patients found that 7% had negative effects.

Massage and aromatherapy

Massage involves the manipulation of soft tissues of the body for therapeutic effect. Aromatherapy massage uses fragranced and volatile oils (essential oils) combined with a carrier oil or cream to manipulate the soft tissues. These treatments are used to relieve stress and improve well-being. One RCT of aromatherapy massage in palliative care demonstrated a significant reduction in pain and anxiety. An observational study of 1920 patients at a tertiary cancer centre in the USA showed an improvement of multiple symptoms including pain throughout the 48 hours of observation. A Cochrane review on the use of aromatherapy and massage for symptom relief in patients with cancer concluded that they provide short-term benefit on psychological well-being, but there was limited evidence on its effect on anxiety.

There is a theoretical risk that massage could spread the cancer, so the tumour site should be avoided. There have been no reported cases of this happening.

Music therapy

Music therapy is the creative and professionally informed use of music in a therapeutic relationship for physical, social, and spiritual help. Music therapists help patients to explore their thoughts and beliefs through music. Patients are encouraged to express their emotions by creating music, singing, or dancing. Through different styles of music, it is possible to trigger relaxation and improve mood. Music therapy is also a form of distraction therapy, increasingly used in palliative care and can potentially alleviate pain.

A Cochrane review showed that music therapy reduces pain intensity levels and opioid requirements in acute, chronic, and cancer pain. The magnitude of these benefits was small, making its clinical significance unclear.

Healing, reiki, and therapeutic touch

Healing often involves the practitioner passing hands over the patient's body either with light touch or just above the body. There are different explanations for this form of therapy, such as the channelling of energy from the healer to the patient and the re-establishment of energy flows. Healing focuses on the improvement of well-being and quality of life rather than cure.

The main forms of healing are spiritual healing, reiki, and therapeutic touch. Spiritual healers seek to stimulate natural healing processes, release tension, and treat the whole person in mind, body, and spirit. Reiki is a Japanese technique involving light touch that is claimed to restore spiritual energy in order to aid well-being. Therapeutic touch, unlike other forms of healing, is not based on the channelling of energy, but on a mutual exchange of energy between the healer, patient, and environment.

Healing has been shown to be helpful with pain, relaxation, and sleep in palliative care patients. Patients undergoing radiotherapy for breast or gynaecological malignancy that had a form of healing were found to have improved quality of life measures for pain and physical functioning. An RCT of reiki healing in patients with advanced cancer reported significant reduction in pain scores and improvement to quality of life scores compared to the control group that had rest periods of similar duration. Touch therapies were a topic of a Cochrane review to evaluate the effectiveness on relieving both acute and chronic pain, including cancer pain. The review concluded that the effect of touch therapies on pain relief is inconclusive, though data suggest a potential analgesic effect, including for cancer pain. No adverse effects were identified.

Conclusion

CAM includes numerous treatments, and whilst some techniques are ineffective, others show promise, or already have a robust evidence base (e.g. acupuncture). Further high-quality research is required to establish whether CAM could be better integrated into healthcare services.

Herbal products are increasingly popular, but patients and practitioners should be aware of the potential for interaction with medical treatments. Healthcare workers need to routinely inquire in a non-judgemental manner about the use of CAM, and advise their patients accordingly. In advanced cancer, a balance needs to be struck between fear of interactions and/or adverse effects and the potential for improving quality of life and well-being for the patient.

CAM therapies are increasingly accessed by oncology patients, often without the knowledge of their doctors, implying a significant unmet need within conventional medicine. Despite the growing demand, accessibility is often limited by a lack of funding, knowledge, qualified staff, or dismissed by some of the whole field as quackery.

Some CAM therapies show potential in the palliative care setting. However expensive and time-consuming conducting clinical trials in this field is, CAM still needs to have a robust evidence base.

Despite the challenges outlined, some CAM modalities appear to be integrating into mainstream medicine, with shared goals of disease prevention, health promotion, improving patient outcomes, and quality of life.

Bibliography

1. Ang-Lee MK, Moss J, Yuan C (2001). Herbal medicines and perioperative care. *JAMA* **286**:208–16.
2. Cassileth BR, Vickers AJ (2004). Massage therapy for symptom control: Outcome study at a major cancer center. *J Pain Symptom Manage* **28**:244–9.
3. Cepeda MS, Carr DB, Lau J, Alvarez H (2006). Music for pain relief. *Cochrane Database Syst Rev* **2**:CD004843.
4. Cohen MH, Eisenberg DM (2002). Potential physician malpractice liability associated with complementary and integrative medical therapies. *Ann Intern Med* **136**:596–603.
5. Ernst E, Casileth BR (1998). The prevalence of complementary/alternative medicine in cancer: a systematic review. *Cancer* **83**:777–82.
6. Ezzo JM, Richardson MA, Vickers A, *et al.* (2006). Acupuncture-point stimulation for chemotherapy-induced nausea and vomiting. *Cochrane Database Syst Rev* 2006; **2**:CD002285.
7. Fellowes D, Barnes K, Wilkinson S (2004). Aromatherapy and massage for symptom relief in patients with cancer. *Cochrane Database Syst Rev* **2**:CD002287.
8. Filshie J, Hester J (2006). Guidelines for providing acupuncture treatment for cancer patients–a peer-reviewed sample policy document. *Acupunct Med* **24**:172–82.
9. Han JS (2004). Acupuncture and endorphins. *Neurosci Lett* **361**: 258–61.
10. Hilgard ER, Hilgard JR (1994). *Hypnosis in the relief of pain*, Revised edn. New York: Brunner/Mazel.
11. Hilliard RE (2005). Music therapy in hospice and palliative care: a review of the empirical data. *Evid Based Complement Alternat Med* **2**:173–8.
12. Kassab S, Cummings M, Berkovitz S, van Haselen R, Fisher P (2009). Homeopathic medicines for adverse effects of cancer treatments. *Cochrane Database Syst Rev* **2**:CD004845.
13. Kwekkeboom KL, Cherwin CH, Lee JW, Wanta B (2010). Mind-body treatments for the pain-fatigue-sleep disturbance symptom cluster in persons with cancer. *J Pain Sympt Manage* **39**:126–38.
14. Martin BR, Wiley JL (2004). Mechanism of action of cannabinoids: how it may lead to treatment of cachexia, emesis, and pain. *J Support Oncol* 2004; **2**:305–14.
15. Molassiotis A, Fernadez-Ortega P, Pud D, *et al.* (2005). Use of complementary and alternative medicine in cancer patients: a European survey. *Ann Oncol* **16**(4):655–63.
16. NIH Technology Assessment Panel on Integration of Behavioral and Relaxation Approaches into the Treatment of Chronic Pain and Insominia (1996). Integration of behavioral and relaxation approaches into the treatment of chronic pain and insomnia. *JAMA* **276**:313–18.
17. Oberbaum M, Yaniv I, Ben-Gal Y, *et al.* (2001). A randomized, controlled trial of the homeopathic medication TRAUMEEL S in the treatment of chemotherapy-induced stomatitis in children undergoing stem cell transplantation. *Cancer* **92**:684–90.
18. O'Regan D, Filshie J (2010). Acupuncture and cancer. *Auton Neurosci* **157**(1–2):96–100.
19. Sayre Adams J, Wright S (2001). *Therapeutic Touch*. London: Churchill Livingstone.
20. Speigel D, Bloom J, Kraemer HC, *et al.* (1989). The beneficial effect of psychosocial treatment on survival of metastatic breast cancer patients: a randomized prospective outcome study. *Lancet* **2**:888–91.

21. So PS, Jiang Y, Qin Y (2008). Touch therapies for pain relief in adults. *Cochrane Database Syst Rev* **4**:CD006535.

22. Sun Y, Gan T, Dubose J, Habib A (2008). Acupuncture and related techniques for postoperative pain: a systematic review of randomized controlled trials. *Br J Anaesth* **101**(2):151–60.

23. White A (2004). A cumulative review of the range and incidence of significant adverse events associated with acupuncture. *Acupunct Med* **22**:122–33.

24. Werneke U, Earl J, Seydel C, *et al.* (2004). Potential health risks of complementary alternative medicines in cancer patients. *Br J Cancer* **90**:408–13.

25. White A, Cummings M, Filshie J (2008). *An introduction to Western Medical Acupuncture.* London: Churchill Livingstone.

Chapter 24

Pain in cancer survivors

Paul Farquhar-Smith

Introduction

Pain associated with cancer is common, and may affect up to 75% of those with advanced disease. Improvements in cancer treatments have lead to a steady increase in the number of cancer survivors either cured or with long-term disease control and it is estimated that rates of survivorship have tripled from 30 years ago. Globally there are now approximately 22.4 million cancer survivors. Chronic pain in cancer survivors also has a high prevalence (up to 50%) and is an under-recognized, inadequately understood, and a growing problem. These pains can have a major adverse impact on quality of life and activities of daily living.

Pain in cancer can be caused by:

- Pain from cancer itself
- Pain from treatment of cancer
- Pain unrelated to cancer, e.g. chronic low back pain.

Pain in cancer survivors is predominantly secondary to cancer treatments:

- Surgery
- Chemotherapy
- Radiotherapy.

Pain after cancer surgery

The presence and the need for treatment of acute pain following surgery are acknowledged. However, the persistence of pain long after surgical healing is more difficult to explain both to patients and practitioners. The second most common cause of pain in chronic pain patients is previous surgery. Pain after cancer surgery is accepted as a type of neuropathic pain. Evidence indicates the underlying mechanisms are similar to other types of neuropathic pain, including peripheral and central sensitization that results in pain without obvious noxious input. Chronic pain has been reported after most types of surgery and is not restricted to cancer surgery. However, it appears the incidence of chronic pain is greater after cancer surgery. The highest incidence of chronic pain occurs after breast surgery, thoracic surgery, and surgery for head and neck cancers (Table 24.1). It remains under-reported and under-recognized. Patients may be reluctant to tell of

Table 24.1 Incidence of chronic post-surgical pain

Surgery	Incidence	Reference	Severe (>5%)
Amputation	60–80%	Nikolajsen & Jensen 2001	5–10%
Thoracotomy	47%	Perkins & Kehlet 2000	10%
	50%	Wildgaard et al. 2009	3–16%
Breast surgery	14–68%	Jung et al. 2003	5–10%
Head and neck	40%	Burton et al. 2007	

their pain from fear of suspicion of recurrence or from assuming it is not important to surgeons. Although awareness is increasing, some surgeons do not accept postsurgical pain as a significant problem.

Chronic pain after breast cancer surgery

Post-breast cancer surgery pain (PBCSP) is a significant cause of pain and occurs in up to 50% of patients, a number repeatedly confirmed by several large studies. Incidence varies due to the lack of consensus on a reliable and universal assessment tool. There has also been a confusion of terms whereby all PBCSP was misleadingly labelled as 'post-mastectomy pain' even after breast conserving treatment.

Pain can occur in the scar area, chest wall, arm, and breast. As one would expect for a type of neuropathic pain, patients may complain of spontaneous pain, loss of sensation, and allodynia (an innocuous stimulus perceived as painful). PBCSP has a greater deleterious effect on function and quality of life measures than other types of pain, which may be compounded by the increased anxiety from the belief that the pain indicates recurrent disease.

Damage to a specific nerve (intercostobrachial nerve) has been postulated as the pivotal mechanism of pain. Indeed preservation of this nerve during axillary dissection is associated with reduced chronic pain. However, there is still a significant incidence of pain even when the nerve is spared and conversely a proportion of patients who do not develop chronic pain after the nerve is cut.

Risk factors

Many patient and surgical factors have been implicated as risk factors for the development of PBCSP.

Patient factors

- Young age of patients: age has consistently been cited as associated with chronic pain. One study found the incidence of PBCSP of 65% in those aged 30–49 compared to 26% of patients aged 70 or older. A recent Danish survey of 3253 women suggested the key age range was 18–39 years.

- Increased acute postoperative pain: poor postoperative pain control has been robustly associated with chronic pain in numerous studies. Effective postoperative pain control (by whatever method) may reduce PBCSP.

- Anxiety and depression prior to surgery.
- Chemotherapy and radiotherapy: both have been identified as risk factors for chronic pain. However, a recent study showed radiotherapy but not chemotherapy was associated with chronic pain.

Surgical factors
- Mastectomy versus breast conserving surgery: some studies state mastectomy is more likely to result in chronic pain than breast conserving surgery such as wide local excision. However, others found the opposite and pain after conserving surgery may be as prevalent as in 40% of patients especially in the young age group.
- Axillary dissection and the intercostobrachial nerve: some studies have identified axillary dissection as an independent risk factor for chronic pain, which may be in part related to interference with the intercostobrachial nerve as above. Compared to sentinel node biopsy, axillary dissection risks a higher incidence of chronic pain.
- Reconstruction: the presence of an implant after mastectomy increases the chance of chronic pain compared to mastectomy alone. Latissimus dorsi reconstruction is associated with a high incidence of PBCSP. Newer reconstructive techniques such as deep inferior epigastric perforator (DIEP) free flaps are associated with less postoperative pain and may result in less chronic pain.

Chronic pain after thoracic surgery

Chronic pain after thoracic surgery for cancer can affect up to 50% of patients. It, too, demonstrates neuropathic pain characteristics often scoring highly with neuropathic pain assessment tools. Analogous to PBCSP, young age, radiotherapy, and poor acute postoperative pain control is associated with more chronic pain. Several retrospective studies noted that high pain scores 24 hours after surgery resulted in high incidence and severity of chronic pain. Amelioration of acute pain reduces chronic pain. One example using thoracic epidural analgesia demonstrated a reduced incidence of chronic pain to only 12%.

As for PBCSP, surgical factors also contribute to the development of chronic pain. There is some evidence that less extensive surgery (video-assisted thoracic surgery (VATS) compared to posterolateral thoracotomy) may be protective and result in reduced long-term pain. Related to this, damage to the intercostal nerve has been postulated as a major contributor to this pain. However, the degree of intercostal nerve damage does not appear to correlate with the incidence or severity of pain. Moreover, others have reported rates of pain 6 months after surgery of approximately 40% for both thoracotomy and VATS.

Chronic pain after head and neck surgery

The incidence of moderate to severe pain after over 6 months after oral cancer surgery has been reported as high—over 30%—with only 40% of patients having no pain. Pain is implicated as the major reason why 40% of patients do not return to work after head and neck surgery. However, pain slowly improves over time and only 15% experience significant pain at 5 years post surgery. Pain may occur not only in the mouth and face but also in the neck and shoulder. Neck lymph node dissection is especially associated with chronic neck and shoulder pain. There are certain similarities to PBCSP and post-thoracic pain such as reduction of chronic pain by good perioperative pain control, less extensive surgery, and by sparing a specific nerve (accessory nerve). This pain also demonstrates neuropathic features.

Treatment of post-cancer surgery chronic pain

Reduction of risk factors may lead to potential prevention. Of prime importance is the need to ensure optimal postoperative pain control. Careful assessment and a multidisciplinary approach are imperative. There is a lack of evidence base concerning the efficacy of treatments for post-surgical pain compared to other types of neuropathic pain. Small trials of the use of amitriptyline, venlefaxine, gabapentin (as part of a multimodal perioperative regimen), and topical treatments (local anaesthetic and capsaicin) have shown modest efficacy in treatment or reduction in incidence of post-surgical pain. Current treatment recommendations are based on data primarily from investigation of post-herpetic neuralgia and painful diabetic neuropathy. However, good randomized controlled trial (RCT) studies are required to investigate post-surgery pain since there is evidence that it may involve mechanisms distinct from other types of neuropathic pain. The lack of information on treatments may explain the low use of analgesic medicines in patients with post-surgical pain.

Chemotherapy-induced neuropathic pain

Many types of chemotherapy and biological anticancer therapy are neurotoxic. The most common neurotoxicity is a sensory peripheral neuropathy which may be associated with pain. The severity of toxicity for some agents can lead to dose reduction or even having to stop the chemotherapy. As with other types of pain in cancer survivors, painful chemotherapy-induced peripheral neuropathy (CIPN) is under-recognized compounded by the lack of specific assessment tools. CIPN can adversely affect quality of life in patients cured or in remission from their cancer. As survival rates for many cancers improve, the problems of survivorship will require understanding and appropriate management.

Risk factors in CIPN

- Type of chemotherapeutic agent—examples most commonly associated with CIPN:
  - Vinca alkaloids: vincristine
  - Platinum analogues: cisplatin
  - Taxanes: paclitaxel
  - Biological agents: bortezomib.
- Combination of neurotoxic therapies can also increase risk of CIPN.
- Cumulative dose of agent: higher cumulative dose and longer duration of therapy is associated with higher risk of most CIPN.

- Pre-existing neuropathy: neuropathy of any origin such as diabetes and also pre-existing CIPN increases risk of incidence or exacerbation of CIPN.
- Variable recovery: recovery and spontaneous improvement of symptoms depends on type of agent and severity of symptoms; more severe CIPN is less likely to recover.
- Type of cancer: certain types of cancer are associated with a higher incidence of CIPN such as myeloma.

Clinical presentation of CIPN

- Symmetrical peripheral sensory (less likely to be motor) neuropathy: if unilateral symptoms are present, other causes of neuropathy need to be carefully excluded.
- Symptoms/signs of peripheral nerve dysfunction: such as numbness, paraesthesias, and pain.
- Length dependence: 'stocking/glove' distribution, distal parts of limbs affected first.
- Onset related to administration of anticancer therapy: depending on agent may present any time after exposure and even after treatment has stopped. The development of CIPN after the cessation of chemotherapy is known as 'coasting'.

These signs and symptoms of a length-dependent sensory peripheral neuropathy are thought to be due to disruption of axonal transport leading to the more distal part of nerves being first starved of nutrients. However, this explanation does not fully account for pain mechanisms identified in animal models, nor does it explain the observation of presence of pain before this final pathway of anatomical damage has occurred. Chemotherapy-induced alterations in biochemical moieties such as inflammatory cytokines contribute to the development of sensitization and other changes in neuronal excitability that result in pain. Although all types of CIPN are often considered collectively, CIPN caused by different agents may have subtle mechanistic and electrophysiological differences. These differences may have implications both for the assessment and the treatment of CIPN associated with each chemotherapeutic agent.

Assessment of CIPN

CIPN is under-recognized by clinicians which may be in part due to a limitation of awareness of the problem and the lack of an accepted and validated assessment tool. Heterogeneity of assessment tools has made standardization of assessment and diagnosis difficult. Several tools are in common usage but apart from their lack of consensus they are also often predominantly physician, rather than patient-based assessments. Even the most commonly used have poor interobserver reliability and few include pain as part of their assessment. More recent tools have emphasized a more patient-centred approach and newer tools have also been developed that assess agent-specific CIPN. There is a need for a robust and validated patient-centred assessment tool that is sensitive enough to identify neuropathy and allow accurate understanding and communication of patients' CIPN.

Quantitative sensory testing (QST) has been used to assess the electrophysiological alterations associated with CIPN. Patients with CIPN exhibit alterations in the function of sensory nerves such as thresholds to modalities such as cold, heat, pain, and touch. The patterns of these alterations have been shown to be agent specific. For example, the threshold to detect skin heating is unchanged with vincristine or paclitaxel CIPN but after bortezomib, this threshold is significantly increased (i.e. less sensitive to heat detection). QST has been used as the outcome measure in several trials although QST changes do not correlate well with clinical symptoms or signs of CIPN. Furthermore, alterations in QST do not precede or predict development of symptoms of CIPN. Currently the use of QST remains predominantly for research.

Agent-specific CIPN (Table 24.2)

Vinca alkaloids

Vinca alkaloids act by disruption of microtubules and directly interfere with axonal transport. Vincristine is associated with a higher incidence of neuropathy compared with vinblastine and vinorelbine. A high proportion of patients develop typical CIPN changes within 3 months with a peak 2–3 weeks after treatment. Paraesthesias predominate in presenting symptoms. Most patients experience spontaneous improvement over months, especially in those with mild symptoms. Motor neuropathies may occur.

Table 24.2 Neuropathies associated with specific chemotherapies and biological therapies. Reproduced with permission from *Cancer Pain Management*, 2010 British Pain Society Consultation Document

Chemotherapy	Type of neuropathy (incidence)	Onset time (coasting)	Duration/recovery	Other differences
Cisplatin (carboplatin)	Chronic	c.1month (+)	Some resolution in 80% over months/years	Carboplatin less CIPN
Oxaliplatin (Cersosimo, 2005)	Acute (90%) and chronic	Acute: hours Chronic: c.1 month (+)	Acute: Chronic: as cisplatin	Acute pain in up to 90% cold induced
Vincristine (Quasthoff, 2002) (vinblastine)	Chronic (30% severe)	Peak 2–3 weeks (+)	Some recovery 1–3 months, longer recovery into years	Paraesthesias common, vinblastine less CIPN
Paditaxel (docetaxel) (Hausheer, 2006)	Chronic	Within days (+)	@6/12 19% complete recovery, 25% no recovery (Verstappen, 2003)	More CIPN with more frequent dosing; docetaxel less CIPN
Bortezomib (Velcade®) (Richardson, 2006)	Chronic (35%)		At 2y 71% some recovery	High incidence of neuropathy before starting bortezomib
Thalidomide	Chronic	Any time (+)	Recovery less likely (Richardson, 2006)	No cumulative dose response, daily dose

Platinum compounds

Cisplatin acts by alkylation of DNA and apoptotic cell death. Sensory neurotoxicity is common especially after higher cumulative dose and may worsen for weeks or months after the treatment has stopped. Indeed CIPN can develop weeks or months after cessation of a platin ('coasting'). Recovery is variable and less likely in more severe cases. CIPN is less likely after carboplatin.

Oxaliplatin can cause chronic CIPN similar to other agents (but less than after cisplatin) with the common features described above. However, oxaliplatin also can also cause an acute neuropathy affecting hands, feet, and perioral region that occurs during or immediately after infusion in up to 60% of patients and usually resolves a few days later.

Taxanes

Taxanes (paclitaxel, docetaxel) also interfere with microtubule function and can cause severe damage to small and large peripheral nerve fibres. The incidence of paclitaxel-induced CIPN has been reported as high as 80% (30% severe) and appears to be associated with higher dose per course as well as cumulative dose. Symptoms often start in the lower limbs. CIPN is less common after docetaxel treatment. As for CIPN after other chemotherapeutic agents, recovery is variable. However, due to changing dose regimens, incidence of paclitaxel-induced CIPN and severe CIPN is reducing.

Biological agents

Bortezomib is a proteosome inhibitor that affects cancer cell division and induces apoptosis. It is used in the treatment of refractory multiple myeloma. This neurotoxicity is dose dependent, can be dose limiting, and in severe cases can result in stopping treatment altogether (8%). In one major study, 35% of patients receiving bortezomib developed a sensory peripheral neuropathy. This study also demonstrated a high proportion of patients (up to 80%) that had evidence of existing neuropathy prior to receiving bortezomib which may be related to the neurotoxicity of previous chemotherapies (including thalidomide) but also be influenced by the myeloma itself. Indeed the use of bortezomib for other cancer types is associated with less pre-existing and less treatment-induced neuropathy. Most CIPN develops after the second cycle with maximum effect after the fourth cycle. Bortezomib-induced CIPN may increase after treatment has stopped and also displays 'coasting' in up to 8% of patients. Recovery ranged from total resolution (approximately a third) to almost none when measured 2 years after bortezomib treatment.

Thalidomide is used in the maintenance therapy of multiple myeloma and has a relatively high incidence of CIPN (up to 40%). Thalidomide differs from other agents in that it does not display a clear cumulative dose response. Symptoms are more closely related to older age and daily dose rather than duration of treatment. Indeed CIPN can occur at any time during treatment, including 'coasting'. Symptoms can be dose limiting and recovery appears to be less common and more protracted.

Prevention and treatment of CIPN

Therapeutic options for CIPN include trying to prevent its development and treating with pharmacological and non-pharmacological approaches after CIPN has developed.

A number of cryoprotectants (amifostine) nutritional supplements (glutamine, glutathione, N-acetyl cysteine, vitamin E), and antineuropathic agents (oxcarbazepine, amitriptyline) have been used, with variable success, to prevent the development of CIPN caused by several agents. The relative lack of evidence has meant their use is sporadic and generally has not been integrated into standard treatment protocols. Vitamin E has some proven efficacy in prevention of paclitaxel- and vincristine-induced CIPN and is the most commonly used.

Treatment of established painful CIPN also has a limited evidence base. Pharmacological treatment of painful CIPN has also been based upon antineuropathic agents with established evidence for efficacy in other types of neuropathic pain. However, as for post-surgical pain, it is possible that mechanistic differences exist. Although many prospective therapeutic targets have been identified from animal models of CIPN such as calcium channels, these as yet have not translated into clinical treatments.

Several antineuropathic agents have been investigated specifically in painful CIPN. Results were mixed with low-quality data showing a potential beneficial effect of gabapentin and venlefaxine. However, RCTs of gabapentin, amitriptyline, nortriptyline, and lamotrigine all failed to show any improvements in pain control. Guidelines for general neuropathic pain are often used for CIPN despite these negative data.

Non-pharmacological treatments such as physiotherapy and occupational therapy have important roles to play in the complete management of CIPN.

Radiation-induced pain

Radiotherapy is a common cancer therapy option both as a primary treatment and adjunct. Radiotherapy can contribute to pain directly by direct effects on nerves causing pain or as a risk factor for pain after surgery or chemotherapy. Moreover, radiation damage in bowel and gynaecological cancer can cause long-term pain.

Brachial plexus neuropathy (BPN)

Brachial plexus neuropathy after radiotherapy for breast cancer is probably the most infamous example of radiation-induced toxicity. Although modification of treatments has significantly reduced the incidence of BPN, it is estimated to affect 1–5% of patients having breast cancer radiotherapy treatment especially in younger women and those also receiving chemotherapy. Tumour-induced BPN is more common (approximately 75% of BPN) and displays some differentiating features compared to radiation induced BPN (Table 24.3). Pain is actually a rarer symptom in radiation-induced BPN. The onset of radiation-induced BPN occurs from 6 months but may not develop for years. One case series demonstrated an increase in prevalence from 2% at 5 years up to 19% 19 years after radiotherapy.

Radiotherapy fraction size and total dose is linked to the incidence of BPN. Using fractions of 2.2–2.5Gy and limiting total dose to between 34–40Gy results in less than 1% BPN. As for the other types of treatment-induced neuropathic pain and neuropathy, therapy is multifactorial including occupational and physiotherapy input for the frequent

Table 24.3 Clinical features of radiation and tumour-induced brachial plexopathy. Using modified lower fraction dose radiotherapy schedules may reduce BPN

	Tumour	**Radiation**
Incidence of pain	75%	25%
Location of pain	Shoulder, upper arm 4th and 5th fingers	Shoulder, wrist, and hand
Severity of pain	Moderate to severe (severe in 90%)	Mild to moderate (severe in 30%)
Course	Progressive neurological dysfunction, atrophy/weakness (more commonly C7/T1)	Progressive weakness of all or predominantly upper plexus
EMG	Segmental slowing	Diffuse myokymia

loss of function associated with BPN. There are anecdotal reports of efficacy of certain surgical approaches including cervical cordotomy. Pharmacological treatment for the pain of BPN is not evidence based but often, as above, follows general neuropathic pain guidelines.

Bibliography

1. Bajrovic A, Rades D, Fehlauer F, *et al.* (2004). Is there a life-long risk of brachial plexopathy after radiotherapy of supraclavicular lymph nodes in breast cancer patients? *Radiother Oncol* **71**(3): 297–301.

2. Burton AW, Fanciullo GJ, Beasley RD, Fisch MJ (2007). Chronic pain in the cancer survivor: a new frontier. *Pain Med* **8**(2):189–98.

3. Cata JP, Weng HR, Lee BN, *et al.* (2006). Clinical and experimental findings in humans and animals with chemotherapy-induced peripheral neuropathy. *Minerva Anesthesiol* **72**(3):151–69.

4. Cersosimo RJ (2005). Oxaliplatin-associated neuropathy: a review. *Ann Pharmacother* **39**:128–35.

5. Dworkin RH, O'Connor AB, Backonja M, *et al.* (2007). Pharmacologic management of neuropathic pain: evidence-based recommendations. *Pain* **132**(3):237–51.

6. Galecki J, Hicer-Grzenkowicz J, Grudzien-Kowalska M, *et al.* (2006). Radiation-induced brachial plexopathy and hypofractionated regimens in adjuvant irradiation of patients with breast cancer—a review. *Acta Oncol* **45**(3):280–4.

7. Gartner R, Jensen MB, Nielsen J, *et al.* (2009). Prevalence of and factors associated with persistent pain following breast cancer surgery. *JAMA* **302**(18):1985–92.

8. Gellrich NC, Schimming R, Schramm A, *et al.* (2002). Pain, function, and psychologic outcome before, during, and after intraoral tumor resection. *J Oral Maxillofac Surg* 2002, **60**(7):772–7.

9. Hausheer FH, Schilsky RL, Bain S, Berghorn EJ, Lieberman F (2006). Diagnosis, management, and evaluation of chemotherapy-induced peripheral neuropathy. *Semin Oncol* **33**:15–49.

10. Jung BF, Ahrendt GM, Oaklander AL, Dworkin RH (2003). Neuropathic pain following breast cancer surgery: proposed classification and research update. *Pain* **104**(1–2):1–13.

11. Nikolajsen L, Jensen TS (2001). Phantom limb pain. *Br J Anaesth* **87**(1):107–16.

12. Perkins FM, Kehlet H (2000). Chronic pain as an outcome of surgery. A review of predictive factors. *Anesthesiology* **93**(4):1123–33.

13. Poleshuck EL, Katz J, Andrus CH, *et al.* (2006). Risk factors for chronic pain following breast cancer surgery: a prospective study. *J Pain* **7**(9):626–34.

14. Postma TJ, Heimans JJ, Muller MJ, *et al.* (1998). Pitfalls in grading severity of chemotherapy-induced peripheral neuropathy. *Ann Oncol* **9**(7):739–44.

15. Quasthoff S, Hartung HP (2002). Chemotherapy-induced peripheral neuropathy. *J Neurol* **249**(1):9–17.

16. Richardson PG, Briemberg H, Jagannath S, *et al.* (2006). Frequency, characteristics, and reversibility of peripheral neuropathy during treatment of advanced multiple myeloma with bortezomib. *J Clin Oncol* **24**:3113–20.

17. Richardson PG, Xie W, Mitsiades C, *et al.* (2009). Single-agent bortezomib in previously untreated multiple myeloma: efficacy, characterization of peripheral neuropathy, and molecular correlations with response and neuropathy. *J Clin Oncol* **27**(21):3518–25.

18. Smith WC, Bourne D, Squair J, *et al.* (1999). A retrospective cohort study of post mastectomy pain syndrome. *Pain* **83**(1):91–5.

19. Stevens PE, Dibble SL, Miaskowski C (1995). Prevalence, characteristics, and impact of postmastectomy pain syndrome: an investigation of women's experiences. *Pain* **61**(1):61–8.

20. Tasmuth T, Kataja M, Blomqvist C, *et al.* (1997). Treatment-related factors predisposing to chronic pain in patients with breast cancer—a multivariate approach. *Acta Oncol* **36**(6):625–30.

21. Tiippana E, Nilsson E, Kalso E (2003). Post-thoracotomy pain after thoracic epidural analgesia: a prospective follow-up study. *Acta Anaesthesiol Scand* **47**(4):433–8.

22. Verstappen CC, Postma TJ, Hoekman K, Heimans JJ (2003). Peripheral neuropathy due to therapy with paclitaxel, gemcitabine, and cisplatin in patients with advanced ovarian cancer. *J Neurooncol* **63**:201–5.

23. Wildgaard K, Ravn J, Kehlet H (2009). Chronic post-thoracotomy pain: a critical review of pathogenic mechanisms and strategies for prevention. *Eur J Cardiothorac Surg* **36**(1):170–80.

24. Windebank AJ, Grisold W (2008). Chemotherapy-induced neuropathy. *J Peripher Nerv Syst* **13**(1):27–46.

Index